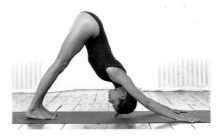

LEARN HOW TO USE

Astanga Yoga
& Meditation

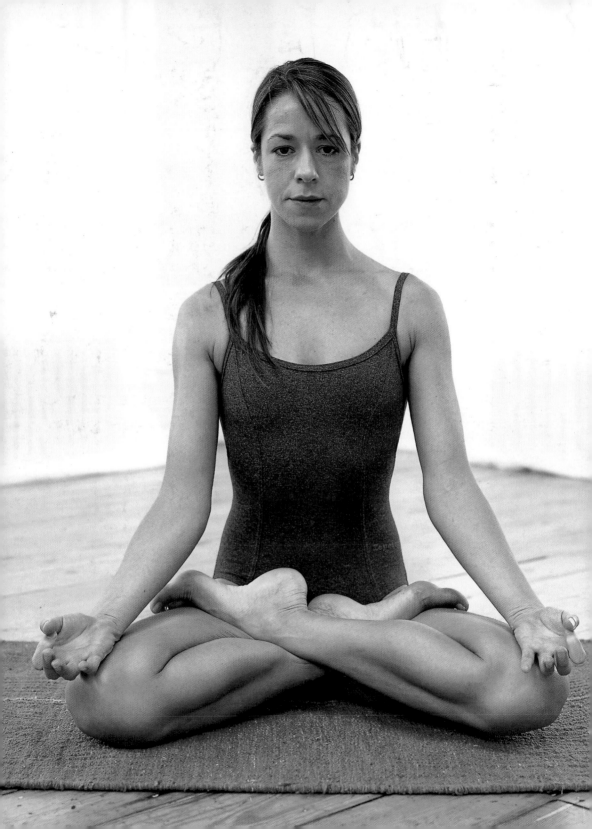

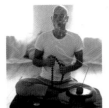
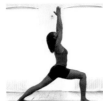
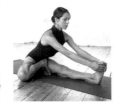
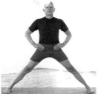
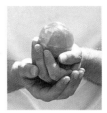

LEARN HOW TO USE

Astanga Yoga & Meditation

A complete sourcebook of yoga and meditation exercises to tone and strengthen body and mind, with more than 900 photographs

Jean Hall and Doriel Hall

southwater

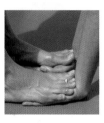
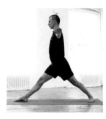
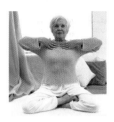
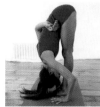
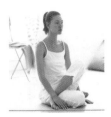

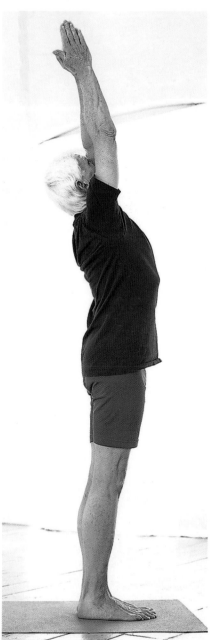

This edition is published by Southwater, an imprint of Anness Publishing Ltd,
108 Great Russell Street, London WC1B 3NA; info@anness.com

www.southwaterbooks.com; www.annesspublishing.com; twitter: @Anness_Books

If you like the images in this book and would like to investigate using
them for publishing, promotions or advertising, please visit our website
www.practicalpictures.com for more information.

A CIP catalogue record for this book is available from the British Library.

Publisher **Joanna Lorenz**
Editorial Director **Helen Sudell**
Project Editors **Katy Bevan**, **Ann Kay** and **Joanne Rippin**
Project Designers **Nigel Partridge** and **Lisa Tai**
Copy-editing and new text for this edition
    (notably pages 6–7 and 20–21) **Beverley Jollands**

Astanga Yoga/pages 8–139
Author **Jean Hall**
Photography **Clare Park**

Meditation/pages 140–225
Author **Doriel Hall**
Photography **Michelle Garrett**

Working with the Chakras/pages 226–49
Authors **Sue and Simon Lilly**
Photography **Michelle Garrett**

Previously published in three separate volumes, *Astanga Yoga*, *Meditation* and
Chakra Healing

PUBLISHER'S NOTE:
The authors and publisher disclaim any liability resulting from the techniques and
information in this book. If you are concerned about any aspect of your physical or
psychological health, always seek professional help. It is advisable to consult a
qualified medical professional before undertaking any exercise routines – especially
if you have a medical condition or are pregnant.

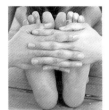
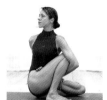
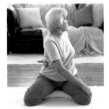
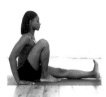
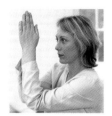

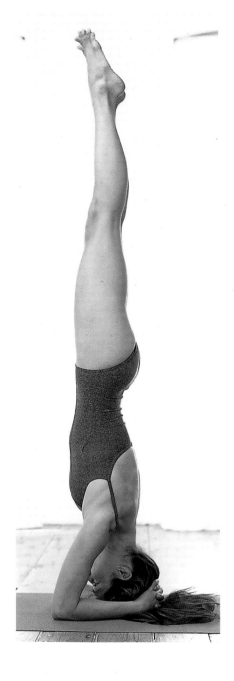

Contents

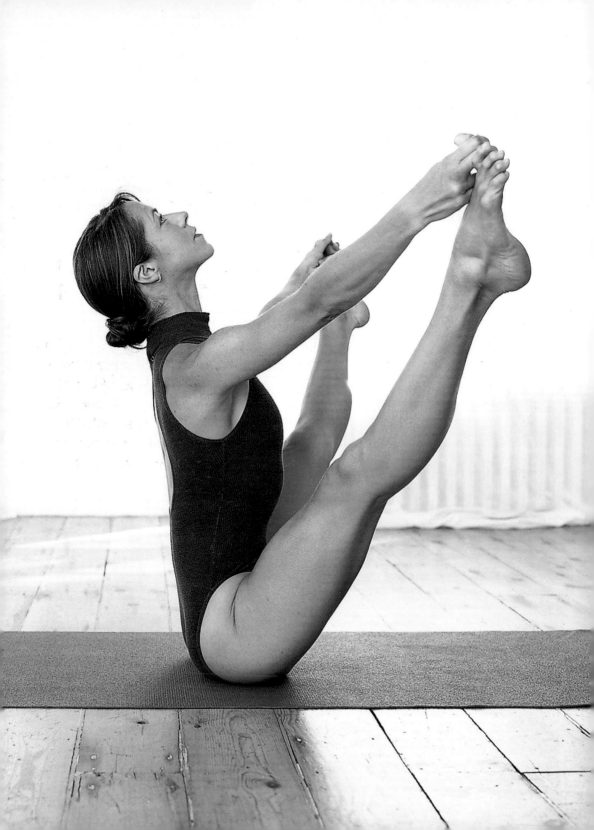

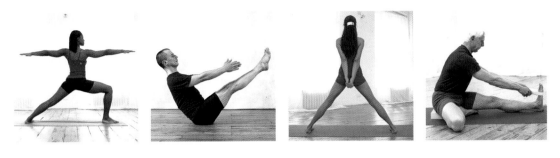

Astanga Yoga

Yoga has its seeds in the beginning of time, yet it still continues to evolve. It is a live, breathing art, inspired from the depths of nature. Astanga is a unique form of physical yoga that places emphasis on the flowing energy of breath, body and mind to cultivate an inner core strength. Its primary instrument is the body, which is led through a sequence of yoga postures (asanas). The following pages form an ideal introduction for newcomers to the subject, and will help to deepen the awareness of anyone who is already practising.

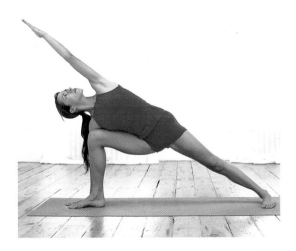

Yoga's History and Philosophy

Yoga has its origins deep in pre-history and slowly evolved through the ancient Tantric civilizations that were in existence more than 10,000 years ago throughout India and in many other parts of the world. In these ancient Tantric times, the *rishis* (seekers and seers), finding inspiration and truth in nature, realized techniques to attain freedom from the burdens and attachments of the world while still living within it. First, recognition of the human limitations of body and mind was needed. Then methods to transcend these limitations in order to open consciousness into higher realms of reality were taught. These skills were then handed down by word of mouth from *guru* (teacher) to pupil throughout the generations.

Tantra, the name given to the sacred books of Tantrism, stems from *tan-oti*, meaning "expansion", and *tra-yati*, meaning "liberation". In Tantric philosophy, the body is regarded as the gateway to the inner temple of the divine. Thus the body and bodily existence was recognized on a manifest level as a wonderful instrument through which the expansion of the unmanifest consciousness (*Siva*) and freedom of energy (*Sakti*) can be realized and united.

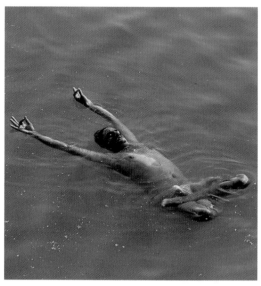

The term "yoga" emerged in written sources over 4,000 years ago in the ancient Sanskrit hymns and poems of the *Tantras* and later the *Vedas*, which refer to ritualistic traditions, folklore, esoteric practices and spiritual awakenings. These scriptures are considered to be sacred, as they were originally revealed to the rishis while they were in deep yogic states of meditation.

Further writings, called the *Upanisads* (literally meaning "to sit near the teachings"), gave clearer definition to the journey of yoga. These texts, 108 authentic books in all, are the final part of the Vedas, and the basis of Vedanta, which is one of the six philosophical systems of Indian thought. The Upanisads are diverse in their varied spiritual teachings, but in essence they reveal that the soul is at the core of us all and that therefore none of us is separate:

The Self is the Ultimate Reality
That which was before creation, And from which creation
    was born
Yet who sees this Self, Sees it resting in the hearts of all.

Katha Upanisad

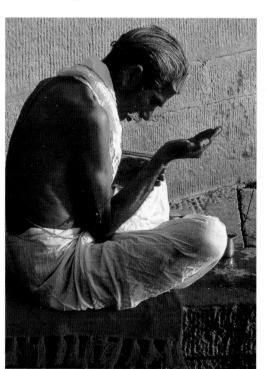

Above A yogi floating in clear green waters of the Ganges, Varanasi, India. The *Gangajal*, or water of the river, is considered a life tonic.
Left Yogis gather on the banks of the Ganges to practise meditation and yoga, and to bathe in the purifying waters. Hindus regard the river Ganges as the most sacred river in India.

This knowledge is realized not through speculation and theory but through duty, inner contemplation and meditation. The Upanisads provide the source of Astanga yoga, but they are more inspirational than instructional, with profound suppositions and revelations, both practical and poetic.

At this point in yoga's history (the Upanisads were written between 400 and 200BC), the instructional methods of yoga were still imparted personally from the guru directly to his pupil. Different teachers taught different techniques and aspects, making its development somewhat random. It was not until the rishi Patanjali (c. 100BC – AD100) systematized and compiled the existing yoga practices that had been handed down to him, along with knowledge contained in the Vedas and Upanisads, that yoga was given a comprehensive format and philosophical shape. Patanjali's *Yoga Sutras*, meaning "yoga threads", create the essential foundations of yoga as we know it today and the work is considered one of the most significant texts on yoga. In the 196 aphorisms of this book, Patanjali provides the aspiring yogi with a profound structure of eight steps, or limbs (*asta* means "eight", *anga* means "limb"), to follow, like a thread, along the yogic pathway in order to reach liberation and enlightenment.

THE EIGHT LIMBS OF ASTANGA YOGA

1 **The five yamas** (Ethical and moral restraints)
Ahimsa: non-violence and non-harming in any form to any living creature. This creates compassionate living, as true non-violence is a state of mind and heart.
Satya: truthfulness in mind, word and action. This is considered to be the highest law of morality.
Asteya: non-stealing, to free ourselves from possessiveness and envy.
Brahmacharya: abstinence and the practice of moderation in all things.
Aparigraha: non-greed in order to simplify life by adopting an attitude of generosity and non-hoarding.

2 **The five niyamas** (Practices to create inner integrity)
Saucha: purity and cleanliness of mind, body, heart and environment.
Santosha: cultivation of inner contentment, in order not to hold others responsible for our happiness.
Tapas: to glow and be illuminated with an inner aim and direction in life for growth. The great yogi Iyengar suggests that a "life without tapas is like a heart without love".
Svadhyaya: study, not only of an intellectual kind but also of oneself, to develop self-understanding of our inner nature.
Isvara-pranidhana: realization, devotion and dedication to the divine presence within all life.

3 **Asanas** (Postures)
Asana means "seat" and refers to the art of body postures that have evolved over many centuries. Apart from cultivating *kanti* (physical beauty) due to the enhanced pranic flow (life energy) through the body, asanas remove fickleness of mind to restore mental and physical health, strength, wellbeing and vitality. Asana practice also reflects the tendencies, strengths, weaknesses and actions in our life.

4 **Pranayama** (Breath regulation)
Prana is the vital life energy within the breath, and so it can also be translated as "the breath of life". *Ayama* means "expansion" or "to stretch", and therefore pranayama is the practice whereby life energy is expanded through the regulation and control of the breath. The natural sound of the breath, *soham* (soh-hum), in Sanskrit means "I am that ... beyond the limitations of body and mind" and resonates unconsciously through the body like a mantra (sacred sound) with each breath taken. In yoga it is believed that by listening into our breath we also become aware of this quiet blessing.

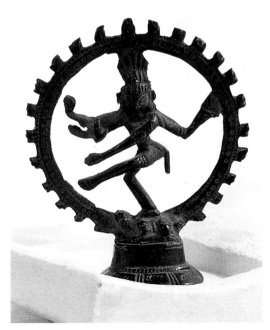

Above Siva, the third god of the Hindu trinity, is here depicted in his reincarnate form of Nataraja – the Lord of Dancers. The circle of fire symbolizes the ever-turning universe in its state of eternal flux.

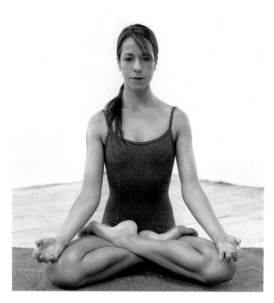

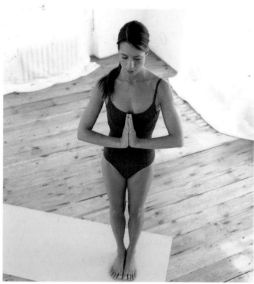

Top Sitting in Padmasana (lotus pose) with the hands in the *chin mudra* position is a comfortable and traditional way to practise meditation, focusing the mind and calming the brain (see pages 22–3).
Bottom A mantra is recited at the beginning of yoga practice. This is traditionally done standing in Tadasana with the hands in Namaste, palms together as if in prayer (see page 32).

5 **Pratyahara** (Sensory withdrawal)

The ancient scriptures suggest that the entire cosmos is situated within the human body, and therefore it is understood that the source of happiness lies within each individual. By withdrawing our senses from external stimulation, we are able to connect to this inner well of contentment, rather than relying on outward sensory stimulus and grasping in order to fulfil our unquenchable desires. The process of introspection and pratyahara, which certain asanas, such as Kurmasana (tortoise posture), induce, also leads to self-understanding and acceptance.

6 **Dharana** (Concentration)

The practice of dharana, or concentration, can take many forms. Methods include being completely attentive to the flow of the breath in harmony with the movement of the body, or focusing on the glow of a candle flame, watching its movements and sharing its light. Whatever technique is used, the aim is the same – to strengthen the mind and gather psychic energies in order to move into a meditative state.

7 **Dhyana** (Meditation)

Through the practice of one-directional flow of the mind, *ekatanata*, or concentration, meditation will begin to follow naturally if time is given to it. Meditation is absolute, it is where we can go beyond time, space, conditions and limitations, allowing our individual core of consciousness to expand and connect with the infinite universal consciousness. The ancient sages described meditation as yoking with nature, as they conceived the infinite universe to be part of the nature of life, death and beyond.

8 **Samadhi** (Enlightenment, bliss state of oneness)

This is the ultimate yoga, and it is the culmination of the previous seven limbs. Samadhi transcends meditation: it is without seed, as it goes beyond beginning and end; it is a state of absolute liberation and bliss in which nothing is needed, desired or required as the self has merged all.

To truly practise Astanga yoga we need to endeavour to incorporate all eight limbs: to practise the physical aspects, which are the asanas and pranayama, and to strive to live the actions of yoga, yama, niyama, pratyahara, dharana and dhyana. By reading and discussing, the concepts of yoga may be intellectually understood, but that understanding needs to be put into practice if we wish to experience the richness of its benefits and bring meaning into our lives. As Sri K. Pattabhi Jois expounded, yoga is 99 per cent practice and 1 per cent theory. This requires practice of all the eight limbs of yoga, not just the asanas.

SRI T. KRISHNAMACHARYA, SRI K. PATTABHI JOIS AND THE YOGA KORUNTA

Two of the most revered yoga gurus of our times rediscovered a forgotten ancient manuscript sitting in the recesses of the national library of Calcutta during the early 1930s. Sri K. Pattabhi Jois, under the guidance of his guru Sri T. Krishnamacharya, helped to date, collate, record and decipher this manuscript, the *Yoga Korunta*, which dates back between 1,000 and 1,500 years. It was written in Sanskrit upon leaves and was still just intact.

In the Yoga Korunta a system of Hatha yoga that was created and practised by its author, a seer called Vamana Rishi, is described. The manuscript comprises hundreds of stanzas and advocates the way of the breath to integrate the eight limbs of Patanjali's Yoga Sutras. In full detail, movement and breath are described as the means into and out of the postures, with counted breaths while in each asana, advising, "Oh yogi, do not do asana without vinyasa." *Vinyasa* means "breath-synchronized movement". It is the practice of moving the body in harmony with the breath to help induce a state of deep concentration.

Within the Yoga Korunta, three series of yoga sequences are imparted:

1 Yoga Chikitsa – yoga therapy, to align and detoxify the body and mind. This is the primary series.
2 Nadi Sodhana – channel cleansing, to purify the subtle body and energy within. This is the intermediate series.
3 Sthira Bhaga – divine stability, to create profound openness, humility and stability. This series came to be divided into four subseries due to its demanding nature.

This is the system of Hatha yoga now taught at the Sri K. Pattabhi Jois Astanga Yoga Institute in Mysore, India, and throughout the world. Through the teaching of Pattabhi Jois, Astanga yoga has reached countless people worldwide. He continued to teach with his daughter and grandson until his death in 2009. Many students still travel to India to study under their personal tutelage. Beginning their day at 4 a.m., they guide devotees through the various yoga series. Only when the first series has been fully understood and achieved is the next one introduced.

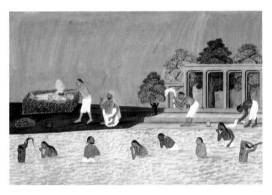

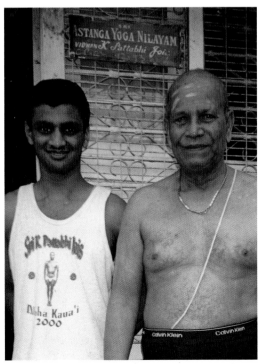

Above This painting from Trichinopoly, India, depicts *varuna snana* – or watery bathing – a component of *niyama*, to cleanse and purify the yogi's body. Bathing in sacred water, ashes, soil, sunshine, and contemplation of the divine are all forms of snana.
Right Sri K. Pattabhi Jois with his grandson, Sharath, outside his yoga shala, Mysore, India, 2001. This is the original home of Mysore-style self-practice, whereby the student flows through the learnt sequence of postures to the rhythm of their own breath.

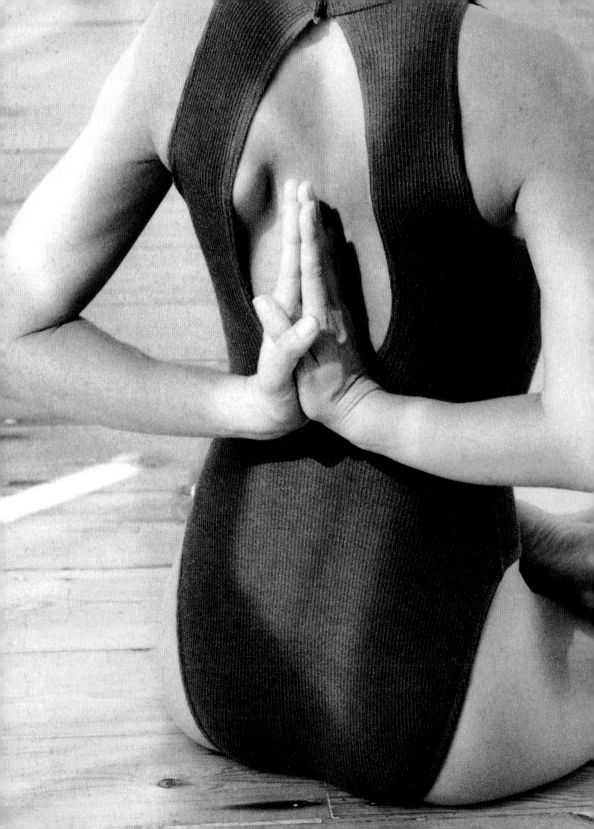

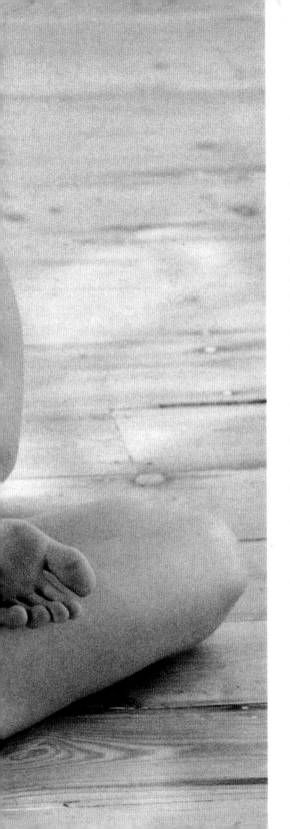

The Elements of Astanga Yoga

The distinguishing elements of Astanga yoga and its practice are woven together with the eight limbs of Patanjali's Yoga Sutras to create *sadhana* – a complete spiritual practice. These elements are:

- *vinyasa* – breath-synchronized motion
- *ujjayi pranayama* – victorious breathing
- the *bandhas* – inner locks
- the *dristis* – gaze points.

As the breath and body flow together as one, *tapas* (internal heat) is generated and begins a process of purification. Through practice, layers of bodily existence are cleansed, transforming deep-rooted patterns to liberate the body, mind and heart.

The outer, physical body in yoga is referred to as *sthula-sarira* – the gross or coarse body. This cage of the physical body houses the *suksma-sarira* – the subtle body, which is the inner, or psychic, realm of our existence. This subtle body is not visible to the eye but is just as real as the physical, and even more powerful and profound. The subtle inner dimension of existence can be felt and experienced through deep internal awareness, pranayama and meditation.

Vinyasa

The motion of breath is the inspiration of the body and propels the body into action, and it is the essence of Astanga yoga. Vinyasa teaches us to move in harmony with the subtle and profound power of our breathing – its movement skywards with the inhalation, and its surrender earthwards on the exhalation. Vinyasa, or "breath-synchronized movement", is the external expression of the internal motion of the breath. Through breath the life energy of prana is carried throughout the body.

Pattabhi Jois describes the system of vinyasa as a yoga *mala*. Mala means "garland" or "rosary", and in this sense, instead of a garland of flowers or rosary of prayers, vinyasa creates a garland or rosary of yoga postures, threaded together through the flow of the breath. Thus each motion of the body is inspired by the motion of the breath.

The natural motion of our breathing carries our body through the practice. The breath, softly lifting us up and releasing us down, motivates our body to flow in and out of the postures. This creates a continuous stream of movement in which body and mind are linked. The uniting of breath and motion symbolizes the union of the individual consciousness with the universal consciousness.

By becoming mindful of our breathing and its natural rhythm, we move into the full realms of yoga. This is because conscious linking of body, mind and breath as we move through the postures cultivates continuous concentration (dharana) on the flow of breath (pranayama) with the flow of asanas. This deep attention to the breath creates a quietening of the senses (pratyahara), preparing the pathway for the meditative state of contemplation and meditation (dhyana), which leads us towards the blissful union of the soul with the divine (samadhi). Yama and niyama can be more readily understood and absorbed as the body and mind become open and liberated through these practices.

On a physical level, vinyasa builds and maintains the heat of the body, allowing for the deep releasing stretches of the body in the asanas, while stoking the digestive fire to further the internal benefits of each posture. Another important aspect of vinyasa is that it enables us to develop our self-practice, so that we may flow at our own pace, moving to the rhythm of our own breath, drawing ourselves on every level deeper and deeper into meditation.

Vinyasa begins with Surya Namaskara (sun salutation); the rise and fall of the breath carries the flow of the body from posture to posture. Through the standing asanas, we surrender into each posture with the exhalation, and move out of the posture with the inhalation. Even as we are in the stillness of each posture, the breath continues to flow, opening and releasing the body further with every breath.

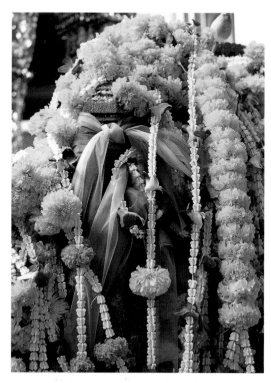

Above Yoga movements with vinyasa are described as being like a *mala*, or garland of flowers, linked together by the breath.

TO PRACTISE VINYASA

Within seated asanas, *a half vinyasa* is practised between each side of the posture in order to neutralize the body. After completing a sitting posture on both sides and before entering into the next new posture, *a full vinyasa* is practised. The full and half vinyasa sequences take their inspiration from Surya Namaskara, which incorporates pranayama (breath control), asanas (postures of body), dristis (focus points) and bandhas (locks or seals). It is for this reason that the flowing sequence of postures that is Surya Namaskara forms the bedrock of the physical practice of Astanga yoga.

As you flow through your practice, pay attention to the detail and alignment of each posture. Just as words are strung together to create a sentence, so the postures are linked to create the vinyasa. However, if the words are not pronounced coherently, the meaning of the sentence is lost. If the postures are not formed correctly, there will be no internal understanding, and your practice will make no sense.

Ujjayi Pranayama

Ujjayi pranayama encourages full breathing, so that oxygen and life can enter into our lungs and permeate every cell of the body. The word *ujjayi* is composed of two Sanskrit roots: *ji*, which means "to conquer or to be victorious", and the prefix *ud*, meaning "bondage". Thus ujjayi is the method of breathing that conquers bondage and liberates the mind. The breathing practice of ujjayi creates a soft resonating sound as the breath is drawn through the back of the throat on its way down into the lungs. This enables us to listen consciously to our breathing, and to tune into our life force and vital energy as our breathing washes in and out of our body. The sonorous sound of ujjayi breathing becomes a gentle mantra (sacred thought or prayer) on which our mind can focus, while creating a rhythm and flow for our body to follow as we move from asana to asana.

TO PRACTISE UJJAYI PRANAYAMA

Sit in any comfortable position, keeping your back straight and your spine lengthened. Now relax your body without slumping, and draw your focus downwards or allow your eyes to close completely. Bring your awareness to your breath entering and exiting through your nostrils. Allow your breathing to become deep, slow, rhythmic and calm. Now take your awareness to your throat: feel your breath softly brushing through the back of your throat on both your inhalation and exhalation.

As your concentration deepens, become aware of the four stages of each breath cycle without exaggerating any one of them. First, there is your inhalation (*puraka*), which pours into your lower body and fills all the way to the brim of your collarbones. Second, there is a moment of suspension when your inhalation is complete but the exhalation has not begun; this is called *antara kumbhaka*. Third, there is the exhalation (*rechaka*), where the breath is released from your upper body and empties down through to your lower body. Finally, there is a gentle retention (*bahya kumbhaka*), when your exhalation is complete but the inhalation has yet to begin. Be careful just to notice antara kumbhaka and bahya kumbhaka and not to accentuate either of them.

Now begin to contract the glottis gently by moving the well of your front throat in towards your back throat, so that a soft internal sonorous sound resonates from the throat to the heart on your inhalation, and from your heart to your throat on your exhalation. The sound will resemble that of a whispering breeze or the gentle breath of a sleeping baby. The resonating vibration of the breath ripples internally rather than being projected or pushed outwards.

If you have difficulty at first in creating the sound of ujjayi pranayama, practise by inhaling and exhaling through your mouth while whispering "hhaaa" at the back of your throat with each in and out breath. As your practice of ujjayi pranayama deepens, be aware of the polarity of energies contained within each cycle. The inhalation draws energy in to inspire our body to flow upwards. The exhalation releases energy downwards, connecting us to gravity and the earth.

Below Sit in Padmasana (lotus posture) to practise ujjayi pranayama. If this is not comfortable, refer to page 24 for alternatives.

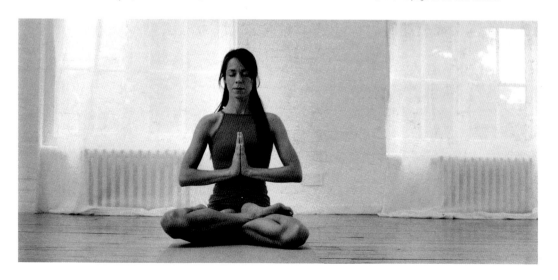

The Bandhas

The Sanskrit word *bandha* means "to bond, catch hold of or lock", and this is exactly the physical action involved in the creation and practice of the bandhas.

There are three primary bandhas: *jalandhara bandha, uddiyana bandha* and *mula bandha*. These bandhas, or locks, are created by gently yet powerfully contracting specific parts of the body to seal in the vital energy (prana) of the breath and redirect the pranic flow into the *susumna nadi,* which is the subtle pathway of the spine. Once energy begins to flow through the susumna, spiritual awakening begins.

Each bandha helps to dissipate psychic knots (called *granthis*) within the subtle body that block the free flow of prana ascending along the susumna, thus hindering meditation and ultimately liberation. On a physical level, the bandhas form the core strength of the body and are engaged throughout the practice to provide internal support.

JALANDHARA BANDHA

The word *jala* means "a net or a mesh". In this bandha, the front of the throat is locked by the chin being drawn down and pressed into the notch at the centre of the collarbones. This throat lock has the effect of regulating the flow of prana to the heart and the heart chakra (see page 25). In various postures, jalandhara bandha occurs naturally through the positioning of the entire body, for example in the Salamba Sarvangasana (supported whole body posture), Halasana (plough posture) and Garbha Pindasana (womb embryo posture). It may also be practised sitting in any comfortable position, such as cross-legged or in Ardha Padmasana or Padmasana (half or full lotus, described on page 126).

- Place your palms down on your knees and sit with your back tall without tensing, and allow your body to relax.
- Inhale slowly and deeply.
- Draw your head forwards, lowering your chin and pressing it down firmly into the collarbone notch. Straighten your arms and press your palms securely downwards on to your knees. This will cause your shoulders to rise.
- Hold this position of jalandhara bandha for only a moment or two, then lift your chin away from your chest, release the pressure of your hands from your knees, bend your elbows and relax your shoulders down. Exhale slowly and fully. Repeat four more times.
- Throughout your asana practice, the throat lock of jalandhara bandha has its subtle form in the gentle contraction of the glottis, while ujjayi pranayama is continuously present.

Below The subtle form of uddiyana bandha strengthens the abdominal muscles, deepens the breath and, at the same time, protects the spine from injury.

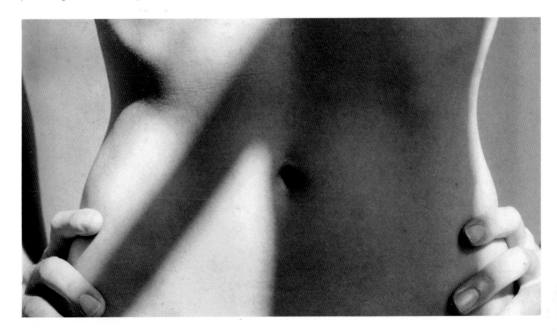

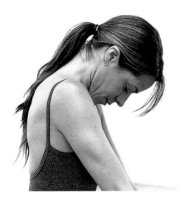

Above Jalandhara bandha

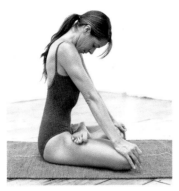

Above Uddiyana with jalandhara bandha

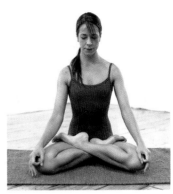

Above Mula bandha

UDDIYANA BANDHA

The word *uddiyana* means "to fly upwards", and it relates to the fact that the drawing in of the abdominal muscles causes the diaphragm to rise. Within the subtle body, uddiyana bandha causes pranic energy to fly, like a great bird soaring upwards, along the susumna nadi into the top chakra, bringing enlightenment and ultimate union. Uddiyana bandha may be practised sitting cross-legged, or in Siddhasana (accomplished posture), or in Ardha Padmasana or Padmasana (half or full lotus).

- Draw your spine up straight and place your hands on your knees. Relax your body and cast your gaze downwards or close your eyes to internalize your focus.
- Breathe in slowly and deeply through your nostrils.
- Now strongly exhale through your mouth, whooshing your breath out to empty your lungs completely.
- Retain the exhalation and scoop your stomach in, contracting your abdominal muscles inwards and upwards while locking your chin down on to your collarbone notch (jalandhara bandha). Allow your shoulders to rise slightly as you firmly straighten your arms by pressing your palms down on to your knees. Do not strain and only hold for as long as is comfortable.
- To release uddiyana bandha, relax your abdomen, bend your elbows, softening your shoulders down, lift your chin and inhale slowly and gently. Let your breathing return to normal before practising uddiyana again.

The above exercise is the full expression of uddiyana bandha. However, during your asana practice it will not be possible to engage this lock to such an extreme, as it would constrict your breathing. A subtler lift upwards and inwards of the abdomen as you practise will enhance your breathing,

helping you to draw your breath deeply into your back and side ribs rather than into your stomach. This will improve your lung capacity and strengthen your entire body. Be careful not to become tense as you engage uddiyana bandha. Let your abdominal muscles softly curve inwards as your breath flows into your back.

MULA BANDHA

The word *mula* means "root, cause or source". The location of mula bandha is at the perineal muscle, which is the muscle of the perineum area between the anus and genitals. For women, however, the contraction of this region goes deeper, so that mula bandha can be located at the cervix.

- Sit in a comfortable position (in Sukhasana, Siddhasana, or in half or full lotus).
- Lengthen your spine and relax your shoulders.
- Lower your focus or close your eyes completely and draw your awareness to the natural flow of your breath.
- Continue to breathe steadily, and take your attention to your perineal muscle or cervix. Contract this area by drawing the perineum or cervix upwards. Then relax the area. Repeat the contraction another four to five times, increasing the duration of each contraction in order to develop your strength to sustain mula bandha while breathing fully.

At first you may find you contract the anal and urinary sphincters, but with practice you will be able to refine the action of contraction into the specific area of the perineal muscle or cervix. As you practise, also be careful not to clench or grip your buttocks.

Mula bandha directs prana from the lower pelvic region upwards, helping to energize the entire body and relieve sexual frustration, guilt and suppression.

The Dristis

Our gaze point, known in Sanskrit as *dristi*, plays an important role in our practice on four different levels: practical, physical, mental and spiritual.

Of all our senses, sight and hearing are the two most compelling, continuously distracting us and drawing our mind outwards. Through our eyes we view the world outside ourselves, but we can also turn our focus inwards towards our inner life and gain insight to our true nature. As we direct our focus outwards through our open eyes, the steady vision of the dristi is a method of introspection. The outward focus is reflected inwards, focusing clearly, intently and softly, so that our open eyes are not aware of the outside world beyond our dristi.

There are nine points of focus, and each one completes the positioning of the body in each asana. The nine dristis are:

Bhru madhya: the space between the eyebrows (third eye centre, may be referred to as the *ajna chakra* or *sambhavi mudra*)
Nasagrai: the nose tip (also referred to as *agochari mudra*)
Nabi chakra: the navel
Padhayoragrai: the toes
Angustha ma dyai: the thumbs
Hastagrai: the hand
Parsva: to the right side
Parsva: to the left side
Urdhva: upwards and skywards

The prescribed dristis allow our eyes to rest on one point, helping to prevent our mental focus from being distracted during yoga practice by other visual stimulations and their associations. This helps us to develop one-pointedness – where the focus is concentrated on one single point. With practice this induces higher states of concentration that promote mental energy, awareness and introspection.

For this reason, dristis are also often used individually as tools in meditation practice. We therefore draw upon this meditative aspect to create tranquillity of mind and purity of inner vision, in order to reflect on our true nature as we move through the yogasanas.

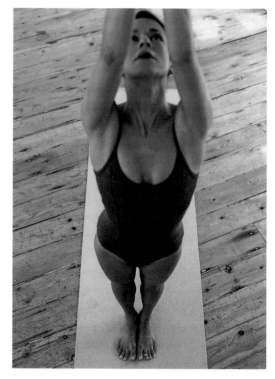

Above Angustha ma dyai (directing the focus to the thumbs) is the first dristi of Surya Namaskara (sun salutation).
Right Specific dristis being used to bring balance and focus.

Having a steady focal point also gives orientation and balance to the body in the postures, and helps to align the neck through the head position. The changes of dristi throughout Surya Namaskara (sun salutation) help the body's directional flow, cultivating physical and mental clarity. Dristis also strengthen the eye muscles and help to improve the eyesight – another practical physical benefit.

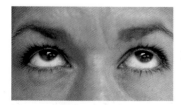

Above Dristi urdhva

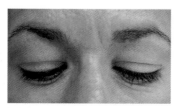

Above Dristi nasagrai

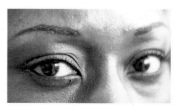

Above Dristi parsva

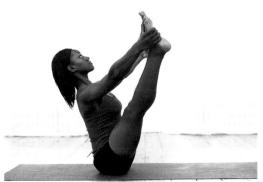

Above Dristi bhru madhya

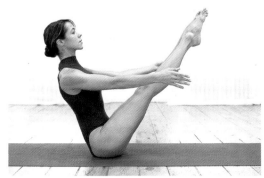

Above Dristi padhayoragrai

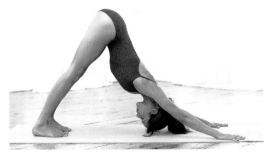

Above Dristi nabi chakra

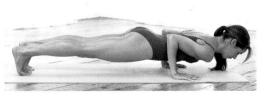

Above Dristi nasagrai

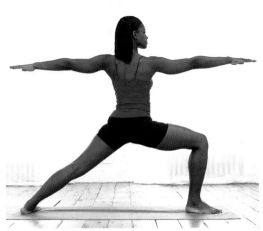

Above Dristi hastagrai

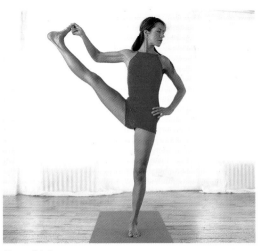

Above Dristi parsva

The Subtle Body

Patanjali's eight limbs of yoga can be seen as steps on a journey inward to the deepest levels of consciousness through the inner dimension of *suksma-sarira*, the subtle body. The breath is considered to be the vital link between the physical and subtle bodies, because it carries the energy of prana, the breath of life. This is why the breath is the essence of our yoga practice, as it bridges the psychic and physical realms of our existence. Within the subtle body there are energy channels called *nadis*. There are thought to be 72,000 such channels forming a complete network of energy pathways through which prana flows.

At the very core of the energy body, and corresponding to the spine of the physical body, is the central spiritual channel of the *susumna nadi* (the most gracious channel), along which there are seven energy centres, called *chakras*.

Weaving through the chakras and around the susumna nadi are two major subsidiary channels, called *ida nadi* (the comforting channel) and *pingala nadi* (the tawny channel). The pingala nadi stems from the right side of the susumna nadi and is associated with the fiery, purifying energy of the sun, while the ida nadi originates from the left of the susumna nadi and is associated with the soothing, cooling influence of the moon. These two pathways feed into the susumna nadi through the chakras, where their dynamic polarities and opposing forces are integrated.

On a physical level, like the susumna nadi, they have anatomical counterparts. The pingala nadi corresponds to the sympathetic (excitatory) nervous system, while the ida nadi corresponds to the parasympathetic (relaxatory) nervous system.

On a spiritual level, the subtle body is believed to remain after death and is thought to be carried into future embodiment and reincarnation.

THE CHAKRAS

Chakra means "wheel" or "circle", and along the length of the susumna nadi there are seven chakras. These chakras, which also correlate with key nerve centres or plexuses of the outer physical body, are like whirlpools of pranic energy, and each one signifies a different level of awareness. They are symbolic stepping-stones along the spiritual path.

Through the practice of the yoga postures; pranayama and meditation, the susumna nadi is cleansed, allowing pure energy to flow freely upwards through it, opening subtle dimensions of the mind and body to induce heightened states of consciousness and spiritual awakening. This is often depicted as a sleeping serpent coiled up at the base of the spine. As the snake is roused from its psychic slumber, serpent power (*kundalini-sakti*) is awakened, which activates the chakras as it ascends through the susumna, raising consciousness from the lower to the higher self.

CHAKRAS AND MEDITATION

Dhyana, the seventh limb of Astanga yoga, is meditation, which has been practised for thousands of years by adherents of many religions. Dhyana is the process whereby the mind is freed from the restlessness of scattered thoughts in order to see clearly and look within to connect to our internal source of wisdom, happiness and divinity.

> The fabled musk deer searches the whole world over for the source of the scent which comes from within ...
> Ramakrisna Paramhamsa

The mind is limitless, like the infinite blue expanse of the sky, but it is made small and foggy by our constant internal chatter of worries, anxieties, regrets, resentments, desires, memories, fantasies, dramas and set patterns of thinking. By releasing these clouds of thoughts, the unending open expansiveness of the inner mind and heart are revealed.

This opening into meditation is beyond words, and for this reason meditation can only be experienced rather than taught. However, there are many wonderful techniques that help to induce meditative states. Be patient in your practice, as meditation will come in its own time when you are open to receive it.

Meditation is not an escape from the stresses and strains of everyday life. It is a meeting with the self in its fullness, and a living exploration of the wondrous life force within.

Primarily there are two categories of meditation: concrete, or *saguna* (with qualities), and abstract, or *nirguna* (without qualities). In saguna meditation, the mind contemplates and focuses on a concrete or definite object or image. In nirguna meditation, by contrast, there is no object; instead, the practitioner is absorbed in contemplating the absolute oneness of the universe. By focusing on the imagery of the chakras, heightened states of awareness can be induced. The image of the lotus is often used to depict the chakras, as it symbolizes the three stages of the spiritual journey:

1 The darkness of ignorance – the roots of the lotus grow in the dark, murky mud of swamps.
2 Aspiration – the stem of the lotus grows upwards away from the darkness towards the water's surface.
3 Illumination – as the lotus pierces the water's surface, its petals open up to the light of the sun, symbolizing spiritual enlightenment.

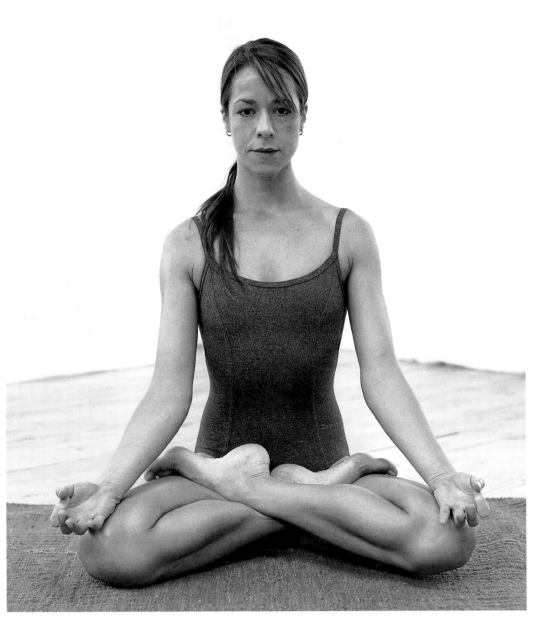

Above Sitting in Padmasana (lotus posture) encourages the body and mind to become still and steady. The folding of the legs creates a secure and firm foundation, providing the spine with a strong base to grow from. Steady stillness is the first step towards meditation. Curl your index finger under your thumb, symbolizing the individual self bowing to and uniting with the universal soul. This is called *chin mudra*.

Meditation

SITTING FOR MEDITATION

For the purpose of meditation, you must ensure that you assume a comfortable posture that you will be able to remain in without moving. Only when the body has been sitting in steady stillness for a while may meditation be experienced. Sit in any of the following asanas:

Sukhasana (easy happy posture)

Siddhasana (accomplished posture)

Ardha Padmasana (half lotus posture)

Padmasana (lotus posture as on the previous page)

Choose one in which you can comfortably maintain a straightness and length in your spine without feeling tension anywhere in your body. Sitting on a cushion or a yoga block is most useful in the beginning stages. As your back becomes stronger you will be able to sit for longer periods of time and without any props. If none of the above postures feels comfortable sit on a chair.

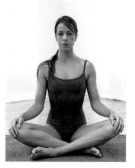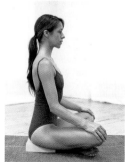

Above Sukhasana (easy happy posture) with and without a block.

Once you have chosen your sitting position:

1 Sit evenly on both buttocks, so your foundation is balanced and steady.
2 Relax in your hips and legs, so your knees may release down towards the floor.
3 Lengthen your spine, drawing your back tall and long and your chest open.
4 Relax your shoulders, letting your arms release down and resting your hands on your knees.
5 Relax your face and jaw, gently lowering your chin slightly to bring length into the back of your neck.
6 Soften your eyes, lowering your focus or closing your eyes completely, and draw your awareness/consciousness to the natural flow and motion of your breath.

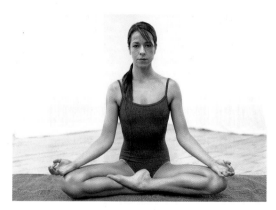

Above Siddhasana (accomplished posture)

As you sit in stillness, notice your chattering thoughts as they arise, but then simply observe them instead of getting caught up and trapped within the drama of them. Once you have noticed these thoughts clouding in, take a moment to breathe them all in. Don't get angry or frustrated by them, or try to suppress them, as this will cause you to get even further bound up with them all.

Let whatever needs to ripple up to the surface of your consciousness do so. See it, observe it, recognize it, feel it, and then slowly and gently breathe it all out, clearing your mind and returning your focus once more to the natural flow of your breathing.

As your mind becomes quieter and calmer, which may take some time and much practice at sitting, let your mind focus on the location, sensation, symbolic imagery and meaning of the various chakras.

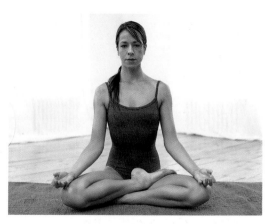

Above Ardha Padmasana (half lotus posture)

CHAKRAS: THEIR LOCATION, ELEMENT, IMAGERY AND MEANING

1 **Muladhara, the base chakra** – root centre

mul = root or source; adhara = place or vital part

Muladhara chakra is the source of all energy available to humanity, whether it be physical, mental, emotional, spiritual or psychic. As this energy (known as kundalini-sakti) is released and drawn up through the chakras, it is purified, and spiritual awakening begins.

Physical location: perineum, pelvic plexus
Element: *prithvi tattva* (earth element)
Seed mantra: *lam*
Symbolism: a lotus flower of four deep-red petals. At the centre of the lotus flower is a glowing yellow square, representing the element of earth. Within the yellow square is an inverted red triangle, whose apex points downwards. This is sakti – the symbol of creative energy.

Internally focusing on the red triangle within the yellow square enhances inner balance and integration of creativity and stability.

2 **Svadhisthana, the sacral chakra** – dwelling place of the self

sva = self or soul; adhisthana = abode or seat

This chakra is associated with relationships, procreation, pleasure and desire. It is the dwelling place of deep-rooted instincts and of all *samskaras* – mental and emotional impressions of the past.

Physical location: two finger widths above muladhara chakra and directly behind the genitals, hypogastric plexus
Element: *apas tattva* (water element)
Seed mantra: *vam*
Symbolism: a lotus flower of six deep-crimson petals. A blue-white crescent moon sits within the lower half of the lotus's circle, symbolizing the moon's influence on the ocean's tides and human emotion.

Concentrating on the image of a silvery blue crescent moon above a deep open ocean helps to restore emotional calm and balance cravings, freeing us from compulsive behaviour and unhealthy habitual patterns of the past.

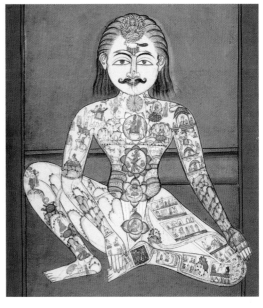

Above A depiction of the body's chakras and energy channels from an 18th-century manuscript.
Below Representations of the seven chakra centres and their symbolic imagery.

3 **Manipura, the navel chakra** – city of jewels

mani = gem or jewel; pura = city

Manipura chakra is the centre of inner power, energy, ambitious drive and assertiveness.

Physical location: situated behind the navel, solar plexus
Element: *agni tattva* (fire element)
Seed mantra: *ram*
Symbolism: a lotus flower of ten petals. Within the circle of the lotus is a downward-pointing fiery red triangle, like a gleaming ruby signifying energy and power.

Visualizing golden light radiating out from the fiery triangle and spreading throughout the body cultivates physical, mental and psychic energy, dynamism and vitality.

| 1 Muladhara chakra | 2 Svadhishthana chakra | 3 Manipura chakra | 4 Anahata chakra | 5 Visuddhi chakra | 6 Ajna chakra | 7 Sahasrara chakra |

4 **Anahata, the heart chakra** – unstruck sound
anahata = unstruck, referring to cosmic sound, which does not arise from
two objects being struck (as with all other sounds) but is always present
in the heart
From this centre the internal vibration and pulsing of the
heart can be heard, sending out waves of compassion,
unconditional love and understanding of equality and
brotherhood.
Physical location: behind the sternum, level with the heart (for
this reason this chakra is often called the "lotus of the
heart"), cardiac plexus
Element: *vaya tattva* (air element)
Seed mantra: *yam*
Symbolism: a lotus flower of 12 petals. At the centre of the lotus
is a star of six points like a hexagram, which is created by
two triangles interlacing, one with an apex pointing up and
the other with one pointing down. The upward and downward
triangles denote the midway balance of the lower chakras of
physical existence and the upper chakras of spiritual and
transcendental levels. Within the star there is a gentle
burning flame – the symbol of the individual soul (jiva).

Focusing on the steadiness of the inner flame of the heart
connects us to our individual soul, internal truth and
compassion, which remain steady and undisturbed by the
external activities of the world.

5 **Visuddhi, the throat chakra** – wheel of purity
suddhi = purification
It is at this centre that all dualities, polarities and dichotomies
of opposites are accepted within ourselves without judgment.
Physical location: behind the well of the throat,
pharyngeal plexus
Element: *akasha tattva* (ether element)
Seed mantra: *ham*
Symbolism: a lotus flower of 16 violet petals. Within the lotus
flower is a white circle like a silvery full moon, with a
teardrop shape of nectar at its centre, symbolizing the
harmonizing and purifying of all polarities and opposites.

Visualizing and sensing a sweet teardrop of nectar, like
calming balm at the level of the throat as you breathe, is
said to help smooth internal conflicts of heart and mind.
This helps to cultivate understanding and a non-judgmental
attitude to mind and heart.

6 **Ajna, the brow chakra** – command centre
ajni = command
This energy centre is the gateway to our intuition, where
communication and command from the internal guru is
heard. At this point the link between the mental and psychic
aspects of our being is created as the three channels of
susumna, ida and pingala converge.
Physical location: behind the space in between the eyebrows,
mid-brain at the medulla and pineal plexuses. Because of its
location at the third eye it may also be referred to as *jnana
chakshu* – the eye of wisdom.
Element: *maha tattva* (cause of the mind element)
Seed mantra: *om*
Symbolism: a two-petalled silver lotus, one petal representing
the sun (pingala) and one the moon (ida). The circle of the
lotus is of a silvery white shade, with a *lingam* (symbol of
masculine creative energy) in its centre, placed within a
downward-pointing triangle, which is a symbol of the
feminine principle (sakti).

Focusing on a glowing circle of light at the centre of your
eyebrows, radiating wisdom and intuition, enhances insight
and inner knowing.

7 **Sahasrara, the crown chakra** – thousand-petalled lotus
sahasrara = thousand-spoked; also known as sunya, the voidless void
of totality
The crown chakra is the dwelling place of our highest
awareness. It is the union of all consciousness and
all energy.
Physical location: crown of the head, top of the skull
Seed mantra: *om*, or the entire Sanskrit alphabet
Symbolism: a circular lotus blossom of a thousand shining
petals overlying one another. Inscribed on each petal is a
letter of the Sanskrit alphabet. In the centre of the lotus
is a full moon (*purna chandra*), and within the full moon is a
jyotirlinga – a lingam of light shining upwards, symbolizing
pure consciousness.

It is said that the experience of sahasrara is beyond
words and all definition – it has to be felt to be understood.
Practitioners of different religions describe it in different
words: Christians refer to it as heaven, Buddhists call it
nirvana, yogis name it *samadhi* and Hindus call it *kaivalya*. It is
the perfect merging of all things – it is yoga itself.

Right The seven chakras lie along the central energy channel of the susumna nadi, with the intertwining
ida nadi (moon energy) stemming from the left side and the pingala nadi (sun energy) from the right.

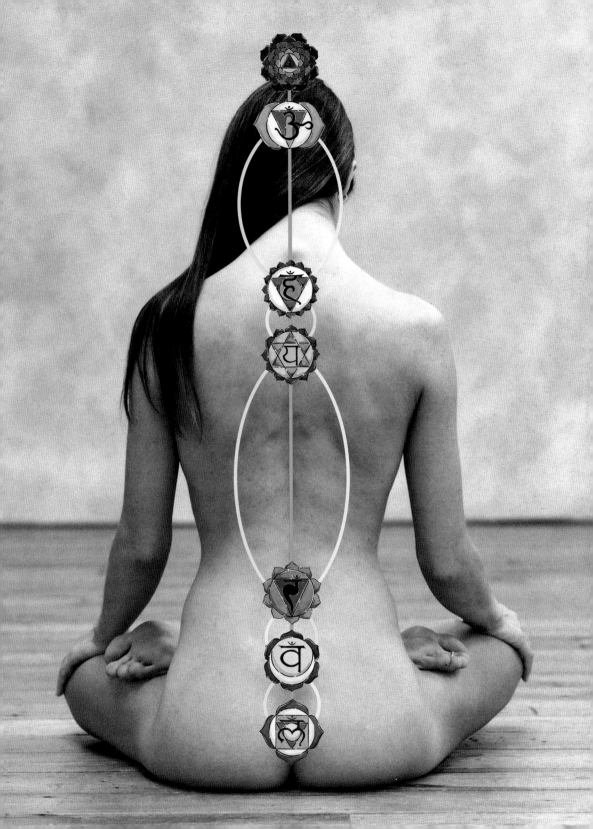

Preparing to Practise Astanga Yoga

Make yoga a part of your daily routine. Your practice is there to enhance your life rather than create stress, so don't worry if on some days you can't fit it in. However, regular, short practice sessions will be more beneficial than the occasional long session.

WHEN TO PRACTISE

• Traditionally, dawn and dusk are considered the most auspicious times of day to practise yoga, as the rising and setting of the sun both charge the atmosphere with spiritual energy. However, if these times are impossible for you, just practise when you can.

• Allow a minimum of three hours after a meal before you begin your practice. It is best to drink before and after your practice, so as not to become dehydrated, but avoid drinking during your practice, as this will interrupt your concentration and flow from one asana to another.

• Make time in your life for regular practice. Even if you can practise for only 15 minutes every other day, this is better than nothing at all. Over time, it is likely that you will want to give more time to your yoga, as your body and mind become revitalized by your practice.

HOW TO PRACTISE

• Never hold a posture – each asana is a moving, breathing experience, an exploration to open, release and strengthen your body and mind. The awakening journey of yoga is the goal, rather than the postures themselves.

• Always practise with awareness, care, attention and patience. Let your awareness extend not only to how you are breathing and moving but also to how you are thinking and feeling. Accept both good and bad thoughts and feelings equally with no judgment and no attachment, and then let them go as you breathe out, so that your yoga becomes a cleansing practice.

• Never push or bully your body to achieve a posture – injury will be sure to follow. Instead, allow yourself to flow with and yield to gravity. The natural force of gravity is far more powerful than ourselves, and if we surrender to it, it will take us deeper into the posture than any of our efforts using brute force.

• Always practise barefoot and wear soft, comfortable, non-restrictive clothing made of natural materials to allow your skin to breathe.

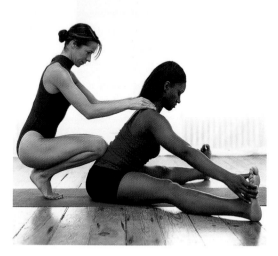

Above Gentle but firm hands-on adjustments can help the body to yield into asanas.

• Clear space for your practice – a clear, uncluttered space will help to create a clear, uncluttered mind.

• Practise systematically through the postures, starting with the sun salutes. With each session, add another posture and commit it to memory, so that you build your self-practice and carry it with you wherever you go.

• The three primary touchstones for you to be continuously aware of at all times are:

  1 The essence of your yoga practice – your breath. It will tell you when you are pushing too hard or when you have lost concentration. The breath is the link between body and mind, and a barometer to your state of being.
  2 Your foundations – your feet. Open and release them down into the ground to receive the upward surge of energy from the earth.
  3 The elongation of your spine – as you move through your practice, breathe length into your back to create space and energy within your body.

• Never confuse flow with rush. Flow steadily and smoothly through your postures, and this will generate dynamic energy, agility and awareness. Rushing through your practice will create a tense body and an agitated mind.

- Familiarize yourself with your body parts – in particular your feet, tailbone, sitting bones, pubic bone, sacrum, back ribs, collarbones, shoulder blades, neck, the crown of your head and the location of your three bandhas. Your bandhas need to be engaged throughout your practice, and throughout the instructions there are reminders.

- Always focus on breathing at least five full, deep, steady breaths in each asana. As you develop strength, concentration and stamina, you may wish to take more breaths in order to sustain the postures for longer. Also, by breathing more deeply and slowly, you will create time and space to explore each asana fully.

- Before practising each posture, carefully study it by reading the instructions and observing the photographs to develop both a mental understanding and visual concept of it. Pay particular attention to the placement of the feet, as they are the foundation of each posture and the roots of your alignment.

- Shortened and moderated sequences are demonstrated in the chapter Abridged Sequences. As you become familiar and confident with the asanas and sequences you may wish to begin to develop your own practice, always closing with the key finishing asanas.

SAFETY IN PRACTICE
- Inversions (upside-down postures), jumps or any asana that feels strenuous should be avoided during recovery

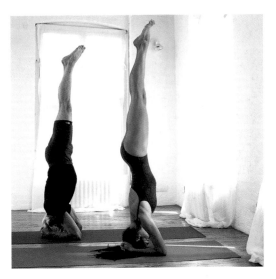

Above As you progress in your practice your body becomes stronger, more supple and agile.

from injury, during menstruation, or by those with high blood pressure, a hernia, a heart condition or a spinal injury such as prolapsed disc.

- Although many of the postures within this book are individually safe and extremely beneficial during pregnancy, the full Astanga primary series is unsuitable for expectant mothers and must not be practised in its complete form. Your yoga practice must be moderated during pregnancy; pre-natal yoga classes are recommended.

- The use of props such as straps, yoga blocks and cushions can be very useful when first learning an asana, or when recovering from injury, but it is unwise to become dependent on them. They are there to aid you initially rather than being a permanent crutch to your practice. A yoga mat, however, is one piece of equipment that you may wish to keep as your constant companion – they are light and easily transportable.

- Most importantly, enjoy your practice, and do not let it become a rigidly imposed ordeal. Instead, let yourself be creative, exploring the wonder of your body and its inner energy and wisdom. Listen to and respect your body, and let it lead you. It is your greatest teacher, and yoga is your inner sanctuary.

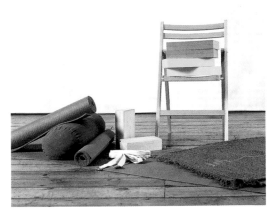

Above Chairs, foam blocks, wooden blocks, straps, bolsters and yoga mats are all props that can aid moderations of the asanas.

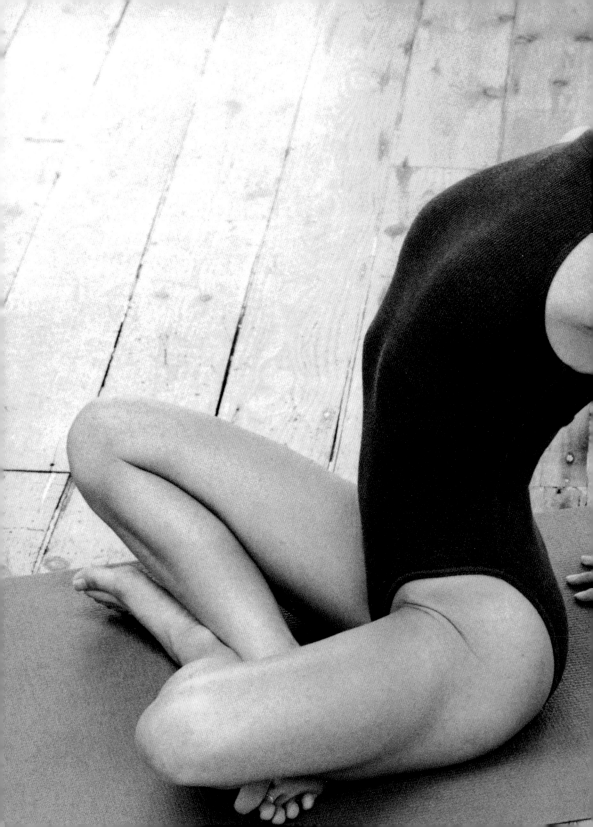

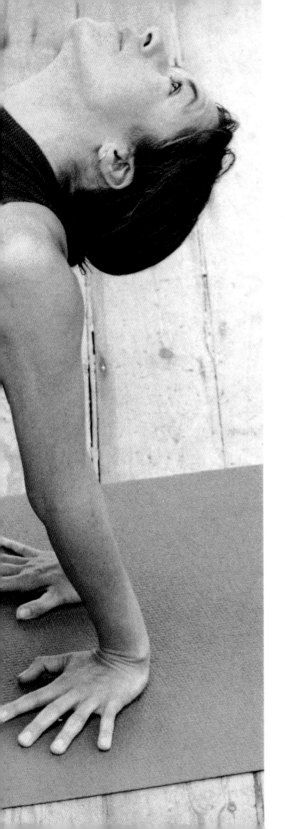

The Primary Series

The Yoga Korunta consists of six series of some forty postures each. The first series, or primary series, is called Yoga Chikitsa (yoga therapy). It is sometimes referred to as the "healing series", as the asanas (postures) within it realign, rebalance and cleanse both the body and the mind, restoring health and vitality. The second series or intermediate level, is called Nadi Sodhana (purification of the subtle channels). It works on harmonizing body and mind by fortifying the nervous system. The advanced series, levels A, B, C and D, develop and intensify vital prana energy.

This book focuses on the first series. Through Surya Namaskara A and B (sun salutations), the body–breath–mind connection is awakened. The standing asanas develop concentration and strength; the seated asanas create suppleness and a sense of calm; and the finishing sequence slows the mind, cultivating clarity and a meditative state.

Yoga Chikitsa

In this chapter the flow form of the primary series is shown in its entirety, leading you through the correct sequential order of asanas. By steadily progressing through the postures you will gain strength, flexibility and a deepened understanding of your body and mind, which will help guide you along the yogic path.

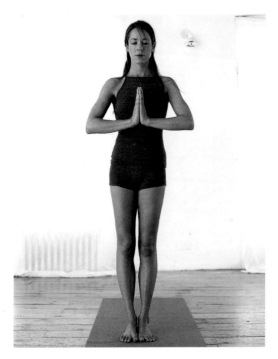

Above While standing in Tadasana, bring the palms together in Namaste and recite your mantra at the beginning of a practice.

Once the primary series is mastered, progression on to the second series, Nadi Sodhana, and eventually the advanced series, follows. It is a natural journey that will unfold with time and practice. There is no need to hurry, as the asanas and the series are purely a vehicle by which you may access your soul.

THE MANTRA

The yoga mantra is spoken at the beginning and end of practice, usually in the original Sanskrit. It should be repeated with an openness of mind to absorb its full meaning, which will become more apparent with time.

Mantras are subtle resonation structures and sacred phrases expressing intention and thought as sound, in much the same way as a prayer. They are the link between consciousness and manifest sound, and have far-reaching powers of transformation, turning negative impulses into positive ones and heightening realms of awareness through their sound vibration.

It is auspicious to open and close your yoga practice with a mantra, and the one at the foot of this page is traditional. Alternatively, reciting silently or aloud the syllable of OM ॐ (the primordial sound, seed of creation and all mantras) will help to channel the body's energy and focus the mind. OM, which forms part of all mantras, is spelt AUM in Sanskrit. Each letter is a sacred symbol:

A represents the individual physical self in the material world
U represents the psychic realms of the mind
M represents the in-dwelling spiritual light of the intuitive self

Repeating this OM mantra for 20 minutes relaxes every atom of the body.

OPENING ASTANGA YOGA MANTRA

~OM~
VANDE GURUNAM CARANARAVINDE
SANDARSITA SVATMA SUKHAVA BODHE
NIH SREYASE JANALIKAYAMANE
SAMSARA HALA HALA MOHASANTYAI

ABAHU PURUSAKARAM
SANKHACAKRASI DHARINAM
SAHASRA SIRASAM SVETAM
PRANAMAMI PATANJALIM
~OM~

TRANSLATION

I pray to the lotus feet of the supreme guru
Awakening the happiness of the inner self revealed
Acting like a doctor of the jungle
Able to pacify the delusion of the poison of conditioned existence

To Patanjali, incarnate of Adisesa, white in colour with
one thousand glowing heads of the divine serpent Anata,
Human in form carrying the sword of discrimination,
the eternal wheel of fire and light and a conch of divine sound,
I prostrate

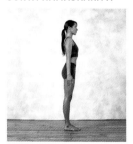

Tadasana Mountain posture p44

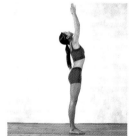

Urdhva Tadasana Upward mountain posture p44

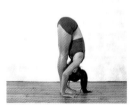

Uttanasana Intense stretch posture p44

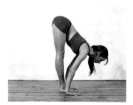

Urdhva Uttanasana Upwards intense stretch posture p44

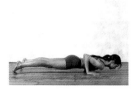

Chaturanga Dandasana Four limbs staff posture p45

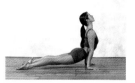

Urdhva Mukha Svanasana Upward facing dog p45

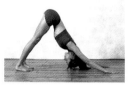

Adho Mukha Svanasana Downward facing dog p45

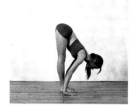

Urdhva Uttanasana Upward intense stretch posture p45

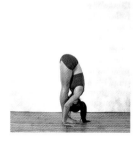

Uttanasana Intense stretch posture p46

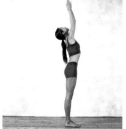

Urdhva Tadasana Upward mountain posture p46

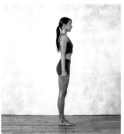

Tadasana Mountain posture p46

SURYA NAMASKARA B

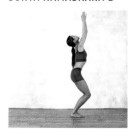

Utkatasana Powerful posture p47

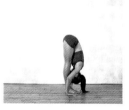

Uttanasana Intense stretch posture p47

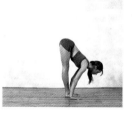

Urdhva Uttanasana Upwards intense stretch posture p47

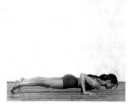

Chaturanga Dandasana Four limbs staff posture p47

▷

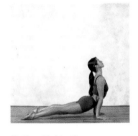

Urdhva Mukha Svanasana
Upward facing dog p47

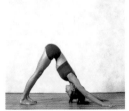

Adho Mukha Svanasana
Downward facing dog p47

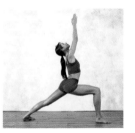

Virabhadrasana I Warrior
posture I p48

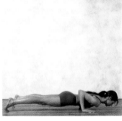

Chaturanga Dandasana
Four limbs staff posture p48

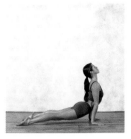

Urdhva Mukha Svanasana
Upward facing dog p47

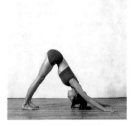

Adho Mukha Svanasana
Downward facing dog p47

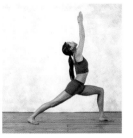

Virabhadrasana I Warrior
posture I p48

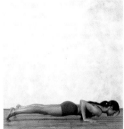

Chaturanga Dandasana
Four limbs staff posture p48

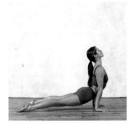

Urdhva Mukha Svanasana
Upward facing dog p49

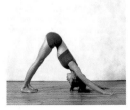

Adho Mukha Svanasana
Downward facing dog p49

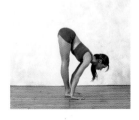

Urdhva Uttanasana Upward
intense stretch posture p49

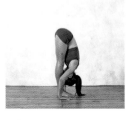

Uttanasana Intense stretch
posture p49

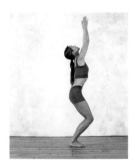

Utkatasana Powerful
posture p49

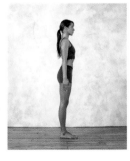

Tadasana Mountain
posture p49

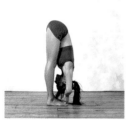

Padangusthasana Foot big toe posture p50

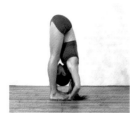

Pada Hastasana Foot hand posture p51

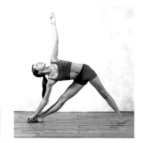

Utthita Trikonasana
Extended triangle p52

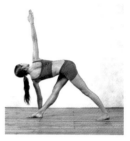

Parivrtta Trikonasana
Revolved triangle p53

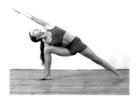

Utthita Parsvakonasana
Extended lateral angle p54

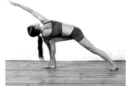

Parivrtta Parsvakonasana
Revolved lateral angle p55

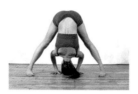

Prasarita Padottanasana A
Expanded leg stretch A p56

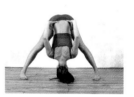

Prasarita Padottanasana B
Expanded leg stretch B p57

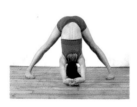

Prasarita Padottanasana C
Expanded leg stretch C p58

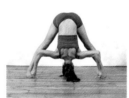

Prasarita Padottanasana D
Expanded leg stretch D p59

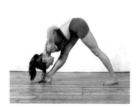

Parsvottanasana Side Intense stretch posture p60

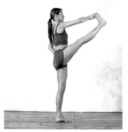

Utthita Hasta Padangusthasana
Extended hand big toe p61

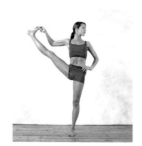

Utthita Parsvasahita A
Extended side posture p62

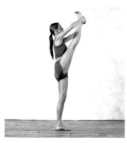

Utthita Parsvasahita B
Extended side posture p63

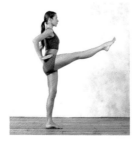

Utthita Parsvasahita C
Extended side posture p63

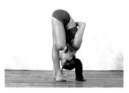

Ardha Baddha Padmottanasana
Half bound lotus stretch p64   ▷

THE PRIMARY SERIES

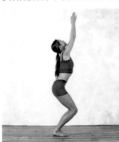

Utkatasana Powerful
posture p65

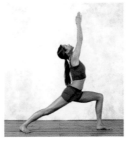

Virabhadrasana I Warrior
posture I p66

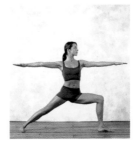

Virabhadrasana II Warrior
posture II p67

SEATED POSTURES

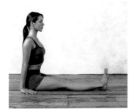

Dandasana Staff posture p72

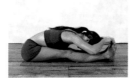

Paschimottanasana A
Stretch of the West A p72

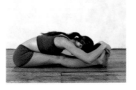

Paschimottanasana B
Stretch of the West B p73

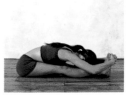

Paschimottanasana C
Stretch of the West C p73

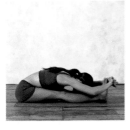

Paschimottanasana D
Stretch of the West D p73

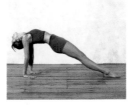

Purvottansana Stretch of the
East p76

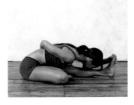

**Ardha Baddha Padma
Paschimottanasana** Half
bound lotus stretch p77

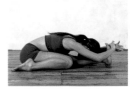

**Triang Mukhaikapada
Paschimottanasana** Three
limbs face one leg stretch p78

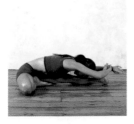

Janu Sirsasana A Knee head
posture A p79

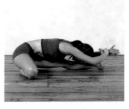

Janu Sirsasana B Knee head
posture B p80

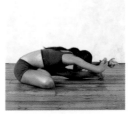

Janu Sirsasana C Knee head
posture C p81

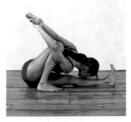

Marichyasana A Sage
Marichi posture A p82

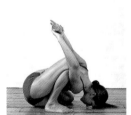

Marichyasana B Sage
Marichi posture B p83

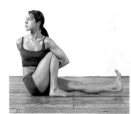

Marichyasana C Sage
Marichi posture C p84

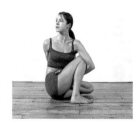

Marichyasana D Sage
Marichi posture D p85

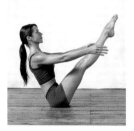

Navasana Boat posture p86

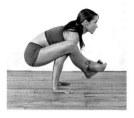

Bhujapidasana A Arm
pressure posture A p87

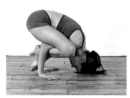

Bhujapidasana B Arm
pressure posture B p87

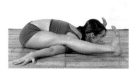

Kurmasana Tortoise
posture p89

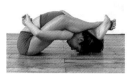

Supta Kurmasana Sleeping
tortoise posture p90

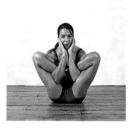

Garbha Pindasana Womb
embryo posture p92

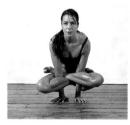

Kukkutasana Rooster
posture p93

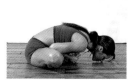

Baddha Konasana A Bound
angle posture A p94

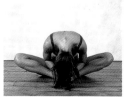

Baddha Konasana B Bound
angle posture B p94

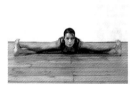

Upavista Konasana A Seated
angle posture A p95

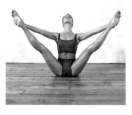

Upavista Konasana B Seated
angle posture B p96

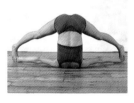

Supta Konasana A Sleeping
angle posture A p97

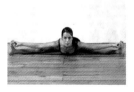

Supta Konasana B Sleeping
angle posture B p98

▷

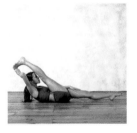

Supta Padangusthasana
Sleeping foot big toe p99

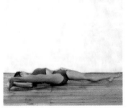

Supta Parsvasahita A
Sleeping side posture A p100

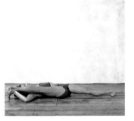

Supta Parsvasahita B
Sleeping side posture B p101

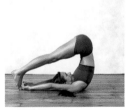

Ubhaya Padangusthasana A
Both feet big toe posture A p103

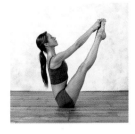

Ubhaya Padangusthasana B
Both feet big toe posture B
p103

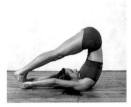

**Urdhva Mukha
Paschimottanasana A**
Upward facing stretch A p104

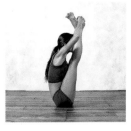

**Urdhva Mukha
Paschimottanasana B**
Upward facing stretch B p104

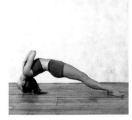

Setu Bandhasana Bridge
posture p105

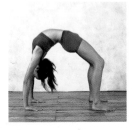

Urdhva Dhanurasana
Upward bow posture p106

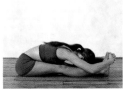
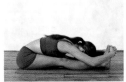

Paschimottanasana C
Stretch of the West C p73

FINISHING SEQUENCE

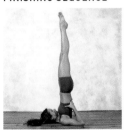

Salamba Sarvangasana
Supported body posture p112

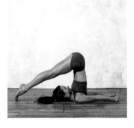

Halasana Plough
posture p114

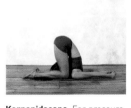

Karnapidasana Ear pressure
posture p115

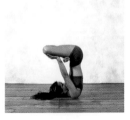

Urdhva Padmasana Upward
lotus posture p116

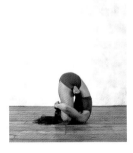

Pindasana Embryo
posture p117

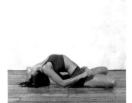

Matsyasana Fish
posture p118

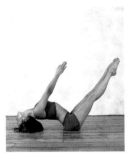

Uttana Padasana Extended
feet posture p119

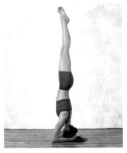

Sirsasana Headstand
posture p120

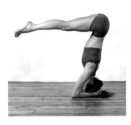

Sirsasana Urdhva Dandasana
Headstand upward staff p123

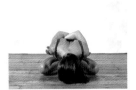

Yoga Mudrasana Yoga
sealing posture p125

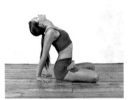

Padmasana A Lotus
posture A p126

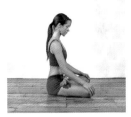

Padmasana B Lotus
posture B p126

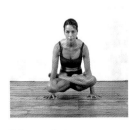

Tolasana Scales
posture p127

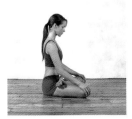

Padmasana Lotus
posture p126

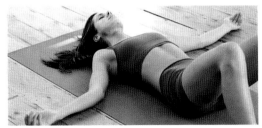

Savasana/Mrtasana Corpse
posture p128

CLOSING ASTANGA YOGA MANTRA

~OM~
SWASTHI – PRAJA BHYAH PARI PALA YANTAM
NYA – YENA MARGENA MAHI – MAHISHAHA
GO – BRAHMANEBHYAHA – SUBHAMASTU – NITYAM
LOKAA – SAMASTHA SUKHINO – BHAVANTHU
~OM~

TRANSLATION

Let prosperity be glorified
May law and justice rule the world
May all divinity be protected and
May people of the whole world be happy and prosperous

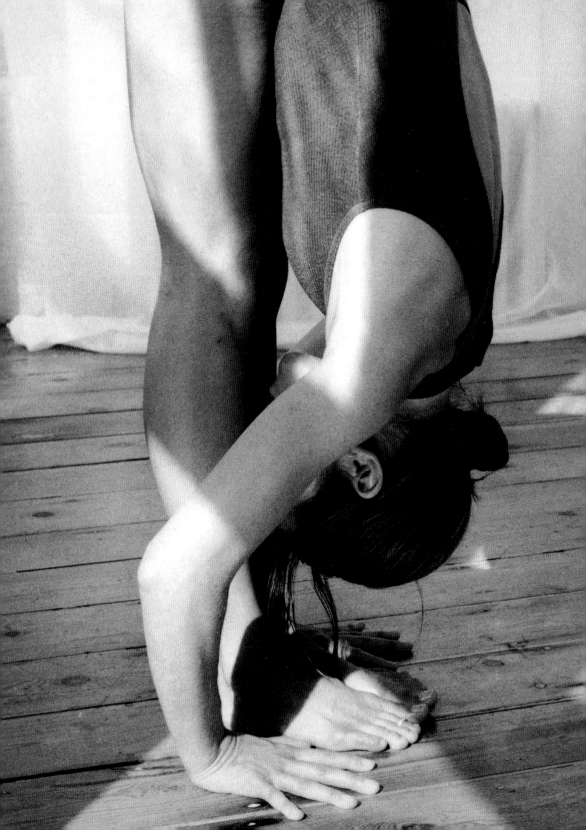

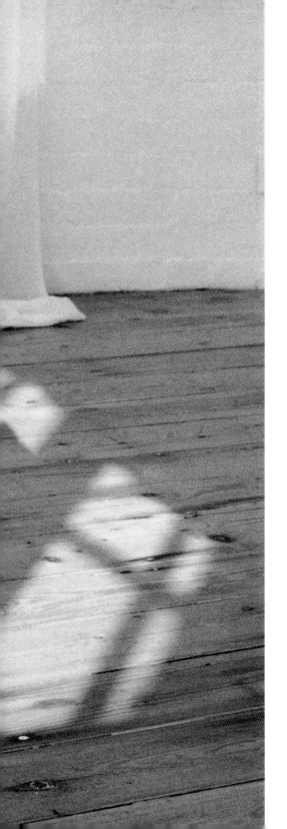

Standing Asanas

Yoga Chikitsa, the primary series, begins
by standing in the stillness of Tadasana.
As you move through Surya Namaskara
and the following asanas, the feet open into
the ground, discovering a sound relationship
with the earth. At the same time, the vital
energy of your breath surges up from the
ground, imbuing your entire body and yoga
postures with life.

Surya Namaskara serves to warm and
awaken the body before moving forwards in
the standing postures. The standing asanas
align the body to develop strength, stamina
and tone.

At the end of the standing sequence we
return to the inspiration of Surya Namaskara
to create a vinyasa flow through the last
standing postures. From here a linking jump
leads us directly into the seated asanas.

Tadasana/Samasthiti | MOUNTAIN POSTURE

tada = mountain
sama = upright
sthiti = still and steady

Through the practice of Tadasana the body is released from bad posture and develops clear alignment through the skeleton. This creates vitality, health and balance within the body, providing the opportunity for standing strong without carrying tension.

1 Stand quietly at the front of your yoga mat with your feet together, feeling the skin of your big toe joints, inner heels and ankle bones touching. Soften the soles of your feet into the floor and let your toes open out like roots.

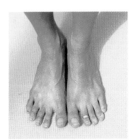

2 Draw your focus inwards, internalizing your awareness, and begin to relax within this standing stillness. Do not tense your muscles, just *breathe softly* and fully, feeling gravity flowing down from the back of your waist through into your tailbone and legs, allowing your weight to drop evenly through your feet into the floor. At the same time, feel energy gently streaming up through your spine, lengthening along the back of your neck and allowing the crown of your skull to float skywards.

With an internal focus, align your hips over your feet and ankles, allowing your sitting bones to release down over your heel bones. Open your shoulders, feeling them directly placed over your pelvis, and balance your head on top of your neck, keeping your throat soft. Allow your bones to fall into alignment without muscular force or tension, which would block the flow of energy and prevent the natural alignment of your skeleton.

In this way, you align from within, stacking your major joints (ankles, knees, hips and shoulders) one above the other like building blocks. Your kneecaps must always follow the same direction as your toes.

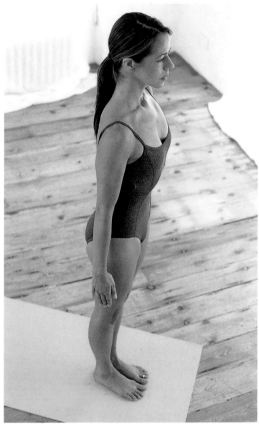

The first building block of yoga

All the standing yoga asanas are born out of Tadasana, and it is from this point of standing in the stillness of mountain posture that the sun salutations begin. Tadasana teaches us how to be still and at ease as we stand alone on our own two feet, and so is central to our practice. As you begin to learn Tadasana, it is important to focus on your internal skeleton, as your bones are the roots of alignment and correct posture. In order for this deep alignment to take place, you need to relax your skin, muscles, mind and heart. By aligning your bones, structural stability and harmony are created from within. Core strength is developed and the muscles can then follow and draw up to support that stability, harmony and movement of your body.

As you stand in Tadasana, allow your mind to become quiet. The quieter we become, the more able we are to listen to, and deepen our awareness of, the energies flowing through our body and existence.

The breath brings new life to these energies, and with the quietness of mind and stillness of body a connection to the rhythmic flow of our breath is made. This connection is our constant backdrop and the inspiration for all existence, which carries and moves us from the inside out through our life and yoga practice.

With improved posture comes ease of movement, confidence, the release of compression on bones and joints, and the creation of internal space for our organs to sit correctly and our lungs to breathe fully.

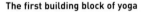

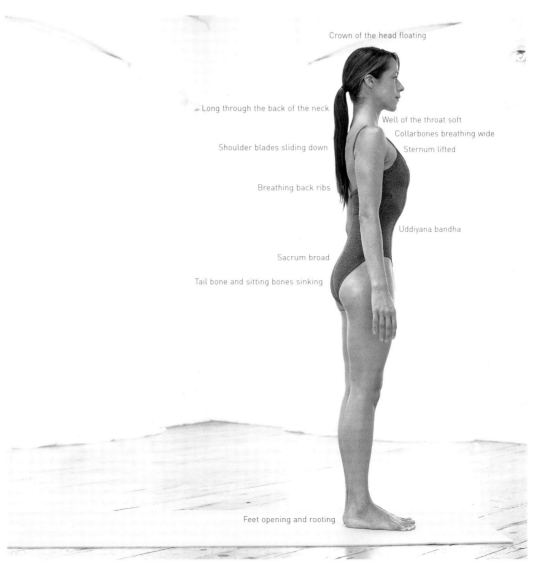

Crown of the head floating

Long through the back of the neck

Well of the throat soft

Collarbones breathing wide

Shoulder blades sliding down

Sternum lifted

Breathing back ribs

Uddiyana bandha

Sacrum broad

Tail bone and sitting bones sinking

Feet opening and rooting

3 Now take your awareness to your perineum and engage mula bandha without gripping your buttocks. Draw your lower abdomen upwards and in, connecting to uddiyana bandha, and softly release your shoulders down and wide. Gently draw in your throat muscles, engaging jalandhara bandha, and guide your breath into ujjayi breathing.

Let your muscles draw in on to your bones, supporting your internal alignment. As you *breathe*, grow into stillness, feeling the subtle internal motion of your breath – both the rising energy of your inhalation (prana) opening you into space, and the down-flowing energy of your exhalation (*aparna*) centring you into the ground.

Once you are in Tadasana
Be aware of and continue the following:
• body breathing
• releasing and opening the feet into the ground
• feeling rebounding energy flowing up through your spine
• yielding the shoulders, tailbone and heels to gravity
• breathing in the sky and breathing it back out again

From breathing in Tadasana, the sequences of Surya Namaskara begin, with each breath moving your body into and out of each asana.

Surya Namaskara A | SUN SALUTATION A

surya = sun
namaskara = respectful greeting
or salute

The flowing sequence of asanas within Surya Namaskara warms and primes the body, building upon the alignment created in Tadasana. With each repetition, prana is generated, helping to deepen awareness and expand consciousness into the practice.

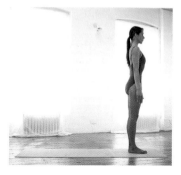

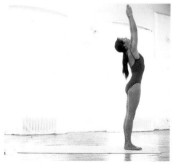

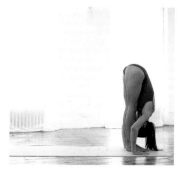

1 TADASANA (mountain posture) Start by quietly standing in this pose. Feel the steady stillness of Tadasana and start to listen to your *breath*, becoming aware of its natural rhythm, and then allow ujjayi pranayama to begin to flow.

2 URDHVA TADASANA (upward mountain posture) *Take a deep inhalation*, as you open your arms out to the sides, stretching up, bringing your palms together into a high prayer gesture. Let energy rise up through your waist to your fingertips and at the same time slide your shoulders and tailbone downwards, opening the soles of your feet into the floor. Lift your gaze up to your thumbs, <u>dristi</u>: angustha ma dyai.

3 UTTANASANA (intense stretch posture) *Slowly exhale*, and fold deeply over your legs. Place your hands on the floor on either side of your feet, and let your head drop down, <u>dristi</u>: nasagrai.

Moderation If your fingers cannot reach the floor with your legs straight, place your hands on your ankles.

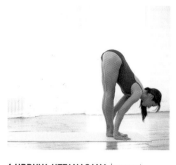

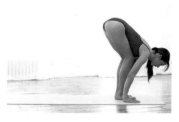

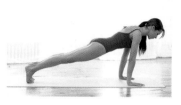

4 URDHVA UTTANASANA (upward intense stretch posture). *Inhale*, lifting and opening your chest and heart forwards as you root your feet downwards. Lengthen through your back, keeping your neck long and in line with your spine. Draw the crown of your head forwards and your shoulder blades down your back. Keep hands on the floor or your ankles. Focus along the nose tip, <u>dristi</u>: nasagrai.

5 PREPARING TO JUMP BACK *Retain your breath*, and bend your knees, keeping your chest lifted and your spine stretching long. Place your hands at the sides of your feet on the floor, if they are not there already, and spread your palms open, pressing them down into the ground. Extend your fingers, with your middle fingers stretching forwards.

6 Keeping your chest opening forwards, softly jump your feet back, allowing them to part slightly. Make sure your shoulders remain aligned over your hands. Feel the body straight and strong in this plank-like position, but do not stay here. Instead, move on smoothly to step 7. Step back if you do not feel confident to jump.

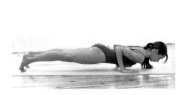

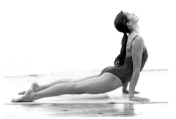

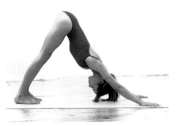

7 CHATURANGA DANDASANA (four limbs staff posture) *Exhale*, bend your elbows, drawing them close into the sides of your body, and lower yourself towards the floor. Keep your spine long and your body straight and parallel to the floor. Broaden your shoulders, engage uddiyana bandha and hover 5cm/2in off the floor. Keep your toes active, pressing into the floor as they are tucked under, spread your palms open and down. Look towards your nose, <u>dristi</u>: **nasagrai**.

Moderation Try bending your knees and lowering your chest in between your hands, keeping the hips lifted.

8 URDHVA MUKHA SVANASANA (upward facing dog posture) *Inhale*, pushing with your toes so that they are stretched long, lift your chest and face skywards, arching evenly through your spine. Gently roll your inner arms forwards and in towards the sides of your waist, without locking the elbows. Draw your shoulders back and stretch your legs long. Press the front of your feet and your palms into the floor, so that the shins, knees, and thighs do not touch the floor, <u>dristi</u>: **bhru madhya**.

Moderation Allow your knees to rest on the floor until you gradually build up the strength to work the full pose.

9 ADHO MUKHA SVANASANA (downward facing dog posture) *Exhale*, roll over the front of your toes and push your hips and buttock bones up and back. Align your feet hip-width apart and extend the outer edges of your feet down while pressing open your big-toe joints into the floor. Spread your toes and fingers, and plant your palms into your mat. Release your shoulders wide, sliding the blades up your back, and gently press your chest towards your legs. Draw your thigh muscles up and on to your upper thigh bones. Sink your heels down into the floor to send your sitting bones higher up. Move your chin in to bring length into the back of your neck, <u>dristi</u>: **nabi chakra**. *Take five long, deep breaths, gathering energy.*

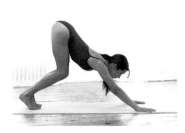

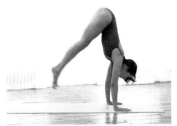

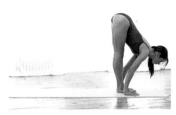

10 JUMP INTO URDHVA UTTANASANA Towards the end of your fifth exhalation, shift your head and shoulders forwards over your hands, allowing your knees to bend slightly and your heels to lift a little off the floor. Keeping your hips well lifted, and still drawing your focus forwards, rock back on to the balls of your feet, bending your knees still further.

11 As you *inhale*, rebound off your toes and lightly jump, projecting your hips upwards and your feet forwards and together in between your hands. At first you may want to step your feet in, especially if you have knee or back injuries.

12 As your feet touch down, keep a lift in your chest and stretch through your spine.

Moderation Place your hands on your ankles and bend your knees, as you stretch your spine forwards.

▷

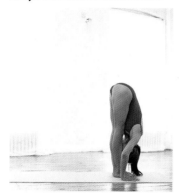

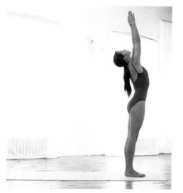

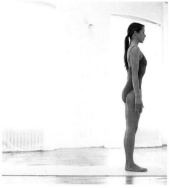

13 UTTANASANA (intense stretch posture) *Slowly and completely exhale*, folding deeply over from your hips. Bring your torso in towards your thighs, and extend the crown of your head down. Make sure your feet are together and that your neck and shoulders are relaxed. Look along your nose tip, <u>dristi</u>: **nasagrai**, and move your chin in towards your chest.

Moderation If you feel any back strain, protect your back by bending your knees and placing your hands on your ankles.

14 URDHVA TADASANA (upward mountain posture) *Inhale*, lifting up through your abdomen and back while pressing your feet firmly into the ground. Raise your arms sideways, bringing your palms together overhead into Urdhva Tadasana. Lift your chest and gaze up to your thumbs and skywards, <u>dristi</u>: **angustha ma dyai**.

15 TADASANA (mountain posture) *Exhale* and turn the palms downwards as you lower your arms down by the sides of your body. Feel your spine lengthening up into Tadasana, and open the soles of your feet broad into the floor beneath you.

• Repeat five to eight times, then move on to Surya Namaskara B.

The importance of Surya Namaskara
• The sun salutation connects body, mind and breath, setting the correct tone and atmosphere to begin your yoga practice. It signifies the worship of the sun god – provider of health and vitality – and is traditionally performed as the sun rises at the dawn of a new day.

• Joints are softly opened, muscles gently stretched, internal organs massaged and the mind–body–breath connection awakened, preparing you for the following journey through the primary series of asanas.

• As the breath and body flow together, an internal heat is created. This begins a process of purification, burning toxins as they are drawn out from the organs, joints and muscles and released through the skin as perspiration.

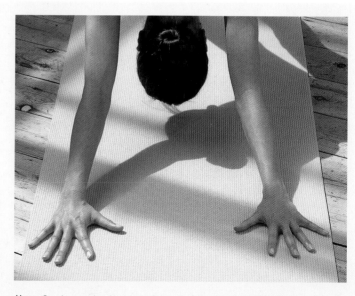

Above Opening your hands generously into the floor with your middle finger stretching forwards develops a secure base in downward facing dog posture.

surya = sun
namaskara = respectful greeting or salute

This second sun salute builds on the first, introducing the posture of Virabhadrasana I (warrior I). This intensifies the internal heat of the body, develops physical stamina and creates a powerful co-ordination of the breath and body in motion.

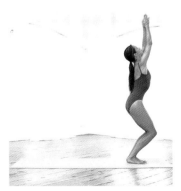

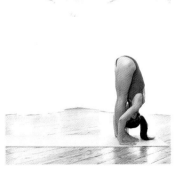

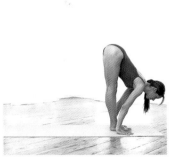

1 UTKATASANA (powerful posture) From Surya Namaskara A, *inhale*, bend your knees deeply and soften at the front of your ankles. Raise your arms sideways and join your palms together arrowing your fingers upwards. Sit your hips low and draw your shoulder blades down your back, raising your focus up to your thumbs, <u>dristi</u>: **angustha ma dyai**.

2 UTTANASANA (intense stretch posture), as in Surya Namaskara A. *Exhale*.

3 URDHVA UTTANASANA (upward intense stretch posture), as in Surya Namaskara A. *Inhale*. Followed by bending your knees to prepare to jump back.

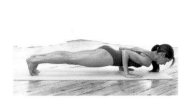

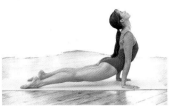

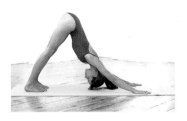

4 CHATURANGA DANDASANA (four limbs staff posture), as in Surya Namaskara A. *Exhale*.

5 URDHVA MUKHA SVANASANA (upward facing dog posture), as in Surya Namaskara A. *Inhale*.

6 ADHO MUKHA SVANASANA (downward facing dog posture), as in Surya Namaskara A. *Exhale*.

Moderation Allow your knees to bend but still focus on tilting your pelvis forwards and your buttocks up.

▷

Surya Namaskara B continued

STANDING ASANAS

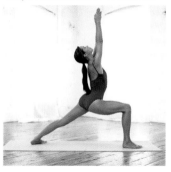

7 VIRABHADRASANA I (warrior posture I)
Pivoting on the ball of your left foot, rotate your left heel in and forwards by 45 degrees towards the arch of your right foot. *Inhale slowly* and step your right foot forwards in between your hands, placing it in line with your right hip. Bend your right knee deeply, drawing it over your ankle, while pressing the sole of your left foot firmly into the floor. Lift up your body, lengthen through your spine and open your arms sideways and then overhead, bringing the palms together. Relax your shoulders and open your chest and face upwards, <u>dristi</u>: **angustha ma dyai.**

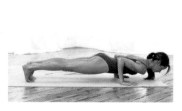

8 CHATURANGA DANDASANA (four limbs staff posture) *Exhale*, placing your hands on the ground on either side of your right foot. Keeping your hips low and your shoulders aligned directly over your hands, take your right foot back parallel to the left and lower yourself down into Chaturanga Dandasana. Look down along the nose tip towards the floor, <u>dristi</u>: **nasagrai.**

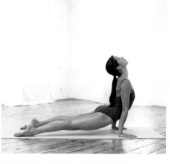

9 URDHVA MUKHA SVANASANA (upward facing dog posture) as in Surya Namaskara A. *Inhale.*

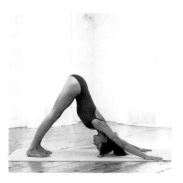

10 ADHO MUKHA SVANASANA (downward facing dog posture) *Exhale*, roll over your toes and lift your hips up and back into Adho Mukha Svanasana. Look towards your navel, <u>dristi</u>: **nabi chakra**, and press your body towards your legs. Do not stay here; instead, flow with your next *inhalation* straight into the next posture.

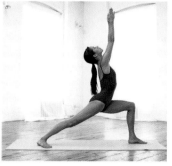

11 VIRABHADRASANA 1 (warrior 1) Inhale and repeat as for step 7, reversing your feet, so that you pivot your right foot to 45 degrees and step your left foot forwards in between your hands.

Moderation If your back heel rises off the floor and your hips swing open out of alignment, lessen the bend of your front leg.

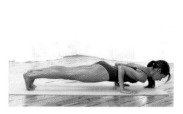

12 CHATURANGA DANDASANA (four limbs staff posture) *Exhale* and place your hands on either side of your left foot and take your left foot back by the right, lowering your body straight to the floor, <u>dristi</u>: **nasagrai.**

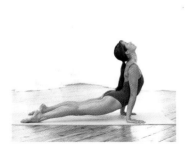

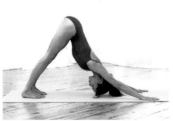

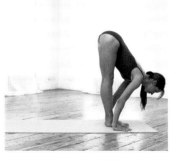

13 URDHVA MUKHA SVANASANA
(upward facing dog posture) *Inhale*, roll
your shoulders back, lift up through your
heart and arch your spine.

14 ADHO MUKHA SVANASANA
(downward facing dog posture) *Exhale*,
roll over your toes and send your hips
back and up. *Take five long, slow, deep ujjayi
breaths*, working deeply into the pose by
pressing your chest open and connecting
the tops of your arms into their shoulder
sockets. Slide the shoulder blades up
away from the ground, and lift your thigh
muscles, abdomen and hips, while
spreading your fingers and toes open
into the floor. Look towards your navel,
<u>dristi</u>: **nabi chakra**.

15 *Inhale* and jump into **URDHVA
UTTANASANA** (upward intense stretch
posture).

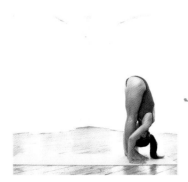

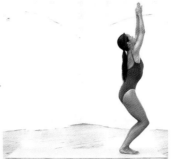

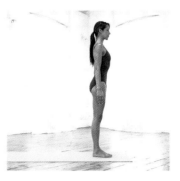

16 UTTANASANA (intense stretch
posture) *Exhale* and fold your torso down
towards your legs.

17 UTKATASANA (powerful posture)
Inhale as you bend your knees and sink
your hips low, lifting up through your
abdomen and back and raising your
arms sideways to bring your palms
together (see step 1).

18 TADASANA (mountain posture) *Exhale*
and gently press your palms downwards
as you lower your arms down by the
sides of your body. Feel your spine
lengthening as you straighten your
legs, and press the soles of your feet
into the floor beneath you to return to
Tadasana. Repeat Surya Namaskara B
five to eight times.

Padangusthasana | FOOT BIG TOE POSTURE

pada = foot or leg
angustha = big toe

This posture teaches the basic mechanics of forward bending from deep within the hip, rather than from the lumbar region. Within this asana, the pelvis is tilted forwards and rotated over the tops of the thigh bones, and the torso is folded over the legs.

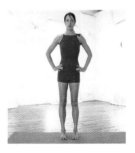
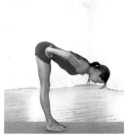
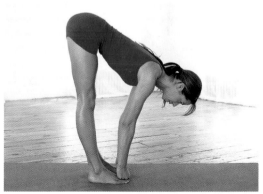

1 From Tadasana, *inhale* while softly jumping your feet slightly apart in line with your hips, aligning your knees to face the same direction as your toes. Sink your heels, big toe joints and outer edges of your feet deeply into the floor. Place your hands on your hips, relax your shoulders down, draw your thighs and lower abdomen up and lengthen your spine.

2 *Exhale slowly*, pivoting your pelvis forwards, and fold from your hips to extend your spine and torso out and over your legs.

3 *Inhale slowly* and catch hold of your big toes. Extend the crown of your head forwards and draw in your abdominal muscles to create length through your spine. Lift your thigh muscles and sitting bones. Root down into your feet while drawing your shoulders down your back and opening your collarbones wide.

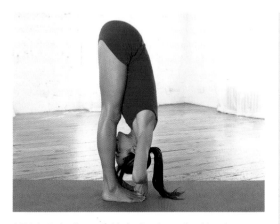

4 *Exhale slowly*, tilt your pelvis further forward and bend more deeply from your hips. Draw your head down and your body close ito your legs. Take your elbows out. Allow your shoulders to release up and away from the floor while lengthening the back of your neck. *Take five deep, slow ujjayi breaths*, allowing your back to yield to gravity. Draw in your abdominal muscles, float your sitting bones and extend your front ribs down. Lift your thigh muscles up and on to their bones. Move your chin in, relax the back of your neck and focus on your nose tip, **dristi**: **nasagrai**. *Inhale*, look up as in step 3 and lengthen your back. Go directly into Pada Hastasana or return to Tadasana, then perform steps 1–3 of Padangusthasana before moving on to Pada Hastasana.

Easing into the pose
Feeling strain, tension or pain is an indication of pushing too hard or of injury. Care must be taken for both. Remember to listen to your body: if you are unable to touch your toes, don't force it. To start with, try practising this pose by holding your ankles instead of your toes, slightly bending your knees. As you tilt your pelvis forwards release your hips over your legs.

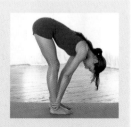

In time, the muscles in your back and legs will gradually become supple enough for you to reach your feet without bending your knees. Practise with patience, and you will be successful.

Deepening the pose
Each time you exhale, feel gravity pouring down through your spine, releasing your back out and down from your hips, while you softly press your buttocks higher and your heels deeper into the floor. Spread your toes open, pressing your big toes down firmly on to your first two fingers. Be lively in the arches of your feet.

pada = foot or leg
hasta = hand

This deepens the stretch of the previous asana, creating release and flexibility in the hips and legs. As the torso is drawn closer into the thighs, focus must be made on lengthening through the front of the torso to help prevent the back rounding over.

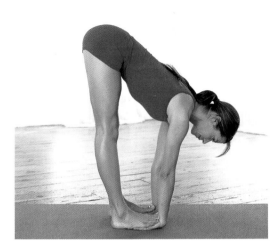

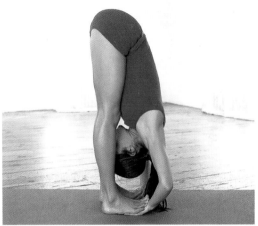

1 *Slowly exhale* and place your hands, palms upwards, under the soles of your feet. *Inhale* here and stretch your spine long, deeply engaging uddiyana bandha.

2 *Slowly exhale.* Hinge from your pelvis to fold your torso down and in towards your legs. Release your neck muscles to allow gravity to flow down through the entire length of your spine as the crown of your head descends. Press the back of your thighs and hips up, drawing uddiyana bandha deeper into your body. *Take five deep breaths.* Broaden across the back of your shoulders and keep your neck long. Open and spread the soles of your feet deeply into the palms of your hands, while sending your sitting bones up and the top of your skull down. Look along your nose tip, <u>dristi:</u> **nasagrai.** *Inhale* and lift your head as in step 1. *Exhale* and place your hands on your hips. *Inhale* and come up to a standing position. *Exhale* and softly jump your feet together to return to Tadasana.

Easing into the pose

If you cannot reach your feet yet, or if your back feels strained when you try, bend your knees, bringing your front ribs on to your thighs. Take your hands on to the floor if standing on them is uncomfortable. From here, gently begin to straighten your legs.

Alternatively, if you are suffering from spinal injuries or a prolapsed disc, stand facing a wall, a little way away from it. Extend your back forwards, lengthening it flat and forming a right angle with your legs. Stretch your arms out straight and press your palms open into the wall. Stay in this position, breathing length into your spine and legs for five breaths.

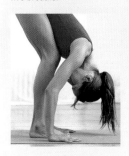

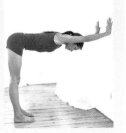

Deepening the pose

To intensify the stretch through the backs of the thighs (the hamstring muscles), press your weight through the balls of your feet into the palms of your hands. Gently draw the outer sides of your knees back to create good alignment; this will keep your knees correctly in line with your toes, which is

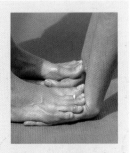

essential for healthy knees and legs.

Utthita Trikonasana | EXTENDED TRIANGLE POSTURE

utthita = extended
tri = three
kona = angle

This posture draws energy up through the legs into the sideways stretch of the back. Strength and flexibility are developed in the feet, ankles, legs and hips, creating a secure foundation for all the following wide-legged asanas.

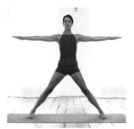 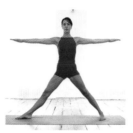

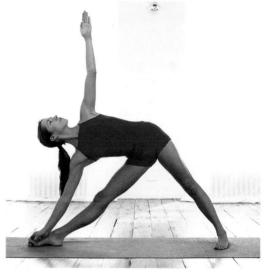

1 From Tadasana, *inhale* and softly jump (or step) to the right, so that you face to the side of your yoga mat, taking your feet about 110cm/45in apart. Keep your legs strong and lift your kneecaps and thigh muscles up. Open the soles of your feet, pressing them down into the ground and aligning them completely parallel to one another. Stretch your arms open and out to the sides in line with your shoulders. Feel your back gently extending up and your shoulders releasing down. Keep your chin level.

2 Begin a *long, slow exhalation*, and turn your left leg, toes and ball of the foot inwards by 10–15 degrees, while turning your right leg outwards by 90 degrees. Place your right heel opposite your left arch, and keep your hips level and your tailbone releasing downwards. Remember to keep your knees aligned over your toes, so that the rotation of your legs occurs within your hip sockets.

3 Continue to *exhale slowly*, and stretch your torso out to the right side over your right leg. Do not lean forwards as you catch hold of your right big toe. Draw your left hip back and outwards. Stretch your left arm up with the hand directly over your left shoulder lengthening through to your fingertips, with the palm facing forwards. Look towards your left hand, <u>dristi</u>: **hastagrai**. *Take five to ten long, steady breaths*, opening your body out like a star. With a *slow inhalation*, draw your body upright, turning your feet parallel. *Exhale slowly*, and repeat step 2, this time turning your right leg in by 10–15 degrees and your left leg out by 90 degrees and stretch over to the left side. *Take five to ten deep, slow breaths*, then *inhale* and draw your body upright, turning your feet parallel. From here, either go directly into the next posture or *exhale* and return to Tadasana. Then jump your feet apart and continue on to Parivrtta Trikonasana.

Easing into the pose

If your torso and hips lean forwards, the benefits of the lateral stretch to the torso will be lost. Instead of trying to grasp your toe, place your right hand lightly on your right shin or ankle instead, or on a wooden yoga block if you have one. Do not abandon the integrity of your practice for the pride of the pose. Work truthfully, and your suppleness will develop, allowing you to catch hold of your big toe in time.

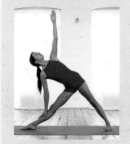 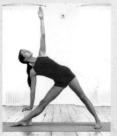

Deepening the pose

Work to draw your left hip back, gently moving the left ribs and shoulder directly over the right ribs and shoulder. Extending your left arm back and taking your fingertips on to your right upper thigh will help in sensing this side stretch.

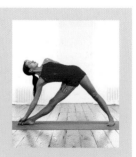

parivrtta = revolved, turned
tri = three
kona = angle

This posture creates a counter-stretch to Trikonasana and introduces the mechanics of twisting, which is essential for spinal health. To twist effectively, the legs and hips have to be firm while the twisting motion flows up through the spine to the head.

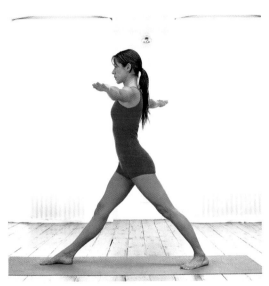

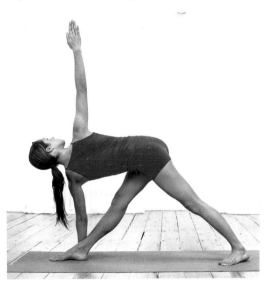

1 Begin to *exhale very slowly*, and turn your left toes, ball of foot, leg and hip in by 45 degrees while rotating your right hip, leg and foot out by 90 degrees. Turn your body to face completely to the right side, squaring both hip bones, collarbones and shoulders evenly, like sets of headlights all shining in the same direction. Stretch your arms out to the sides at shoulder height, and align your feet with their respective hips.

2 Continue to *exhale slowly*, and gently sweep your left arm and the left side of your torso forwards and down towards your right leg. Cross your left wrist over your right ankle, and open your left palm down on to the floor by the little-toe edge of your right foot. Revolve your right shoulder and the side of your right torso back. Extend your right arm up and over your right shoulder. Softly draw both shoulders down away from your ears, keeping your legs active (kneecaps and thigh muscles lifted) and your bandhas engaged. *Take five to ten breaths*, lifting and opening your chest skywards and looking towards your raised hand, <u>dristi</u>: **hastagrai**. With *an inhalation*, lift your torso up, turning your feet parallel, then *exhale* and repeat the pose to the left. *Take five to ten deep, smooth breaths*, then *inhale* and draw your torso upright, turning your feet parallel. *Exhale* and jump into Tadasana.

Easing into the pose
If your hand cannot reach the floor at first, rest it on your shin or ankle or a wooden yoga block, and work the rotation of your torso from here, taking the lifted hand on to the sacrum. With practice, the hand will gradually be able to touch the floor.

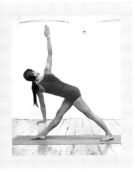

Deepening the pose
The stability of this posture is developed by the rooting of your feet into the ground. Open the sole of your back foot and outer heel deeply into the floor. Draw the muscles of your front thigh up and move your front hip back and your back hip forwards to balance your pelvis. Deepen the twist in the back by opening your right collarbone away from the left. Roll the right side of your torso up and back to align directly over the left side of your torso. On the second side to the posture, focus on drawing the left side of your torso over your right side.

STANDING ASANAS

Utthita Parsvakonasana | EXTENDED LATERAL ANGLE POSTURE

utthita = extended
parsva = side or lateral
kona = angle

This posture furthers the fundamental principles of Utthita Trikonasana with an extended side stretch. The deep lunging in one leg and the stretch through the other creates a dynamic balance of leg strength and flexibility.

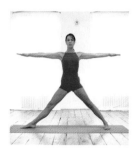 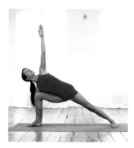 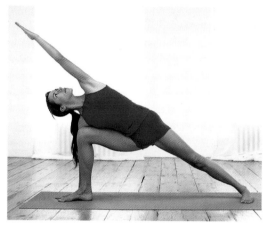

1 From Tadasana, *inhale* and softly jump (or step) to the right, taking your feet parallel and about 140cm/55in apart, with your arms extending out to the sides. Feel your legs stretching long and your spine lengthening up. Begin to *exhale very slowly*, turning your left foot and leg in by 15 degrees and rotating your right leg and foot out by 90 degrees (as in Utthita Trikonasana, step 2), and align your right heel opposite your left arch.

2 Continue to *exhale slowly*, and deeply bend your right knee, drawing the back of the knee completely over (but not beyond) your ankle to create a right angle through the right leg. Lengthen your body over to the right side, taking your right hand on to the floor by the little-toe edge of your right foot. Raise your left arm and extend it up over your shoulder.

3 As you complete your *exhalation*, soften your left shoulder down and rotate your left arm within its socket, then stretch the arm diagonally over by the side of your head, with the palm facing down. Look up towards the little-finger edge of your raised hand, **dristi: hastagrai**, and *take five to ten even, deep breaths*, drawing the entire length of the left side of your torso up and open to turn your chest skywards. Inhale slowly, straightening your knee and lifting your torso upright. Turn your feet parallel, then repeat Parsvakonasana to the left side. *Take five to ten deep, slow breaths*, then *inhale very slowly*, drawing your body upright and turning your feet parallel. From here, either go directly into Parivrtta Parsvakonasana as you begin your next *exhalation*, or *exhale* and lightly jump back into Tadasana. From here, *inhale* and lightly jump your feet 140cm/55in apart to the right, with the arms stretching to the sides at shoulder level, then continue on into Parivrtta Parsvakonasana with the next *exhalation*.

Easing into the pose
This posture creates a very deep and challenging stretch. If reaching for the floor causes your torso to lean forwards, avoid this by bending your elbow and placing your forearm on your thigh. This will also help in keeping the pelvis and hips open, your chest lifted and your waist

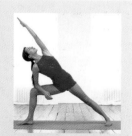

toned. You will gradually advance into the full posture.

Deepening the pose
Work your legs evenly and stretch them away from one another to create a balance of energy in the posture. Feel the legs releasing out from the pelvis and inner groin, then press your right knee and outer thigh back into the right arm, while stretching down through your left leg into left outer heel and little toe. (Reverse for other side.)

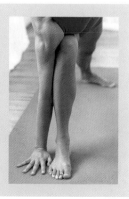

parivrtta = revolved, turned
parsva = side or lateral
kona = angle

In this strong twist, the ribcage is fully rotated, deepening the breath and improving respiration. As the torso is turned blood circulation is stimulated to the internal organs, flushing them of toxins and boosting digestion. Leg strength is developed.

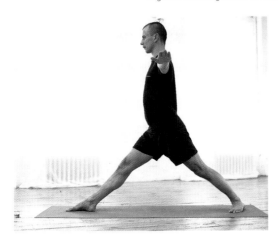

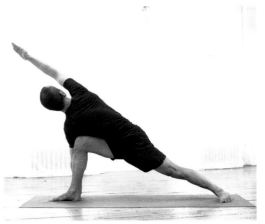

1 Begin to *exhale very slowly* as you rotate your left toes, ball of foot, leg and hip in by 45 degrees, and rotate your right hip, leg and foot out by 90 degrees (as in Parivrtta Trikonasana). Turn your body to face the right side, squaring your shoulders and hip bones evenly while stretching your arms out to the sides at shoulder height. Align your feet with their respective hip sockets.

2 Continue to *exhale slowly* and bend your right knee fully, taking it directly over your right ankle into a right angle. Turn your torso towards your right leg, drawing the left side of your ribcage over your right thigh. Extend your left armpit and arm over the outer side of your right knee and shin. Place your left hand on the floor by the outer side of your right foot. Revolve the right shoulder and side of your body back and up. Rotate your right arm within its shoulder socket to turn your palm to face over head, and stretch your arm diagonally over by the side of your head. Softly draw your shoulders down and press your chest open upwards as you root your back foot down. *Take five to ten breaths*, and look towards your raised hand along the outer edge, <u>**dristi: hastagrai**</u>. With a *slow inhalation*, return your torso upright and straighten your right leg, turning your feet parallel. Start to *exhale slowly*, and repeat steps 1 and 2, with the body turning to the left. *Exhale*, softly jump back into Tadasana.

Easing into the pose
This is a strong posture. If you feel any straining or twisting in your back knee, release the heel off the floor and let the knee touch down to the floor. Alternatively, if the knee feels strong but the chest caves in or the shoulders hunch up, work the back heel down into the floor, and hook your elbow

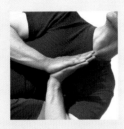

over the opposite thigh, then bring your palms together at the centre of your chest.

Deepening the pose
Cross your arm and shoulder completely over the opposite thigh. Focus on pressing the outer side of your knee and shin against the outer side of your shoulder and arm to help secure this powerful rotation of your torso. As you move into this pose, be sure to stretch the spine while opening the chest upwards.

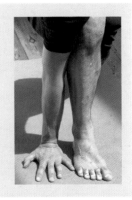

Prasarita Padottanasana A | EXPANDED LEG STRETCH POSTURE A

prasarita = expanded or spread
pada = foot or leg
uttana = extended or intense
stretch

The four variations of this posture each work deeply on strengthening and stretching the legs, and the four work together to stimulate and cleanse the digestive organs. The first pose opens the hip joints and allows energy to flow from the pelvis to the feet.

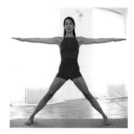
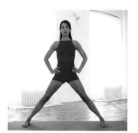

1 From Tadasana, *inhale* and softly jump (or step) to the right, taking your feet parallel and about 140cm/55in apart, with your arms lengthening out to the sides. Take your feet wide to align them directly under your wrists, with your arches strongly lifted.

2 *Exhale slowly*, opening the soles of your feet down into the floor, and place your hands on your hips. *Inhale slowly* and lengthen up through your spine, breathing openness into your back and pelvis. Draw your thigh muscles up, and be especially aware of uddiyana bandha now and throughout this whole series of the four Prasarita Padottanasanas.

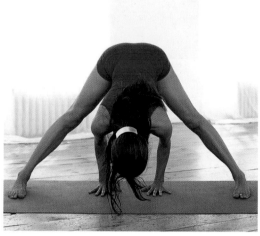

3 *Exhale slowly* and extend your back forwards, folding deeply from your hips. Place your hands on the ground, in between your feet if possible. Spread your fingers and look at your hands, checking that they are shoulder-width apart and that your middle fingers are extending forwards. Keep your chest open and your shoulders relaxed.

Easing into the pose
If you experience strain in your back or over-pulling through the hamstring muscles, you can practise by bending your knees directly over your toes and placing your hands on the floor in line with your shoulders. Using yoga blocks or a pile of books can also be helpful, and in this way you can begin to work your legs straight without causing stress in your back.

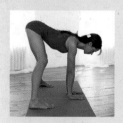
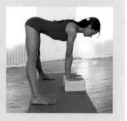

Deepening the pose
Spreading and opening your hands and feet into the floor will create a firm anchor for you, so that you can strongly float your sitting bones upwards. This will begin to increase the flexibility in your hips and legs. Keep long in your neck and open in your shoulders, releasing them up from the floor.

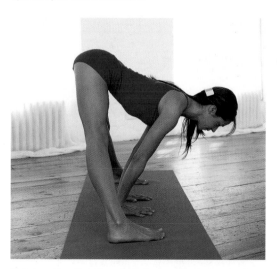

4 *Inhale* and lengthen through the front and back of your spine, drawing your chest and focus forwards while keeping your neck long and in line with your spine. Release your shoulder blades down your back and firmly lift your thigh muscles up.

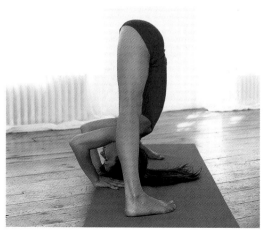

5 *Exhale slowly* into the full posture by pivoting your pelvis further forwards to deepen the rotation within your hip sockets. Step your hands back, so that your fingertips are in line with the heels of your feet, and lower the top of your head to the floor. Bend your elbows over your wrists and slide your shoulders up away from the floor. *Take five to ten slow, even breaths*, yielding your back to gravity, while keeping your legs strong and active by drawing up your thigh muscles. Move the skin of the outer edges of your knees back to prevent your knees misaligning or locking. Look to your nose tip, **dristi: nasagrai**, and open the soles of your feet. *Slowly inhale* and lift your focus and chest forwards. *Exhale*, extend your back flat and parallel to the floor, hands on your hips. *Inhale* and lift your torso up to standing position. From here, either move into posture B, or *exhale*, and jump back into Tadasana. Then *inhale*, jump to the right, parting your feet wide, and continue on to the B variation.

Prasarita Padottanasana B | EXPANDED LEG STRETCH POSTURE B

prasarita = expanded or spread
pada = foot or leg
uttana = extended or intense
stretch

In this variation, the hands remain on the hips, allowing the spine to cascade forwards freely without pulling through the arms to draw the body low. This releases compression on the vertebrae, creating space in the spine and replenishing the inter-vertebral discs.

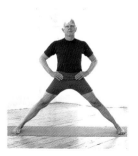

1 *Exhale* and, with your hands on your hips, feel your feet connecting down into the floor while drawing your thigh muscles up. *Inhale*, breathing length into your spine and openness into your chest and collarbones.

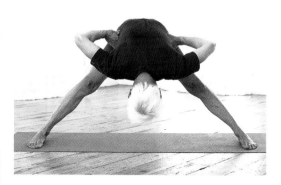

Easing into the pose
If your back rounds, bend your knees to help develop straightness and length through your spine and to facilitate a deeper pivoting of your pelvis forwards.

Deepening the pose
Be careful not to strain or push in this posture: as with all postures, suppleness comes not from straining but from releasing. Keeping this in mind each time you breathe out, feel gravity streaming down through your spine, helping to release your back and head lower. Do not allow your shoulders to press down to your ears; instead, gently slide them up and away.

2 *Exhale* and slowly fold your torso down by pivoting your pelvis forwards. Lengthen through your spine and extend the crown of your head to the floor. Keep your hands on your hips and *take five to ten deep, slow breaths*, again focusing on the dynamic energy in your legs. Be careful not to lock your knees; instead, gently but firmly press your inner thigh muscles away from one another. Look along to your nose tip, **dristi: nasagrai**. *Inhale* and lift from your abdominal muscles to return your torso up to standing position. *Exhale*, relax your shoulders and deepen uddiyana bandha. *Inhale* and lengthen your arms out to the sides at shoulder level. From here, either move straight into posture C, or *exhale* and lightly jump back into Tadasana. From Tadasana *inhale* and jump to the side, taking your feet wide apart and your arms open, then continue into posture C.

Prasarita Padottanasana C | EXPANDED LEG STRETCH POSTURE C

prasarita = expanded or spread
pada = foot or leg
uttana = extended or intense
stretch

This posture creates an intense joint-opening stretch in the hips and legs and through the shoulders and arms. Creating a full rotation inside the shoulder sockets helps to loosen and prevent stiffness in the arms, shoulder girdle and upper back.

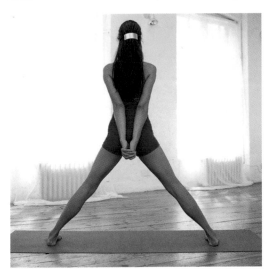

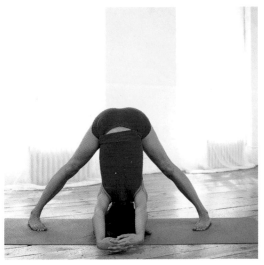

1 *Exhale*, take your hands behind your back and interlace your fingers. *Inhale*, draw your shoulders back and lengthen through your arms, rotating your inner arms forwards. Gently press your knuckles down and open across your chest and collarbones.

2 *Exhale slowly* and fold forwards from your hips, drawing your arms up and over behind your shoulders. Expand your chest, stretching your arms long and directing your little fingers down towards the floor. Feel your shoulder blades drawing inwards and allow your arms to rotate softly within their shoulder sockets. *Breathe* into the posture for *five to ten slow breaths*, looking along to your nose tip, <u>dristi: nasagrai</u>. *Inhale*, draw your abdominal muscles in to move your back upright, then draw your arms down behind your back. *Exhale* here relaxing your shoulders. *Inhale*, release the interlace of your fingers and stretch your arms out to the sides at shoulder level. From here, you can either flow into posture D as you begin your next *exhalation* or you can *exhale* and lightly jump back into Tadasana. From Tadasana *inhale* and jump to the right side, parting your feet wide, and then continue into the final variation of this posture.

Benefits of the pose
The muscles between the upper spine and shoulder blades (intraspinatus) are strengthened by this posture, as circulation to this region is stimulated. The chest and front ribs are expanded, improving respiration and helping to maintain the openness of the front torso.

Easing into the pose
As well as developing flexibility in your legs and hips, this variation creates suppleness in the shoulders and arms. If either your shoulders or arms, or both, feel unable to yield, use a belt or yoga strap to link your hands and then gently work to extend your arms over and you can still benefit. Keep moving your

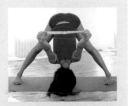

shoulder blades in at the same time as drawing the shoulders back, as this will release tension from the shoulder girdle.

Deepening the pose
Softly move your chin in to bring length to the back of your neck. This also creates space for the rotation and movement of your shoulders needed to release your arms over. Press down through your heels while firmly lifting your front thigh muscles up and on to your thigh bones. Keep your feet active and lift your arches.

prasarita = expanded or spread
pada = foot or leg
uttana = extended or intense
stretch

The final variation of Prasarita Padottanasana strongly stimulates the digestive fire (agni), thereby aiding the digestive process and internal cleansing. The space created between the shoulder blades opens the pathway through the spine into the brain.

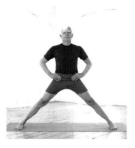

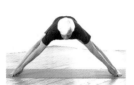

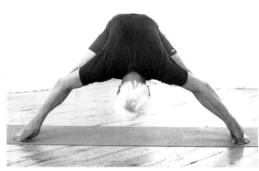

1 *Exhale slowly* and place your hands on your hips while opening the soles of your feet down into the floor. *Inhale slowly,* keeping your hands on your hips, and lengthen up through your spine. Breathe openness into your chest and collarbones as you focus on drawing your thigh muscles up on to the thighbones. Fully engage uddiyana bandha.

2 *Exhale slowly* and extend your back forwards, folding deeply at the hips. Catch hold of your big toes using the index and middle fingers of both hands as in Padangusthasana (foot big toe posture page 44). *Inhale* and lengthen through your spine, drawing your chest and focus out and forwards. Extend your back long, keeping your neck in line with your spine, and stretch the front of your torso. Move your shoulder blades down your back away from your ears, and firmly lift your thighs.

3 *Exhale slowly,* bending your elbows outwards and hinging more deeply within your hip sockets. Release your neck muscles to allow the top of your head to drop towards the floor. Feel the flow of gravity moving down through your spine. Soften your shoulders wide in the same direction as your elbows, and be careful to slide your shoulder blades up and away from your ears. *Take five to ten steady, even breaths,* looking along to your nose tip, <u>dristi</u>: **nasagrai**. *Slowly inhale,* lengthening your spine and lifting your focus and chest forwards, while keeping the back of your neck long. With your fingers still holding your toes, straighten your arms as in step 2. *Exhale* and place your hands on your hips. Extend your back long, stretching the front of your torso parallel to the floor. *Inhale,* lifting up from your abdominal muscles, and draw your torso up to standing position, while opening the soles of your feet down into the floor. *Exhale* and lightly jump your feet together into Tadasana, facing the front of your mat.

Easing into the pose
Bend your knees to release any strain or pressure in your back, and hold your ankles if you are initially unable to take hold of your big toes.

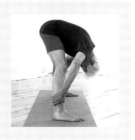

Deepening the pose
Soften the fold at the front of your hips and focus on sending your tailbone, sitting bones and pubic bone back and up to release your spine, and the crown of your head down towards the floor. Keep your legs active, and strongly press your inner thighs away from one another, extending energy down through to the soles of your feet into the floor. Work uddiyana bandha throughout these four poses to increase the benefits and to support and protect the back.

Parsvottanasana | SIDE INTENSE STRETCH POSTURE

parsva = side or lateral
uttana = extended or intense
stretch

This posture develops the alignment, symmetry and balance of the pelvis and hips while strengthening the leg muscles. It stimulates circulation, deepens breathing, improves posture – especially hunching of the back – and unlocks tension.

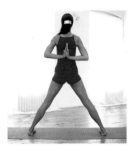

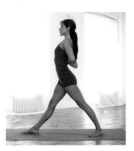

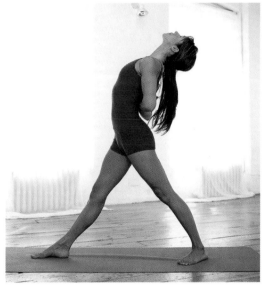

1 From Tadasana, *inhale* and softly jump (or step) to the right, taking your feet about 110cm/45in apart, and open your arms out to the sides in line with your shoulders. Open the soles of your feet and align them parallel to one another. Feel your back gently extending up and your shoulders releasing down. Begin to *exhale slowly* and draw your palms together behind your back into a prayer gesture (Paschima Namaste).

2 Continue to *exhale* and turn your left toes, ball of foot, leg and hip in by 45 degrees, while rotating your right hip, leg and foot out by 90 degrees. Turn your body to face completely to the right side, squaring both hip bones, collarbones and shoulders.

3 *Inhale* and roll your shoulders back and down. Raising your focus and heart, look up, while pressing your palms together.

Easing into the pose
If taking your palms together into Paschima Namaste is not yet possible, hold your elbows behind your back. Gradually your shoulder flexibility will develop so your hands can come together.

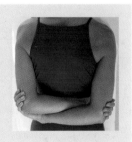

Deepening the pose
In the full posture, roll your elbows backwards and draw your shoulder blades in, to create an openness in your heart and chest. The legs and hips need to be correctly aligned to gain the full benefits of this posture. Focus on strongly drawing

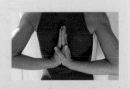

your front kneecap and thigh muscle up to the right hip, while pressing the ball of your front foot down.

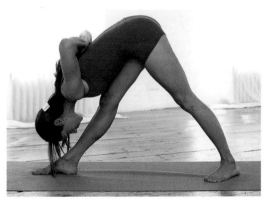

4 *Slowly exhale* and pivot your pelvis forwards to extend your torso out and over your right leg, bringing your face towards your shin. As you *take five to ten deep, even breaths*, elongate the front and back of your spine and lengthen through the back of the neck, releasing your head down. Focus your gaze towards your nose tip, **dristi: nasagrai**. With a *slow inhalation*, lift from uddiyana bandha, returning your torso upright and bringing your feet parallel. Repeat steps 2–4 turning to the left. *Exhale* and softly jump into Tadasana, releasing the arms down.

utthita = extended
hasta = hand
pada = foot or leg
angustha = big toe

This and the three following extended postures flow consecutively into one another creating dynamic power in the muscles of the supporting leg to maintain the balance effectively for the duration of these four asana variations.

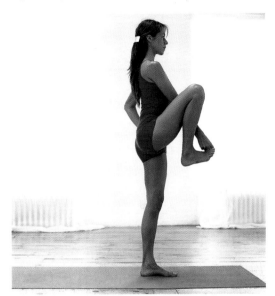

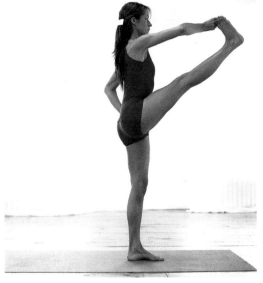

1 From Tadasana, *inhale*, gently swing your right knee up, and, using your right index and middle fingers, catch hold of your right big toe. Press your right big toe into your fingers and draw your right hip down to keep it level with the left. Place your left hand on your left hip, and balance.

2 With a *slow, steady exhalation*, press your right foot up, lengthening your leg straight and up towards your chest. Release the front of your right hip down, creating a seesaw action to raise your right foot and shinbone higher. Roll both your shoulders back and down, and bend your right elbow outwards to help keep your chest open. *Breathe steadily* here, connecting uddiyana bandha deeply into your body, and align your lifted foot directly forwards. Gaze steadily to your right toes, <u>dristi</u>: **padhayoragrai**. *After five to ten full breaths, inhale*, straighten your right arm and flow into the next posture.

Deepening the pose
Do not over-focus on your raised leg: it is really your standing foot and leg that deserve your awareness, since they create your base and support in this posture. Consciously stretch your standing leg, rooting the sole of your open foot into the floor and drawing your knee and thigh up. Focus on aligning the knee and toes forwards and keep the right

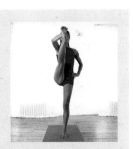

side of your right hip softening down level with the left hip. Press your lifted heel directly forwards.

Easing into the pose
If straightening your leg causes your back to round and your shoulders to hunch, practise this posture at first with your knee bent, as in step 1. With each practice, press your lifted foot slightly forwards to gradually stretch your hamstring. Over time and with practice, you will develop both the strength and flexibility to lengthen the leg straight without compromising the alignment of your back.

Utthita Parsvasahita A | EXTENDED SIDE ACCOMPANIED POSTURE A

utthita = extended
parsva = side or lateral
sahita = accompanied

Opening the raised leg to the side in this asana further enhances balance, co-ordination and mental concentration. Keeping the back straight develops the strength of the muscles on either side of the spine. The legs and buttocks are also toned.

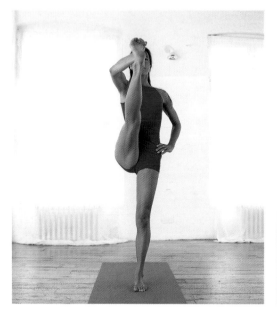

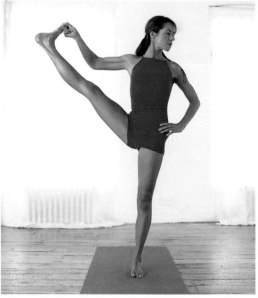

1 From the previous posture as pictured above, take a *long, even exhalation*, open your right arm and leg out to the right side, rotating your inner thigh forwards and releasing your right buttock and tailbone downwards. Open your chest and slide your shoulder blades down your back to create length through your spine and neck.

2 Turn your head to the left, moving your chin over your left shoulder, and *take five to ten breaths* here, levelling your collarbones open and extending your focus out to the right side, **dristi: parsva**. *Inhale*, and return your right arm, leg and focus forwards, then flow into the next posture.

Easing into the pose
As in the previous posture, you can work this pose with your leg bent, focusing on gradually lengthening and straightening it a little more with each practice. Be patient, and, with practice and a calm approach, the full posture will soon be achievable.

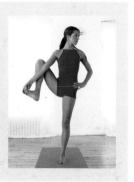

Deepening the pose
Feel the whole pose opening out from your centre in three flowing energy lines:
1 From the back of your waist upwards along your spine through to the very top of your head.
2 Down from the back of your waist through into your tailbone and standing leg, sending the sole of your foot deeper into the floor.
3 Out from the inner thigh of your raised leg through to the heel.
Breathe into these three energy lines and let the posture grow and expand.

utthita = extended
parsva = side or lateral
sahita = accompanied

This creates an amazing stretch through the legs and hips. Pressing down through the supporting leg and foot is crucial for stability. An awareness of gravity and the energy rising up through the body will help to centre and balance the mind and body.

STANDING ASANAS

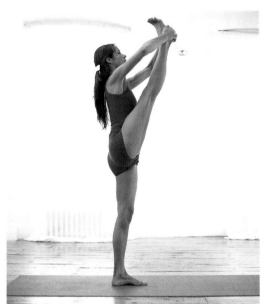

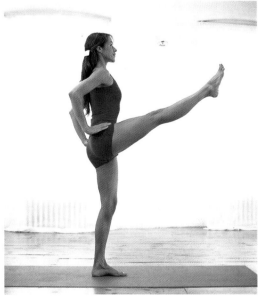

1 With a *smooth exhalation*, catch hold of your right foot with both hands. Root down through your standing foot to lift your raised foot higher. If your standing leg begins to feel weak or tired, focus on sending the energy of your breath down through to your foot, and open your foot into the floor to receive the energy pouring up into your muscles, providing them with strength and vitality. Do not straighten your arms, instead keep your elbows bent. *Take five to ten slow breaths*, looking towards your right toes, <u>dristi</u>: **padhayoragrai**, and then *exhale*, releasing the hold on your foot without dropping your foot to the floor.

2 With your hands on your hips, keep your leg lifted and float your foot to 90 degrees or higher without straining or hunching your back. *Take five full, steady breaths*, stretching up through your back and releasing your shoulders down. Softly gaze towards the toes of your right foot, <u>dristi</u>: **padhayoragrai**. *Exhale* and slowly lower the foot, returning to Tadasana. Repeat Utthita Hasta Padangusthasana, and Utthita Parsvasahita A and B/C on the left side.

Easing into the pose
Maintaining a length and energy flow through your spine is essential for spinal alignment and health. Yoga postures are intended to develop and enhance this energy and health, so do not at any time during your practice sacrifice length and alignment of your spine for the grandeur of a posture. There are no benefits to be gained by straining and hunching your back in an attempt to lift your leg high. In fact, it is more beneficial not to lift your leg so high, or practise initially with the lifted knee bent instead to maintain a strong, straight back. Practising in this way will gradually develop your strength, alignment and flexibility.

Deepening the pose
As you draw your right leg and your foot up, feel the opposite end of the same leg, i.e. the top of your thigh bone, connecting down into its hip socket. In this way, a seesaw motion is created, helping to float the lifted foot further up. Feel the right sitting bone drawing down in line with the left to keep the pelvis aligned. Open the sole of your standing foot deeply down into the floor.

Ardha Baddha Padmottanasana | HALF BOUND LOTUS INTENSE STRETCH

ardha = half
baddha = bound or caught
padma = lotus
uttana = extended/intense stretch

Here the beginnings of the lotus posture are introduced. In the full posture, the heel presses into the lower abdomen, stimulating blood circulation through the intestines. Strength is promoted through the standing leg, and the binding arm creates openness.

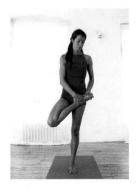

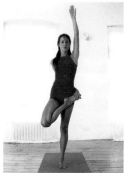

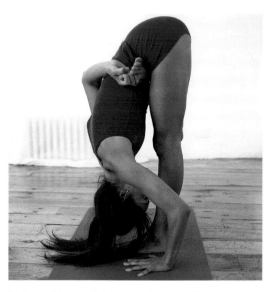

1 *Inhale*. Bend your right knee, lifting your foot up. Use both hands to place your foot at the very top of your left front thigh. Move the little-toe edge of your right foot up to the left hip socket, and gently direct the right kneecap downwards. This is Ardha Padma (half lotus).

2 Continue to *inhale*. Stretch your right arm behind your back and reach your right hand to your right foot, catching hold of the right big toe with your index and middle fingers. Release left hand from your foot and stretch your left arm up. (If you need to steady your balance here, do so, and *breathe out and then in* as you raise your left arm; otherwise move directly on.)

3 *Exhale*, and extend your torso forwards, bending your left knee slightly, and softly fold your back down over your left leg. Place your left hand on the floor next to your left foot and keep your right hand holding your right big toe.

Inhale, breathing length into your spine, and softly roll your shoulders back and press your chest forwards. *Fully exhale*, and fold your torso deeply in towards your left leg, relaxing your neck muscles and releasing your head low. Move your face towards your left shin and *breathe steadily here for five to ten breaths*, looking towards the nose tip, <u>**dristi: nasagrai**</u>. *Inhale* and lift your chest forwards, then *exhale* and slightly bend your left knee. *Inhale* and lift from your abdominal muscles to bring your torso up to stand tall, straightening your left knee as you arrive upright. *Exhale* and release your right leg from the half lotus, then place your foot on the floor, returning to Tadasana. *Inhale*, lift the left foot into half lotus and repeat the posture on this side. After 5–10 breaths, *exhale* and return to Tadasana.

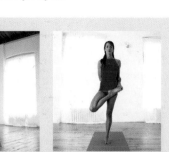

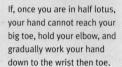

Easing into the pose
If your knees feel strained, begin to practise this pose by placing your lifted foot to the inside of the other thigh.

If, once you are in half lotus, your hand cannot reach your big toe, hold your elbow, and gradually work your hand down to the wrist then toe.

Deepening the pose
Press your lower abdomen towards your raised heel while drawing the thigh muscle of your standing leg firmly upwards. Broaden the sole of the standing foot strongly down to create a stable foundation. Once your balance is secure, try furthering the pose by

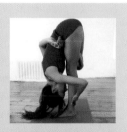

taking your hand off the floor and placing it on the back of your standing ankle.

utkata = powerful or fierce or uneven

The following sequences create a wave of energy as the body flows through the sun salutations to link the last standing postures together through vinyasa. Utkatasana opens the knee joints and helps to remove ankle stiffness.

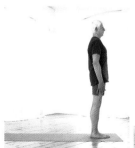

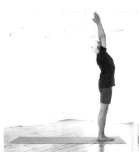

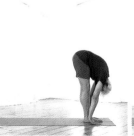

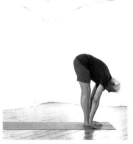

From Tadasana, flow through **Surya Namaskara A**, as follows.

⟶ *Inhale*, drawing the breath deep into your lungs, and lift the arms into **Urdhva Tadasana** (upward mountain).

⟶ *Exhale* and draw your body deep down to your legs into **Uttanasana** (intense stretch posture).

⟶ *Inhale* and open your chest forwards into **Urdhva Uttanasana** (upwards intense stretch posture).

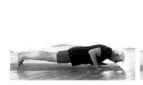

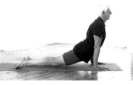

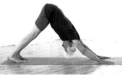

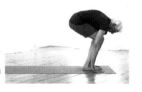

⟶ *Exhale* and jump back into **Chaturanga Dandasana** (staff posture).

⟶ *Inhale* and arch up into **Urdhva Mukha Svanasana** (upward facing dog), lifting your heart.

⟶ *Exhale* and press your hips up into **Adho Mukha Svanasana** (downfacing dog) releasing your neck and head.

⟶ *Inhale* and lightly jump your feet together in between your hands.

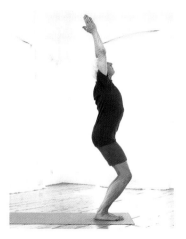

⟶ *Continue to inhale* raising your arms up and deeply bending your knees. Fully engage uddiyana bandha and sink your hips and buttocks low. Stretch the sides of your waist up to your fingertips, creating a counter-balance to gravity. Bring your palms together overhead. Soften the fold at the back of your knees and in the front of your ankles to increase the depth of the posture. *Take five to ten deep, slow breaths*, drawing your focus softly up beyond your thumbs towards the sky, <u>dristi</u>: urdhva. From this posture of Utkatasana, move directly into a vinyasa, as overleaf.

Easing into the pose
If you feel tension in your shoulders when raising your arms, try parting your hands and taking your arms a little wider to make more room for your shoulders to drop. Slide your shoulder blades down, direct your focus down and lower your chin slightly towards your chest.

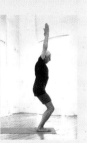

Vinyasa into Virabhadrasana I | WARRIOR POSTURE 1

Virabhadra = a warrior hero
created from the hair of Siva,
third god of the Hindu trinity

There are three warrior postures, which are all dedicated to Virabhadra. The first two are practised here in the primary series and the third is introduced in the third series. They cultivate stamina, co-ordination and transitional smoothness of motion.

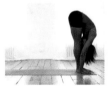 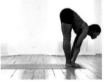 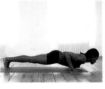 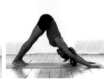

1 *Exhale* from the previous asana of Utkatasana and fold into **Uttanasana** (intense stretch).

⟶ *Inhale* and open your chest forwards into **Urdhva Uttanasana** (upwards intense stretch posture).

⟶ *Exhale* and jump back into **Chaturanga Dandasana** (staff posture).

⟶ *Inhale* and arch up into **Urdhva Mukha Svanasana** (upward facing dog posture), lifting your heart.

⟶ *Exhale*, press your hips up into **Adho Mukha Svanasana** (downward facing dog posture) and release your neck low.

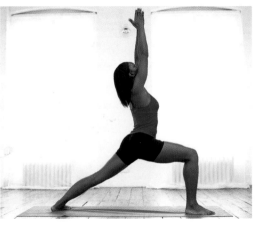

2 *Slowly inhale* and pivot on the ball of your left foot, rotating your heel inwards and forwards by 45 degrees towards your right arch. Step your right foot forwards in between your hands and align it with your right hip. Deeply bend your right knee, drawing it over the ankle, while pressing the sole of your left foot firmly into the floor. Bring your torso upright, opening your arms sideways and then up overhead with your palms together. Lift your face up and look towards your thumbs, <u>dristi</u>: **angustha ma dyai**. *Take five to ten breaths* in Virabhadrasana I.

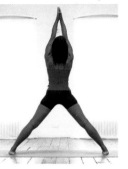 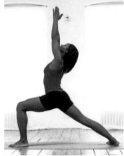

3 *Inhale*, straighten your right leg and turn your feet parallel to face the left side of your mat.

4 *Slowly exhale*, rotate your right toes, ball of foot, leg and hip in by 45 degrees, and turn your left hip, leg and foot out by 90 degrees, squaring your body to face the back edge of your yoga mat. Align your left foot with your left hip and deeply bend your left knee directly over the ankle into Virabhadrasana I. *Take five to ten long breaths* and then move on into Virabhadrasana II.

Easing into the pose
Keeping the hips equally aligned is of prime importance in this posture, so if you feel the hip of your back leg swinging backwards, decrease the bend in your front knee and focus on drawing your hip bone forwards. It can help to place your hands on your hips to steer them in the same direction. Keep the back foot firmly pushing down, especially the outer edge.

Deepening the pose
Allow your tailbone, hips and pelvis to release down with gravity, and feel your front thigh stretching long as your front knee draws forwards over the ankle to create a right angle (your shin vertical and your thigh parallel to the floor). Take care not to let the front knee fall inwards, and move the outer knee over your little toe. Lengthen both sides of your waist evenly, lifting your lower abdomen and raising your chest. Soften your shoulders down and let them align directly above and over your hips.

Virabhadra = a warrior hero created from the hair of Siva, third god of the Hindu trinity

Here, the hip joints are opened, releasing energy and blood circulation from the pelvis into the legs and increasing the muscular power of the lower body. The arms are toned and strengthened as they are drawn wide, helping to open the chest and ribcage.

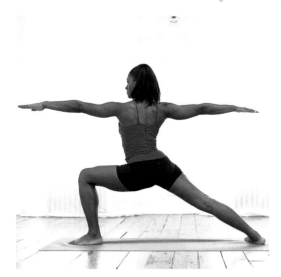

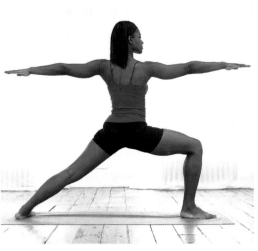

1 From Virabhadrasana I, maintain the deep bend of your left knee. *Exhale*, opening your arms wide out to the sides and stretching through to your fingertips at shoulder level. Draw your right hip bone and right collarbone open outwards away from the left. Align your feet so that your right foot is rotated in at a 15-degree angle and your left foot is open by 90 degrees, with the heel opposite the right arch, as in Parsvakonasana. *Take five to ten steady breaths*, breathing openness into your whole body and looking towards your left hand, <u>dristi</u>: **hastagrai**. *Inhale*, straighten your left leg, lengthen your spine and turn your feet parallel.

2 *Slowly exhale*, turn your feet (rotating your left foot inwards by 15 degrees and your right leg outwards by 90 degrees, with your right heel opposite your left arch), and bend your right knee over its own heel into a right angle, so repeating Virabhadrasana II to the right side. *Take another five to ten breaths*, this time looking over your right hand, <u>dristi</u>: **hastagrai**.

3 *Exhale* and place your hands on the floor. Step your right leg back, lowering into **Chaturanga Dandasana**.

⟶ *Inhale* into **Urdhva Mukha Svanasana**.

⟶ *Exhale* into **Adho Mukha Svanasana** and move straight to the jump through (overleaf).

Easing into the pose

The Virabhadrasana sequence challenges the strength of your legs, so be sure to breathe deeply to supply them with oxygen. If fully bending the knee causes the opposite foot to lose its connection with the floor, ease out of the bend slightly and re-root the opposite foot firmly down

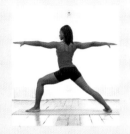

through the outer edge of the foot and heel.

Deepening the pose

Centre your torso directly over your pelvis, relax your shoulders and broaden your collarbones. Feel your legs opening wide and out from the pelvis, and move the pubic bone down to be at the same level as your bent knee. As always, pay attention to aligning the knees in the same direction as your toes and to rooting your feet.

Jump Through

The vinyasa into the jump through develops muscular and mental co-ordination while harnessing the power of the bandhas. This sequence of movement creates a transitional flow from standing to sitting, allowing your practice to become a continuous stream of flowing motion.

The vinyasa is based upon Surya Namaskara (sun salutation), the cornerstone of Astanga practice. The breath links each movement to create a flowing whole. This carries us through the sitting postures all the way through to the end of the practice. The vinyasa helps to maintain the internal body heat so that your muscles can yield and deeply stretch into the floor postures.

Learning the following jump through may take time, patience and practice, but it is integral to developing the fluidity of each vinyasa. It will also cultivate continuity of motion and build complete body and mind co-ordination, strength and a sense of flight while harnessing the power of the bandhas.

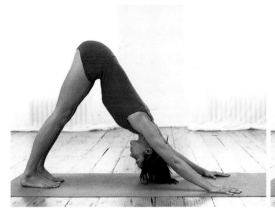

⟶ From exhaling into **Adho Mukha Svanasana** (downward facing dog posture), deeply engage uddiyana bandha.

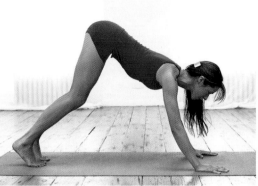

⟶ Continue to *exhale* as you shift your weight forwards on to your hands, letting your heels rise. Direct your focus at the space between your hands. Move your shoulders over your wrists and open your chest.

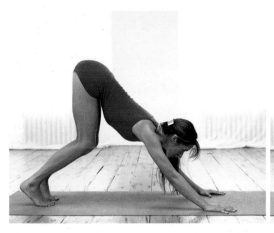

⟶ Bend your knees and take a gentle rebound back on to your feet. This will act as a springboard now for the jump/float through of your legs.

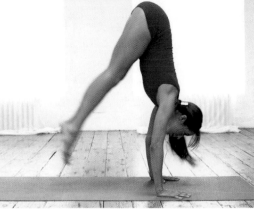

⟶ As you *inhale*, softly jump, moving your shoulders over your hands and swinging your hips in an arch over your shoulders. This will transfer all your weight and centre of balance into your hands, allowing your feet and legs to float up. Lift up out of your shoulders and press your palms down.

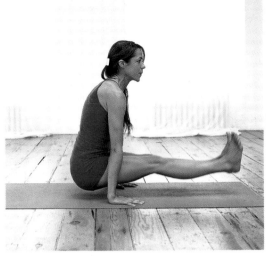 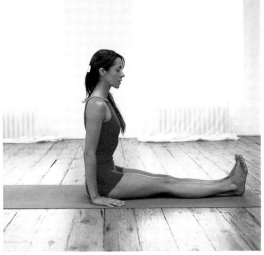

⟶ Continue to *inhale*, while keeping uddiyana bandha strong, and now swing your legs forwards through your arms, extending your feet out, and float your hips forwards. As soon as your legs start to descend, extend your focus forwards to and beyond your toes. Press your palms firmly down and lift your abdomen up to hover your hips, for a moment, just above the floor.

⟶ Keeping uddiyana bandha engaged, lower your buttocks completely down to sit. As your buttocks touch down, lift uddiyana bandha again. Lengthen your back and sit tall in **Dandasana** (staff posture). *Exhale.*

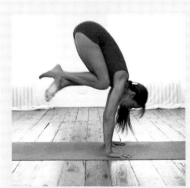 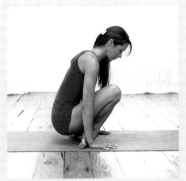

Easing into the pose
This vinyasa jump through may take much time and practice to perfect, so at first try as you jump to cross your ankles and tuck your knees up and into your chest. Press your palms strongly into the floor and lift your shoulders, to help find a moment of suspension before the legs start to lower.

Land softly on to the front of your feet just behind your hands. Roll back on to your buttocks and straighten your crossed legs into Dandasana. Once this becomes easy, slowly work towards swinging your legs straight through to land softly on your buttocks.

Deepening the pose
If you keep practising you will master this jump through. You will find that you can begin to focus on suspending your hips over your hands and finding a point of balance at the highest point of the jump up, that is just before beginning the descent. Engaging your bandhas is crucial, as this will create control and lightness in your pelvis, enabling you to suspend and balance here and helping you to develop a smooth, floating quality to your jump through.

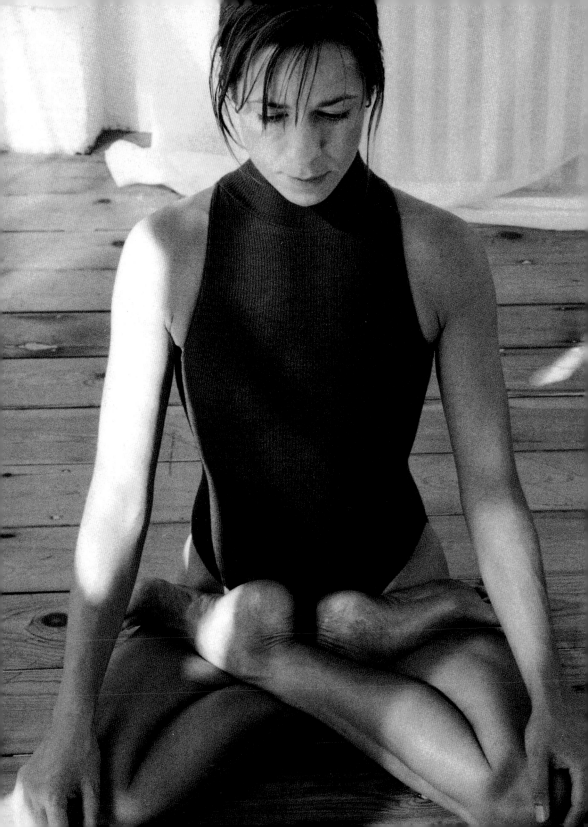

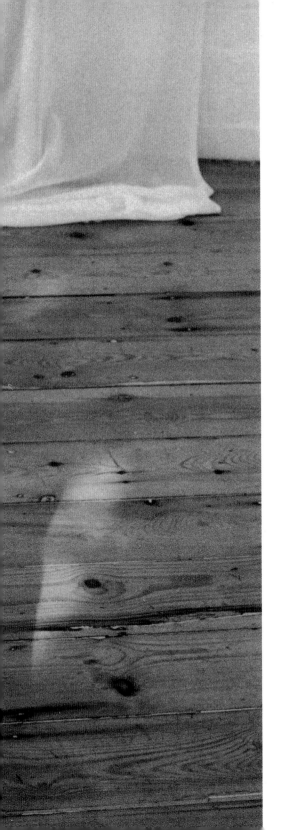

Seated Asanas

The seated asanas provide us with the chance to take the alignment and balance created in the standing sequence into a broader range of postures. The heat that has been generated will enable deep stretching, and the vinyasas between each side of each pose and each asana will help to maintain this internal heat.

The following seated postures, which form the central part of the primary series, purify the internal organs (including the heart) and the muscles while deeply articulating the joints of the body. They release physical, mental and emotional tensions and unlock energy to create physical strength, suppleness and openness of mind. Tightness and rigidity on all levels are challenged.

Focusing on the fullness of each breath will help you to move through these asanas and, as you do so, listen to all that arises within your mind and heart. In this way, we begin to cleanse the body and free the mind from past experiences, letting the breath wash through, bringing in new energy with each in-breath and releasing old energy with each out-breath.

By practising these asanas, a calmness of mind is brought about, an openness of heart and body is rediscovered and a secure connection with the ground is achieved.

Dandasana | STAFF POSTURE

danda = staff, rod or stick

This is the foundation from which all other seated asanas stem. Dandasana teaches us to sit in stillness. The subtle motion of breath flows through the limbs to bring this posture alive, activating and exercising every muscle of the body.

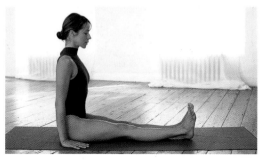

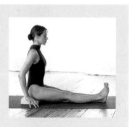

Easing into the pose
If you have tight hamstring muscles or any stiffness or injury in your back, practise this posture sitting on a yoga block or firm cushion to provide extra lift and support for your lower back.

Inhale, anchor your sitting bones into the floor, then lengthen from your lower spine to the crown of your head. Gently press your palms down and feel your shoulders descend. Lift your chest, keeping the back of your neck long, and open your collarbones. Focus on your nose tip, **dristi**: nasagrai, while fully engaging your bandhas to stretch your abdomen up. Press your legs away and draw the front thigh muscles upwards to your hips. Feel the backs of your legs long and open against the floor. *Take five to ten breaths*, then move into the next posture.

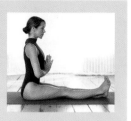

Deepening the pose
As your back gains strength, release your hands from the floor and bring them together in front of the chest in Namaste (prayer position). Maintain the lift through the entire length of your spine.

Paschimottanasana A/B/C/D | INTENSE STRETCH OF THE WEST A/B/C/D

paschima = west (which represents the back in yoga)
uttana = extended or intense stretch

This seated position allows the mechanics of the standing forward bends to be deepened as the torso rests down on the legs, developing flexibility and removing tension and stiffness. Each hand hold moves the body deeper into Paschimottanasana.

Paschimottanasana A

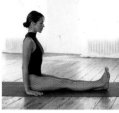

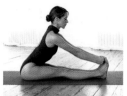

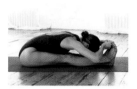

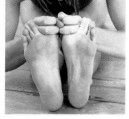

1 Start in Dandasana.

2 *Inhale* and raise your arms gently, extending your back forwards from your hips. Catch hold of your big toes, maintaining openness across your chest and length through the front and back of your spine and neck. Take care not to round your back or shorten the front of your body. Lifting the abdominal muscles (uddiyana bandha), opening your chest and rolling your shoulders back will help to prevent this collapse in the torso.

3 *Exhale* and pivot your pelvis forwards, folding your torso out and over your legs. Send your pubic bone back and down into the floor and lengthen your spine forwards. Feel your sitting bones anchoring down and the crown of your head floating towards your toes. Bend your elbows softly and slide your shoulder blades down your back. Lower your head but keep energy and focus extending out to your feet. *Take five deep breaths* in Paschimottanasana A, then *inhale*, draw your chest up, straighten your arms, and roll your shoulders back.

Paschimottanasana B

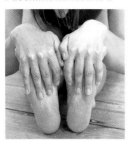

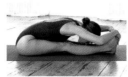

1 *Exhale* and change your hand position by taking your hands over your toes, pointing your fingertips towards your heels and pressing your palms and the soles of your feet together. *Inhale,* breathing length into your back.

2 *Exhale* and hinge deeply in the front of your hips, extending your chest further forwards towards your knees and drawing the elbows wide. This is Paschimottanasana B. Release tension in your neck and shoulders and allow your torso to surrender with gravity down over your legs. *After a full five even breaths, inhale* and draw your chest up, straightening your arms and lengthening your back diagonally forwards. Now continue into Paschimottanasana C.

Paschimottanasana C

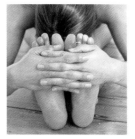

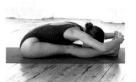

1 *Exhale,* release your hand position from the soles of your feet and interlock your fingers behind the balls of your feet. *Inhale,* lengthen your spine, look forwards and relax your shoulders.

2 *Exhale* and extend the front of your torso long, out and over your legs. Bring your chin on to your shins and move your forehead towards your ankles. Softly bend your elbows wide and focus on fully pivoting your pelvis forwards and deepening the fold in your hips. This is Paschimottanasana C. *Take five steady breaths* and, with your *sixth inhalation,* draw your chest up, lifting your head away from your legs and straightening your arms as you do so.

Paschimottanasana D

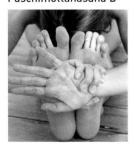

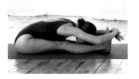

1 *Exhale,* release the interlock of your fingers and take the right hand to clasp your left wrist gently (or vice versa). *Inhale* as you extend your back long and lift your chest open.

2 *Exhale* and fold completely over your legs, sliding your pubis back and down and extending your breastbone forwards and out. Soften the back of your legs down into the floor and rest the entire length of your front torso on the front of your legs. Bend your elbows outwards and relax your shoulders. *Take five deep, slow breaths* in this final variation, Paschimottanasana D, then *inhale,* lifting your chest and head up.

• *Exhale,* release your hands from your feet and place your palms down just in front of your hips. From here, move into **jump back** and **vinyasas** as described overleaf.

Easing into the pose
A and B If you have back stiffness or pain, wrap a strap around the balls of your feet and take your hands as close as possible to your feet. Lengthen your back and keep your legs and feet together.
C and D If you need a strap to reach your feet, continue working as in posture A and focus on surrendering into the posture with each exhalation rather than forcing your torso down. If you are kind to your muscles, they will be more responsive and supple.

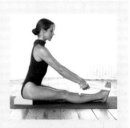

Deepening the pose
A and B Draw your lower abdominal muscles up and in. Work softly and deeply, and do not pull sharply on your arms or shoulders to increase the depth of the posture – this will cause either injury or tension, not flexibility.
C and D Draw the tops of your arms deep into their shoulder sockets and soften your shoulder blades down away from your ears. In all four asanas relax your neck muscles and lower your head while sending energy and focus out through the crown of your head to your feet, **dristi: padhayoragrai.**

Jump Back into Full Vinyasa or Half Vinyasa

The full vinyasa between each completed posture and the half vinyasa between each side of the posture are essential for maintaining the internal heat of the body, which allows the muscles and joints to be deeply stretched and opened safely. The jump back cultivates co-ordination between the body and mind, and develops upper body strength.

Jump Back

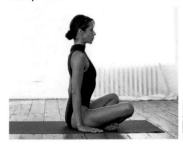
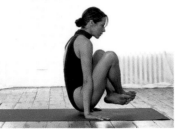
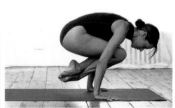

From **Dandasana** (staff posture), cross your ankles and *exhale*, placing your palms down on the floor by the sides of your hips. Deepen uddiyana bandha to prepare for the next step, and shift your shoulders forwards over your wrists.

→ *Inhale* and press your hands strongly into the floor. Use the power and strength of uddiyana bandha to curl the front of your torso up slightly. Press through your arms into your palms and raise your buttocks and feet off the floor into **Lolasana** (tremulous posture).

→ Continue to *inhale* and without touching the floor, swing your feet back and your head and chest forwards into advanced **Lolasana** (tremulous posture) moving your shoulders forwards of your wrists right over your fingertips.

Full Vinyasa

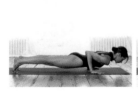
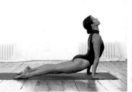
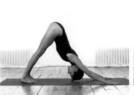
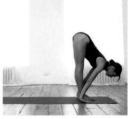

Exhale, jump your feet back into **Chaturanga Dandasana**.

→ *Inhale* to stretch into **Urdhva Mukha Svanasana**.

→ *Exhale* and move into **Adho Mukha Svanasana**.

→ *Inhale*, jump your feet into **Urdhva Uttanasana**.

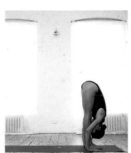
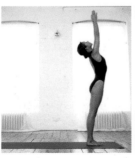
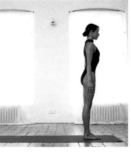
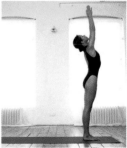

→ *Exhale* and fold into **Uttanasana**.

→ *Inhale* stretching into **Urdhva Tadasana**.

→ *Exhale*, lowering your arms into **Tadasana**.

→ *Inhale*, stretch up into **Urdhva Tadasana**.

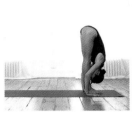

→ *Exhale* and fold forwards into **Uttanasana**.

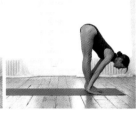

→ *Inhale* and lift your chest into **Urdhva Uttanasana**.

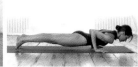

→ *Exhale* and jump into **Chaturanga Dandasana**.

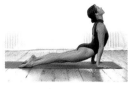

→ *Inhale* and stretch into **Urdhva Mukha Svanasana**.

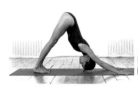

→ *Exhale* and move into **Adho Mukha Svanasana**.

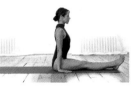

→ *Inhale* and jump through into **Dandasana**.

Benefits of the vinyasa

The sequence of the full vinyasa is practised after having completed a seated posture on both sides. The half vinyasa is practised in between sides of each posture. As well as sustaining the heat of the muscles and the flow of the body, vinyasas neutralize and align the body, preparing it for the next posture. You may wish to refer back to Surya Namaskara for extra details of the transition through the postures of vinyasa.

Jump Back into Half Vinyasa

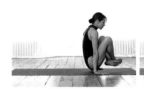

Inhale, press down through your arms and raise your seat off the floor.

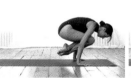

→ Continuing to *inhale*, move into **Lolasana** (see step 3 of jump back).

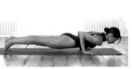

→ *Exhale* and jump your feet back into **Chaturanga Dandasana**.

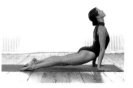

→ *Inhale* and stretch into **Urdhva Mukha Svanasana**.

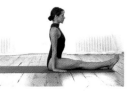

→ *Exhale* and move into **Adho Mukha Svanasana**.

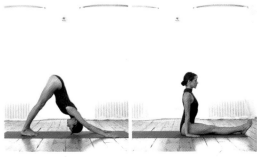

→ *Inhale* and jump through into **Dandasana**.

Easing into the vinyasa

The swing into Lolasana is a very challenging movement, so initially begin to practise this by crossing your ankles and placing your hands on the ground in front of your shins. From here, softly roll forwards over your feet to take your weight into your hands, and then jump or step back into Chaturanga

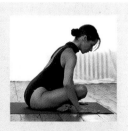

Dandasana. Once you have gained confidence, try to lift your buttocks off the floor.

Purvottanasana | STRETCH OF THE EAST POSTURE

purva = east (which represents the front in yoga)
uttana = extended or intense stretch

In this complete counter-posture to Paschimottanasana the front of the body is lengthened and stretched open, lifting the heart above the level of the spine. This increases the blood flow to the brain, refreshing and revitalizing body and mind.

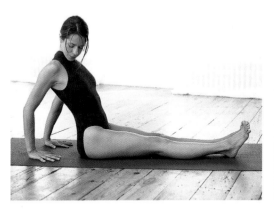

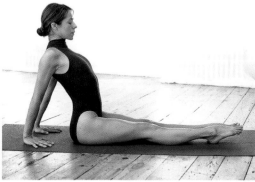

1 From Dandasana, *exhale* and step your hands back behind your hips, planting your palms into the floor with your fingers pointing inwards towards your buttocks.

2 Draw the back of your waist up and in, while strongly lifting your chest up to your chin and rolling your shoulders back. Stretch your legs long, extending out to your toes.

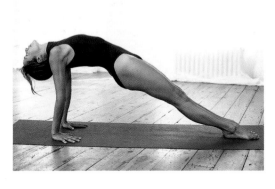

3 *Inhale* and press your hands deeper into the floor, propelling your hips upwards as you extend your toes and the balls of your feet downwards. Raise your heart higher and release your neck, allowing your head to drop softly back. Stretch your legs long and together, keeping them active and rooting your big-toe joints down. *Take five to ten breaths*, expanding your chest and focusing towards your nose tip, <u>**dristi**</u>: **nasagrai**. *Exhale*, lower your buttocks to the floor and lift your head up, returning to Dandasana.

• *Inhale*, press your hands into the floor, tuck your knees up, crossing your ankles, and lift your hips off the floor to swing your feet back into a **full vinyasa**. Flow through the vinyasa and then softly **jump through** and return to Dandasana.

Deepening the pose
Make sure your hands are placed shoulder-width apart and spread your fingers open. Work the rotation in your shoulders and broaden across your chest. Lift your tailbone in and up towards your pubic bone and feel your spine pressing up into the front of your torso.

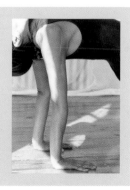

Easing into the pose
If at first you can't get a good lift bend your knees and step your feet apart, both flat on the floor. From here, raise your pelvis and create a parallel line to the floor with your torso.

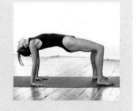

Ardha Baddha Padma Paschimottanasana | HALF BOUND LOTUS INTENSE STRETCH OF THE WEST POSTURE

ardha = half
baddha = bound or caught
padma = lotus   paschima = west
uttana = extended or intense stretch

The full folding of one leg at a time opens the knee joints, preparing them for Padmasana (lotus posture), which forms part of the seated sequence. This posture massages the abdominal organs, improving both digestion and elimination.

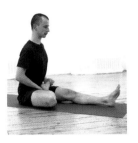
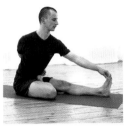

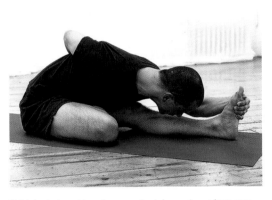

1 From landing in Dandasana from your full vinyasa, continue to *inhale*, folding your right knee and using your hands to draw your right foot up and on to your left upper thigh. Place the little-toe edge of your foot into the crease of your left hip socket. Align your heel just above your pubic bone and move your right knee forwards and in, to create a 45-degree angle with your left leg. Keep your left leg actively lengthening out through its heel, as your right leg is now in Ardha Padma (half lotus).

2 *Towards the end of your inhalation*, stretch your right arm behind your back and catch hold of your right big toe with the first two fingers of your right hand. Extend your left hand to hold your left foot and lengthen your spine.

3 *Exhale slowly* and lengthen your back forwards out from your hips, moving your chest towards your left knee and your chin towards your left shin. Softly bend your left elbow wide to the side, drawing your abdomen long over your right heel, and *breathe five to ten long, even breaths* while sending energy and focus out to your extended foot, <u>**dristi: padhayoragrai**</u>. *Inhale*, lift your chest up, *exhale* and release the bind of your hands from your feet and stretch your right leg forwards into Dandasana.

• *Inhale*, press your hands into the floor, tuck your knees up, crossing your ankles, and lift your hips off the floor to move into a **half vinyasa**. Return to Dandasana. Repeat this posture, this time folding your left leg into half lotus. After *five to ten breaths*, take a **full vinyasa** and **jump through** to Dandasana.

Easing into the pose
If strain is felt in your knees, do not force the posture. Instead, either remain upright and work on relaxing your hips to allow the knee to release and drop closer to the floor, or take your foot to the ground and softly extend your body forwards from here. Use a strap in either of these positions if you are not yet able to reach hold of your foot.

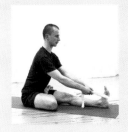
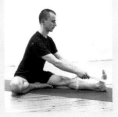

Deepening the pose
Soften the skin over your bent knee to allow the joint to fully bend. Now gently press your knee downwards to further the rotation of your leg and the opening in your hip. Move your lower abdomen forwards and down on to the lotus heel (of your bent leg) to stimulate the abdominal organs.

Triang Mukhaikapada Paschimottanasana | THREE LIMBS FACE ONE LEG INTENSE STRETCH OF THE WEST POSTURE

tri = three
anga = limb
mukha = face
eka = one

pada = foot/leg
paschima = west
uttana = intense
stretch

The three "limbs" referred to are the feet (stretching forwards and backwards), the knees (which are opened) and the buttocks (which are drawn wide as the back extends forwards). This posture also provides a counter-stretch to the previous half lotus.

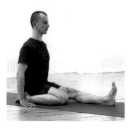
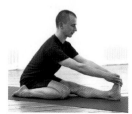
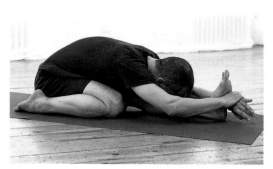

1 From landing in Dandasana from your full vinyasa, continue to *inhale* and bend your right knee, taking your right foot back. Place your heel against your right hip, with the front of your right foot, ankle and shinbone pressing on the floor. Join your knees together and root down evenly into both sitting bones, pressing both buttocks firmly down.

2 At the *end of your inhalation*, open your chest wide, extend your back long and tilt your pelvis forwards, stretching your arms out and catching hold of your left foot with both your hands.

Benefits of the pose
Triang Mukhaikapada Paschimottanasana is particularly helpful for releasing tightness in the back of the pelvis. It also opens the sacrum area to stimulate and improve circulation throughout the nerves (especially the sciatic nerve) of the spine and the muscles of the back.

3 *Exhale* and fold more deeply from your hips, sending your pubic bone back and down and lengthening your torso out and over your left leg. Stretch along your spine and draw the top of your head towards your toes, bending your elbows outwards. Sink your right buttock and hip downwards to maintain an even base for this posture. *Take five to ten breaths* and focus on sending energy out to your extended foot, <u>**dristi: padhayoragrai**</u>. *Inhale*, maintaining the hold of your foot, and draw your chest up, rolling your shoulders back. *Exhale*, release your hands from your foot and bring your body upright, extending your right leg forwards into Dandasana.

• *Inhale*, press your hands into the floor, tuck your knees up, crossing your ankles, and lift your hips off the floor to swing your feet back. Move smoothly through a **half vinyasa** and then **jump through**, landing gently in Dandasana. Repeat this posture, this time bending your left leg. After *five to ten breaths*, take a **full vinyasa** and **jump through** to land softly in Dandasana.

Easing into the pose
Always be aware of pain in the knees, as this may be an indication of working too deeply too quickly. If this is the case, place a firm cushion, folded blanket or yoga block under the buttock of your straight leg. This will not only help to protect the knee but will also assist in rooting both buttocks squarely. Again, with this pose use a strap to

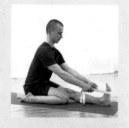

catch your foot if you tend to bend your leg or hunch your back in order to hold it with your hands.

Deepening the pose
To deepen the openness across your sacrum, roll your inner thighs together and downwards; this will also develop the full range of leg rotation. As you do this, be sure to engage uddiyana bandha to support your lower spine.

janu = knee
sirsa = head

This posture provides the foundation of the following two variations and continues to open the pelvis and develop the suppleness and freedom of the hips and knees. It balances and tones the liver and spleen, so improving the digestive system.

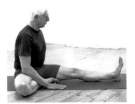 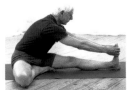

1 From landing in Dandasana out of your full vinyasa, continue to *inhale* and bend your right knee back in line with, or slightly behind, your right shoulder (at 90–95 degrees to your left leg). Place your right heel so that it touches its own inner upper thigh, as this will ensure a full opening in your right hip. Square your body to face your left leg, with your navel in line with your left knee.

2 At the *end of your inhalation*, extend your back forwards from your pelvis and reach your hands out to catch hold of your left foot, keeping your collarbones open and your shoulders relaxed.

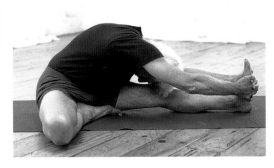

3 *Exhale* and deepen the fold at the level of your hips, extending your torso out over your left leg. Gently press your right knee and outer thigh down on to the floor, and stretch your left heel away to lengthen through your left leg. Draw your shoulders away from your hands, and softly bend your elbows wide, pressing your chest forwards to your left knee. *Take five to ten even breaths* and direct focus and energy out to your extended foot, <u>dristi</u>: **padhayoragrai**. *Inhale*, maintaining hold of your foot, straighten your arms and draw your chest up, drawing your shoulders back and down. *Exhale*, release the hold of your foot and bring your torso upright, extending your right leg forwards into Dandasana.

• *Inhale*, press your hands into the floor, tuck your knees up, crossing your ankles, and lift your hips off the floor. Move smoothly through a **half vinyasa** and **jump through**, landing gently in Dandasana. Repeat this posture, this time bending your left leg. After *five to ten breaths*, take a **full vinyasa** and **jump through** into Dandasana.

Easing into the pose
It is better to work initially with a strap to link your hands to your foot if you feel that you are not yet able to hold your toes with a straight back and leg. Using a strap will help to prevent you from straining your shoulders and rounding your back.

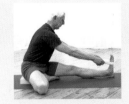

Concentrate on lengthening your spine at all times within this pose.

Deepening the pose
Focus on both sides of your torso being level so that your back expands open and receives an even stretch. This will help to balance the kidneys and the muscle flexibility of the back. With each exhalation, yield the open expanse of your back to gravity.

Janu Sirsasana B | KNEE HEAD POSTURE B

janu = knee
sirsa = head

In this variation of Janu Sirsasana, the heel is pressed underneath the perineum, helping to maintain the activity of mula bandha. Sitting on the foot also helps to tilt the pelvis forwards, thus enabling a deeper forwards stretch through the body.

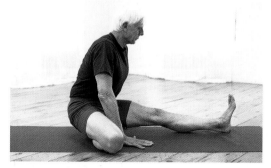

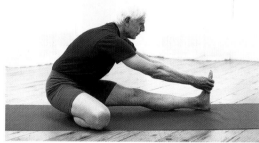

1 From Dandasana, continue to *inhale* as you bend your right knee back, moving your right foot towards the pubis. Press down on your hands to raise your hips, then shift your pelvis forwards, placing your perineum on top of your right heel. Direct the toes of your right foot forwards to your left heel and place your right knee at an 80-degree angle to your left leg.

2 At the *end of your inhalation*, widen your collarbones and extend your back forwards, pivoting from your pelvis and holding your left foot with both hands.

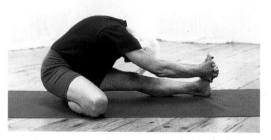

3 *Exhale* and softly fold from your hips to stretch your torso forwards over your left leg, bending your elbows wide and lengthening through the back of your neck. Keep centring the front of your body directly over your left leg. Extend your left heel away and draw your left thigh muscle upwards and in towards your hip. Focus on sending energy out to your extended foot, <u>dristi</u>: **padhayoragrai**, and move your abdomen in. *Inhale* and draw your chest up, keeping your hands held around your foot, and straighten your arms. *Exhale* and bring your torso upright, extending your right leg into Dandasana.

• *Inhale*, press your hands into the floor, tuck your knees up, crossing your ankles, and lift your hips off the floor. Flow through a **half vinyasa** and then softly **jump through** into Dandasana. Repeat this posture, this time bending your left leg. After *five to ten breaths*, take a **full vinyasa** and **jump through** to land softly in Dandasana.

Benefits of the pose
In addition to the overall positive effects of the Janu Sirsasana variations for both men and women, this posture is of particular benefit to men. The placement of the heel against the perineum and the stretch through the pelvis helps to regulate the prostate gland, protecting against its enlargement. Those who have this condition are advised to stay longer in this asana.

Easing into the pose
Use a strap if you have difficulty in reaching your extended foot. If the underside of your foot feels uncomfortable, folding your mat under it may help to cushion the bones.

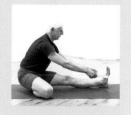

Deepening the pose
Feel the connection of your perineum with your heel at all times throughout this asana. Anchor into this point and release your torso forwards and out, away from this base of mula bandha.

janu = knee
sirsa = head

In this final and deepest posture of the Janu Sirsasana variations, the entire leg, and its potential mobility and power, is fully stimulated from the hip to the toes, improving circulation and energy flow from the pelvis through the hips down into the legs.

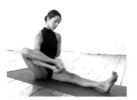

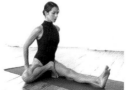

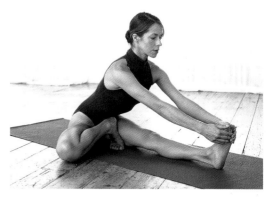

1 From Dandasana, continue to *inhale* as you bend your right leg, taking your right elbow under your right knee and holding your right toes. With your left hand, press your right heel forwards, then place your right toes and ball of the foot by your left inner thigh at a 45-degree angle. Keep your right heel lifting up and move the arch of your right foot to your left inner thigh.

2 With your foot in place, release your hands from your right foot and gently rotate your right knee forwards and down to the floor.

3 At the *end of your inhalation*, lengthen your back forwards, folding from your pelvis, and stretch your abdominal wall long to create length from your pubis to your navel. Raise your abdomen and navel up and over your right heel, extending your hands to hold your left foot.

Benefits of the pose
This particular placement of the foot opens the toe joints, stretches the muscles of the soles and creates suppleness in the ankle joints. As the bent knee descends, an opening of the hip and knee is created and the Achilles tendon and calf muscle are lengthened.

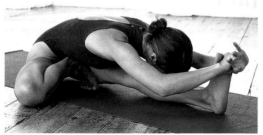

4 *Exhale* and extend your torso out along your left leg, bending your elbows out. Maintain length throughout your spine and back of your neck as you direct the top of your head towards your left ankle. Be active in your left leg and softly open the back of your left thigh, knee and calf down into the floor. *Take five to ten deep breaths*, fully engaging uddiyana bandha, and focus on sending energy out to your extended foot, <u>dristi</u>: **padhayoragrai**, while rooting into both sitting bones. *Inhale* and draw your chest up, rolling your shoulders back and straightening your arms while still holding your foot. *Exhale* and bring your back upright, releasing your right leg into Dandasana.

• *Inhale*, press your hands into the floor, tuck your knees up, cross your ankles and lift your hips off the floor. Move smoothly through a **half vinyasa** and then softly **jump through** into Dandasana. Repeat this posture, this time with your left leg bending in. After *five to ten breaths*, take a **full vinyasa** and **jump through** to land softly in Dandasana.

Easing into the pose
This is a strong posture and so must be approached with care, patience and intelligence. The rotation of the leg and knee originates within your hip socket, so do not strain or force your knee down. With careful practice the hips will gradually release, allowing your knee to descend and your torso to lean over your straight leg. Be content to work just at stage 1 or 2 until your body is ready to go further.

Deepening the pose
As your bent knee descends, it is easy for your base to become unbalanced, which will distort the alignment and posture of your body. Focus on cultivating an even awareness of gravity rooting you into both sitting bones.

Marichyasana A | POSTURE A DEDICATED TO THE GREAT SAGE MARICHI

Marichi = the son of Brahma (the creator) and grandfather of Surya (the sun god)

In this forward extension of the torso, the hands are bound behind the back. This means that the movement of the abdomen inwards to deepen uddiyana bandha and the yielding to gravity are both essential to extend the torso forwards and down.

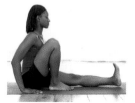
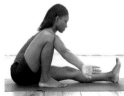

1 From Dandasana, continue to *inhale* slowly, and bend your right knee up towards your right shoulder. Place your right heel firmly on the ground in line with your right sitting bone, with your right toes pointing directly forwards.

2 Continue to *inhale*, and reach your right arm and hand out, with the palm facing away from your body. Move your right outer shoulder to the inside of your right knee, and place your left hand on the floor by your left hip.

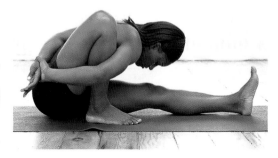

3 Towards the *end of your inhalation*, sweep your right arm around to the right side, opening your right armpit against the front of your right shinbone. Take your hands back to clasp behind your back. Lengthen your spine and open your chest while squaring your shoulders forwards.

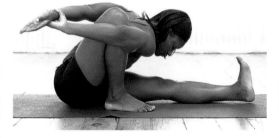

Easing into the pose
When you first learn this posture you may not be able to bind your hands, so instead use a strap to link your hands behind your back. As you practise, gradually walk your fingers closer together along the strap until they touch.

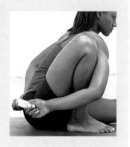

Deepening the pose
Bind your hands securely, as this will create a loop of energy through your arms and help to seal you into the posture. As the binding of your fingers becomes easier and your body more supple, on the first side of this asana use your right hand to hold your left wrist, and on the second side use your left hand to hold your right wrist. Once this is possible, stretch your arms, raising your hands up and away from your back.

4 *Exhale* and extend your torso out and over your left leg, folding deep within your hips. Stretch your left heel away and press your right inner thigh against the side of your right ribcage. Point your right knee directly up. Breathe length into your back and draw your chest open towards your left knee, extending your arms out behind you. *Take five to ten breaths*, deeply engaging uddiyana bandha and focusing energy out to your extended foot, <u>dristi</u>: **padhayoragrai**. *Inhale*, raise your chest and open your shoulders wide. *Exhale* and release the bind of your hands, bringing your body upright and stretching your right leg forwards into Dandasana.

• *Inhale*, press your hands into the floor, tuck your knees up, cross your ankles and lift your hips off the floor. Move smoothly through a **half vinyasa** and then softly **jump through** into Dandasana. Repeat this posture, this time folding your left knee in. After *five to ten breaths*, take a **full vinyasa** and **jump through** to land softly in Dandasana.

Marichi = the son of Brahma
(the creator) and grandfather of
Surya (the sun god)

This asana intensifies the benefits of Marichyasana A, as the heel of the lotus leg applies pressure to the abdomen, helping to stimulate, massage and tone the internal organs. The pose also releases tension from the shoulders.

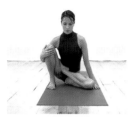
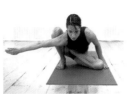

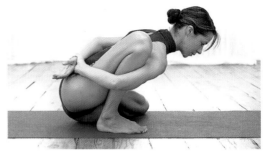

1 From landing in Dandasana from your full vinyasa, continue to *inhale*, bending your left leg, and use your hands to draw your left foot up and on to your right upper thigh into half lotus. Move the little-toe edge of your left foot into the crease of your right hip socket, then release your left hand on to the floor. Sit on your left buttock, drawing your left knee and thigh down. Bend your right knee up towards your right shoulder and place your right heel on the ground in line with your right sitting bone. Direct your right toes to point forwards.

2 Continue to *inhale* and extend your torso forwards over your left foot, moving your right shoulder to the inside of your right knee and beyond. Stretch your right arm out to the side to place your right armpit on the front of your right shin.

3 Towards the *end of your inhalation*, fold your right arm around your right leg, taking both hands backwards to catch hold together behind your back. Extend out through your spine, lifting your chest and squaring your shoulders.

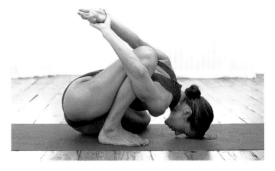

Easing into the pose
Progress through this posture slowly, being extremely careful of your knees. If you experience any pain, ease off and release the lotus foot on to the floor and practise the posture here.

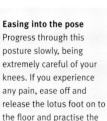

4 *Exhale* and stretch your torso forwards and over your left heel, drawing your head down towards the floor and directing your chin in between and beyond your knee and foot. Press your right inner thigh into the right side of your ribcage, directing the kneecap upwards. *Take five to ten full, even breaths*, releasing the back of your neck long and looking towards your nose tip, <u>**dristi**</u>: **nasagrai**. *Inhale*, raise your chest and open your shoulders wide. *Exhale* and release the bind of your hands, bringing your body upright and stretching your legs forwards into Dandasana.

• *Inhale*, press your hands into the floor, tuck your knees up, cross your ankles and lift your hips off the floor to swing your feet back. Flow through the **half vinyasa** and then **jump through** into Dandasana. Repeat this posture, this time folding your right knee into half lotus. After *five to ten breaths*, take a **full vinyasa** and **jump through** to land softly in Dandasana.

Deepening the pose
As you progress in this posture, concentrate on fully engaging uddiyana bandha, which will help you to extend your torso further forwards and your head lower. As this begins to happen, you will be able to bind at your wrists and raise your hands as in Marichyasana A.

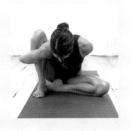

SEATED ASANAS

Marichyasana C | POSTURE C DEDICATED TO THE GREAT SAGE MARICHI

Marichi = the son of Brahma (the creator) and grandfather of Surya (the sun god)

The two previous asanas have increased the blood flow to flush through the internal organs, and now these two twists of Marichyasana C and D squeeze out any toxins from the abdomen, which can create imbalances and sluggishness of digestion.

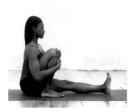
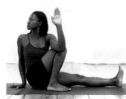
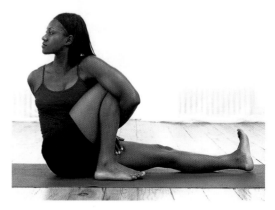

1 From landing in Dandasana from your full vinyasa, continue to *inhale*, and bend your right knee up towards your right shoulder. Place the heel firmly on the ground in line with your right sitting bone, with your right toes pointing directly forwards, as in Marichyasana A. Lengthen your back and softly press your torso forwards to your right thigh.

2 Continue to *inhale*, stretching your back taller, and take your right hand on to the floor behind your pelvis. Open your right shoulder back and draw your right knee inwards to the centre of your chest. Turn your chest to your right leg, then hook your left elbow and armpit over your right knee and move the left side of your ribs into your right inner thigh. Roll the right side of your ribs back.

3 Continue to *inhale* and extend your left hand out so your palm turns down and your elbow rolls up. Now wrap your bent left arm around your bent right leg. Take your right hand off the floor to catch hold of your left hand. Draw your right shoulder back, turning your head to bring your chin over your right shoulder. *Take five to ten breaths*, looking over your right shoulder, <u>**dristi**</u>: **parsva**. With each *inhalation*, breathe length into your spine and openness into your chest. With each exhalation, draw your right shoulder back and down, turning your collarbone and side ribs further around to the right. *Exhale*, release the clasp of your hands and return your body to face forwards, stretching your legs out into Dandasana.

• *Inhale*, press your hands into the floor, tuck your knees up, cross your ankles and lift your hips off the floor to swing your feet back. Flow through a **half vinyasa** and then **jump through** to land gently in Dandasana. Repeat this posture, this time bending your left leg up. After *five to ten breaths*, take a **full vinyasa** and **jump through** to land softly in Dandasana.

Benefits of the pose
Twists are a wonderful tonic for the spine, bringing about spinal health, balance and mobility, as well as helping to alleviate back stiffness and pain.

Easing into the pose
Binding in this posture takes time, as it requires and develops not just full mobility and suppleness but also a good deal of strength throughout the back muscles. Be prepared, therefore, to work this posture only to stage 2 until the body develops sufficient flexibility and control. If you suffer from particular tightness in the back, you may find sitting

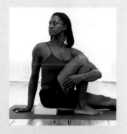

on a firm cushion or yoga block beneficial to help prevent your back from collapsing and dropping backwards.

Deepening the pose
As the rotation through your spine develops, you will be able to bind at your wrists and so rotate further. Note that the left hand holds the right wrist and the right fingers stretch to the left inner thigh (and vice versa on the second side).

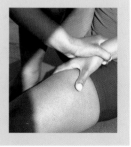

Marichi = the son of the Brahma (the creator) and grandfather of Surya (the sun god)

This final twist develops the flexibility and mobility of the spine and back muscles that were introduced in Marichyasana C. One side of the back and abdomen is squeezed, while the other side is stretched, releasing tension and stress from the spinal nerves.

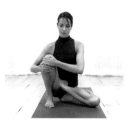
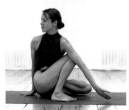
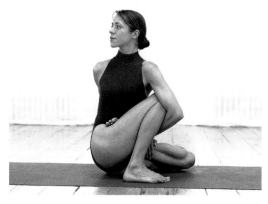

1 From landing in Dandasana from your full vinyasa, continue to *inhale*, drawing your left leg and foot up into half lotus. Sit on to your left buttock and draw your left knee and thigh down. Bend your right knee up and place your right heel on the ground in line with your right sitting bone, as in Marichyasana B. Strongly draw your back tall and your chest up.

2 Continue to *inhale*, lengthening your spine and drawing your right knee across to the centre of your chest, then move your chest to your right knee. Now lean forwards and rotate through your back to hook your left upper arm firmly over your right knee and move your left armpit over on to your right outer knee. Press the left side of your ribs into your right inner thigh, rolling the right side of your torso back. Place your right hand on the floor behind your pelvis, rolling your right shoulder open and extending your left hand forwards.

3 Towards the end of your *inhalation*, twist fully through your spine, and, while pressing your left ribs forwards into your right leg, wrap your left arm around your right leg and then reach your left hand to the left side of your waist. Draw your right shoulder open and stretch your right hand back to grasp your left hand. As you *exhale*, open your right shoulder, turning your head to look over your right shoulder, <u>**dristi: parsva**</u>. *Take five to ten breaths*. Focus on lifting through the entire length of your spine, drawing your chest skywards and sliding your shoulder blades down your back. *Exhale*, release the bind of your hands, returning your body to face forwards, and stretch your legs into Dandasana.

• *Inhale*, press your hands into the floor, tuck your knees up, cross your ankles and lift your hips off the floor to swing your feet back. Flow through the **half vinyasa** and then **jump through** to land gently in Dandasana. Repeat the posture, this time bending your left leg up. After *five to ten breaths*, take a **full vinyasa** and **jump through** to land softly in Dandasana.

Easing into the pose
If initially you are unable to clasp your hands, build up to the binding by hugging into your leg. If your knees are not strong enough for deep lotus work, you can moderate the posture by placing your left foot on the floor close to your right buttock, as in Marichyasana B, and

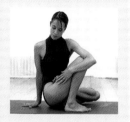

practise twisting your spine from this moderated positioning of your legs.

Deepening the pose
To deepen the rotation of your spine, focus (while on the first side) on moving your left ribcage forwards into your right thigh to close any gap between the two, and draw your right ribcage backwards. This will also enable you to bind at the wrist, taking your fingers on to the shin. In turn, this will

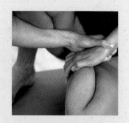

increase the heel pressure against your abdomen, so intensifying the benefits.

Navasana and Lolasana | BOAT POSTURE AND TREMULOUS POSTURE

nava = boat
lola = dangling or swaying like a pendulum

Individually, these postures cultivate bandha awareness and develop bandha control. When practised together, they develop abdominal and leg tone, back strength, and power in the arms, wrists and shoulders.

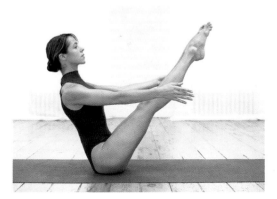

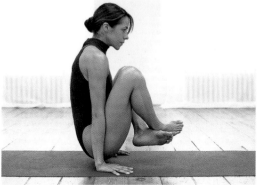

1 From landing in Dandasana from your full vinyasa, continue to *inhale*, reclining your chest back and upwards at the same time as lifting your legs up, with your inner thighs, ankles and big-toe joints pressing together. Stretch your legs and ankles long, raise your arms horizontally and reach your hands forwards beyond your knees. Float your feet upwards as high as your head, and balance on your buttocks, not allowing your back to collapse down on to the floor. *Take five breaths* in Navasana, looking towards your toes, <u>dristi</u>: **padhayoragrai.**

2 *Exhale* and move into Lolasana by placing your palms down on the floor by the sides of your hips and deepening uddiyana bandha to curl and contract the front of your torso. Shift your shoulders forwards over your wrists. *Inhale* and press your hands strongly into the floor, then, using the power and strength of uddiyana bandha and the pressure down through your arms into your palms, raise your buttocks and feet off the floor, tucking your legs in tightly. This is Lolasana. *Exhale softly*, lower your buttocks back down on to the floor and stretch in to Navasana, and *take five breaths*. *Exhale*, place your palms down on the floor by the sides of your hips and lift up into Lolasana. Repeat three more times so that you practise Navasana and Lolasana five times in all.

Easing into the pose
These two poses are challenging. Pace yourself by breathing slowly and deeply. If your lower back feels strained in Navasana, bend your knees, lowering your feet so that your shins are parallel to the floor.

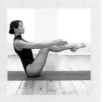

• From your fifth Lolasana jump your feet back into Chaturanga Dandasana and move through a **full vinyasa**. From the Adho Mukha Svanasana of the vinyasa, instead of jumping through to land into Dandasana, jump and gently land on your feet in front of your hands, as shown in Bhujapidasana.

Deepening the pose
As you become proficient in Lolasana, try swinging your feet back, raising your hips over your shoulders and hands, and then stretching your legs up into a full handstand balance as you inhale. To return to Navasana, slowly exhale, tuck your legs in and, with bandha control, gently swing your pelvis back down to Lolasana, then place your buttocks down into Navasana. Practise this five times. This deeper pose combats fatigue and refreshes the nervous system.

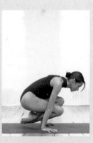
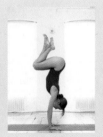
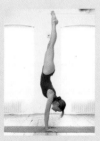

bhuja = arm or shoulder
pida = pressure

This pose creates strength in the hands and wrists, leanness in the muscles of the arms and increased flexibility in the shoulder joints. When the legs are drawn up towards the torso, this helps to balance the pancreas and the secretion of insulin.

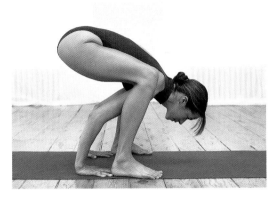

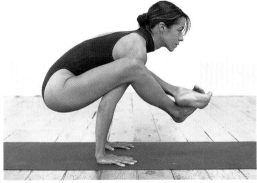

1 From the Adho Mukha Svanasana of your full vinyasa, *inhale* and jump your feet forwards of your hands, with your legs to the outside of your arms and your knees by your shoulders. Continue to *inhale* and deepen the bend of your knees, lowering the back of your thighs towards your inner upper arms. Spread your palms and fingers open, and extend your middle fingers to your heels.

2 Towards the *end of your inhalation*, place the back of your thighs on to your upper arms. Shift your weight back on to your hands, without dropping your buttocks down, and lift your feet from the floor, crossing your ankles. Lift your face and softly gaze towards your nose tip, <u>dristi</u>: nasagrai.

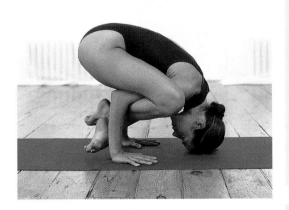

Easing into the pose
In order to get your shoulders far enough back, bend your knees deeply, then step your hands on to the back of your ankles and move your shoulders towards the back of your knees. Work gently and with patience, gradually building confidence to take your full weight on your hands. If at first you cannot

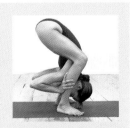

lift both feet at once, practise lifting one foot at a time, then lift both and work to cross your ankles.

3 *Exhale*, tip your head and shoulders forwards and down, bringing your forehead towards the floor, and, at the same time, strongly work uddiyana bandha to send your feet and buttocks back and upwards. This is like a seesaw action into a balance point. *Take five to ten breaths*, looking to your nose tip, <u>dristi</u>: nasagrai. From here, *inhale*, raise your face and chest and return to step 2. Then cross your ankles, and either place your feet on the floor and **jump back** into Chaturanga Dandasana to enter into a **full vinyasa** or stretch your legs into Tittibhasana and then Bakasana, as overleaf, to enter into a **full vinyasa**.

Deepening the pose
Instead of landing on your feet, jump your legs directly into Tittibhasana, then bend your knees, cross your ankles and lower your head into Bhujapidasana. As you gain strength, extend your chin to the floor.

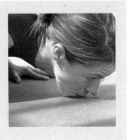

Tittibhasana and Bakasana | FIREFLY POSTURE AND CRANE POSTURE

tittibha = firefly
baka = crane bird

These asanas together create a seamless transition from Bhujapidasana into a full vinyasa. Tittibhasana stretches the spinal cord and back while extending length and power into the legs. Bakasana helps to develop the strength required for a handstand.

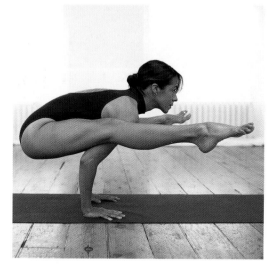

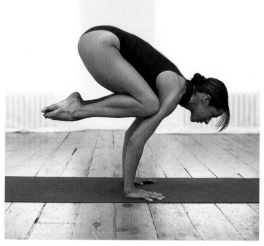

1 From Bhujapidasana, *inhale*, raise your face and chest, uncrossing your ankles and stretching your legs forwards. Extend out through the balls of your feet into Tittibhasana. Maintain the pressure of your inner thighs against your upper arms and press your palms strongly down into the ground. Deeply engage uddiyana bandha. Draw strength up through your arms, lift your buttocks, chest and face so that you hover parallel to the floor. Look towards your nose tip, <u>dristi</u>: **nasagrai**.

2 Begin to *exhale*, and engage uddiyana bandha even more deeply. Raise your hips, keeping your chest open and your head forwards as you fold at your knees, and take your shins, ankles and feet back into Bakasana. Bring your big toes together and lift your heels towards your buttocks. *Inhale*, feeling the support of your arms and uddiyana and mula bandha. Roll your shoulders back and lengthen the back of your neck. Look towards your nose tip, <u>dristi</u>: **nasagrai**.

• *Exhale* and shoot your feet backwards, bending your elbows as your feet land into Chaturanga Dandasana. From here flow into a **full vinyasa**. Do not jump throgh into Dandasana, but as in the vinyasa after Navasana and Lolasana jump your feet on to the floor by your hands (page 87).

Benefits of the pose
The linking together of these two asanas enhances co-ordination, grace and dynamic energy. They harness the energy of the bandhas and tone the abdominal muscles, internal organs and inner thighs to create a sense of poise and balance.

Easing into the pose
This transition may take some practice to accomplish and complete, so as always be patient. At first you may wish to focus on attaining Tittibhasana before attempting Bakasana. Once you feel strong and confident in the first posture, then work towards Bakasana. Try bending one leg back at a time, gradually building the strength to take both feet back together in a smooth motion.

Deepening the pose
As you become more adept in this sweeping, bird-like transition, before springing back into Chaturanga Dandasana raise your knees off your arms with an inhalation and then shoot your feet back to continue into the full vinyasa with your next exhalation. As you practise this transition physical lightness and agility is cultivated and the entire body is toned and strengthened.

Kurma = tortoise incarnation of Visnu, preserver of the universe, second deity of the Hindu trinity

This posture intensely lengthens the back muscles and releases tightness in the lumbar region and sacrum, allowing energy to flow freely through the spine. If uddiyana bandha is fully engaged, respiratory and digestive systems are improved.

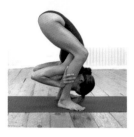

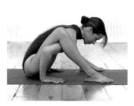

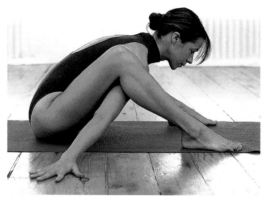

1 From the Adho Mukha Svanasana of your full vinyasa, *inhale* and jump your feet on to the floor forwards of your hands, with your legs to the outside of your arms and your knees by your shoulders, as you did to enter into Bhujapidasana. Take your hands to the backs of your ankles and move your shoulders to the backs of your knees.

2 Continue to *inhale* and bend your knees deeply and soften in your hips. Place your hands on the floor and lower your buttocks on to the floor. Deepen your engagement of uddiyana bandha to control the lowering of your hips into a gentle descent.

3 Stretch your arms out underneath your knees, extending through your fingertips out to the sides, and gently draw the backs of your knees over to the very tops of your arms.

4 As you *complete your inhalation*, deepen the fold in the front of your hips, stretch your legs long while firmly pressing your heels forwards. This straightening of your legs will press down on the backs of your upper arms and shoulders, which will help descend your torso closer to the floor. Open your chest wide and forwards along the floor and move your pubic bone back and down as you reach out through your arms. Draw your abdomen wall long, and lengthen through the front of your spine and throat to lay your ribs and chin on the floor. Look towards your third eye, <u>dristi</u>: **bru madhya**, and *take five to ten full, deep breaths* in this asana, before moving into the profound posture of Supta Kurmasana.

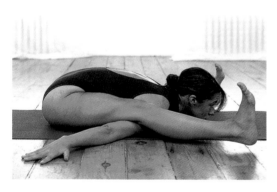

Easing into the pose
Work step by step to press your heels away gradually in order to straighten your legs. If this causes a sensation of overpulling in your back, keep your knees bent and softly release your torso forwards. Then, each time you practise this pose, gently move your feet further forwards until sufficient suppleness is developed within your hips and leg muscles to allow you to extend your legs forwards into the complete posture.

Deepening the pose
Each time you exhale in this asana, feel the fold at the front of your hips receding further backwards and in towards your buttock bones. Send energy out along the backs of your legs through into your heels, while drawing your thigh muscles up and in towards your front hips. This will help to create full length and strength in your leg muscles so that your legs straighten and your heels rise off the ground as the front of your torso opens into the ground.

Supta Kurmasana | SLEEPING TORTOISE POSTURE

supta = sleeping
Kurma = tortoise incarnation of
Visnu, preserver of the universe,
second deity of the Hindu trinity

This asana is physically completed by bowing the head low, and mentally completed by the drawing in of the mind, inducing introspection, stillness, inner calm and a quiet surrender to universal flow.

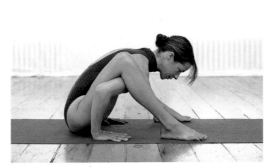

1 From Kurmasana, *inhale* and raise your head from the floor, bending your knees to release your arms and pressing your palms down under your shoulders to draw your torso up.

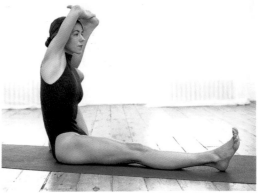

2 *Exhale* and, bringing your body upright, catch hold of your left foot with your right hand, bending your left knee up and back behind your left shoulder. *Inhale*, opening your chest. Press your left shoulder back to help move your left thigh and knee back.

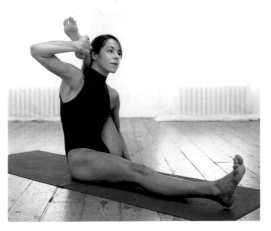

3 *Exhale*, softly rotate your left leg within its hip socket, and move your left knee back even more. Using your right hand, draw your left shin and ankle across behind your head and then your neck. Press your left side ribs forwards and lengthen up through your whole torso. Lift your face and press the back of your head backwards against your left ankle, drawing your chest up and shoulders wide to secure your left leg and foot in place.

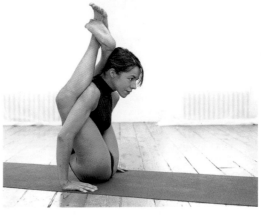

4 *Inhale* and bend your right knee, drawing it deeply back, with your right hand, and up behind your right shoulder. With an *exhalation*, rotate your right knee outwards, and with your right hand again work your right shin and ankle behind your head and neck, crossing it over your left ankle. *Inhale* and place both hands on the floor on either side of your hips, lifting your chest and rolling your shoulders firmly back. This will help in taking the knees further back and securing your ankles in a crossed position behind your head. Press the back of your neck against your ankles and lift your face to look forwards.

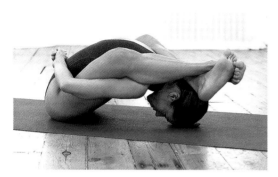

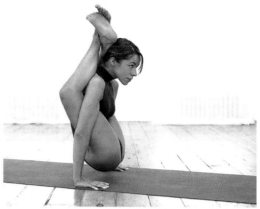

5 *Exhale*, step your hands forward and bend your elbows to lower your body forwards and down, placing your forehead on the floor. Thread your arms underneath your knees, turning your palms to face upwards and allowing your elbows to roll outwards. Now reach your hands back and clasp them together behind your waist. *Breathe five to ten full, deep breaths*, and gaze softly towards your third eye centre, <u>dristi</u>: **bhru madhya**.

Pratyahara

This sacred yogasana prepares us for pratyahara, or sensory withdrawal, which is the fifth limb of astanga yoga. Sensory withdrawal is symbolized here by the form of a tortoise drawing into its shell, moving attention away from the outer world and towards the inner life of the soul.

Easing into the pose

From step 1, rest your arms over your shinbones, bring the soles of your feet together and release your head forwards and down, so that your forehead is cradled in the arches of your feet. Once this is comfortable, progress on to slipping your arms under your knees and use a strap to link your hands. From here, enter your full vinyasa by raising your face and chest and placing your hands on the floor by the sides of your hips. Draw your feet in, crossing your ankles and tucking your knees up into your body to then jump back into Chaturanga Dandasana.

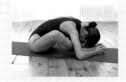 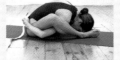

6 *Exhale*, release your hands and place them on the floor under your shoulders. Press down with your hands to raise your head and chest off the floor and so bring your torso upright. Straighten your arms with your ankles still strongly crossed behind your neck. As your torso rises, roll on to your buttocks and sit tall. *Inhale*, place your hands on the floor by the sides of your buttocks and lift your seat up off the floor as you press down through your arms and open your palms down into the ground. As you *breathe five steady breaths*, draw your chest open and move your shoulders and head back, looking forwards to your third eye centre, <u>dristi</u>: **bhru madhya**. After five breaths, *inhale*, uncross your ankles and stretch your legs into Tittibhasana. *Slowly exhale* as you fold your feet back into Bakasana and *inhale* here.

• On your next *exhalation*, softly jump your feet back into Chaturanga Dandasana and continue to flow into a **full vinyasa**. If you feel that the last five steps are too intense or strong at first, follow the instructions for easing into the posture.

Deepening the pose

This is a deep and intense posture, so work slowly and carefully into it, progressing gradually through the stages. As you place your forehead on the ground, gently extend your chin away from your chest and press your shoulders back to help prevent your feet from slipping forwards off the back of your head. When you have managed to catch hold of your hands, work towards deepening the bind by catching hold of the wrist, which will help to draw your shoulders further back and your chest and torso further forwards through your legs.

Garbha Pindasana A | WOMB EMBRYO POSTURE A

garbha = womb
pinda = embryo

Both Garbha Pindasanas and Kukkutasana are linked through breath and motion, one flowing into the other with no vinyasa. Garbha Pindasana A gently massages and tones the organs of the abdomen, particularly the liver.

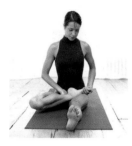 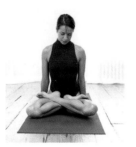 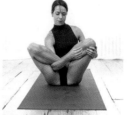 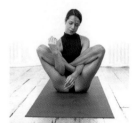

1 From Dandasana, *inhale very slowly*, bend your right knee and draw your right foot across on to the top of your left upper thigh into Ardha Padma (half lotus).

2 Continue to *inhale slowly* and bend your left knee, placing your left foot over on to your right upper thigh to come into the full lotus posture of Padmasana.

3 Still *inhaling*, draw your knees up and slide your right hand and forearm through the space between the front of your left ankle and the back of your right calf. Reach your hand along your left shinbone to feed your right elbow all the way through.

4 At the *end of your inhalation*, lift your right hand upwards to keep the right elbow in place, then slide your left hand and forearm through the gap between your right ankle and left calf. Slide your left forearm through until your left elbow is completely drawn through the gap.

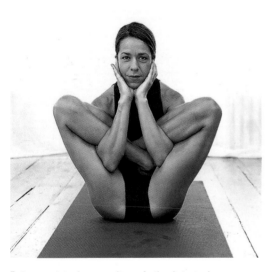

5 As you *exhale*, draw your knees further in towards your shoulders and bend both elbows strongly to lift your hands up under your chin and cradle your face, with your fingertips resting by your ears. Deepen your connection to uddiyana and mula bandha to help balance on your buttocks, and *take five to ten steady, deep breaths*, focusing forwards to your nose tip, <u>dristi</u>: **nasagrai**, before moving into Garbha Pindasana B.

Easing into the pose
If pain or strain is felt in your knees, proceed with caution and alternate the full lotus with a half lotus or with Sukhasana (cross-legged; see page 24). Wrap your arms around the outsides of your folded legs, clasping your hands around your ankles. To achieve the full posture, it may be useful to apply oil or water

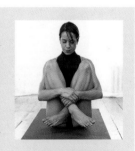

to your hands up to your elbows to help your arms slip through your legs.

Deepening the pose
As your fingertips reach your ears, gently press the ears shut to withdraw your hearing. In this way, Garbha Pindasana furthers the preparation of pratyahara (the fifth limb of astanga yoga) as experienced in Supta Kurmasana, where you withdraw your focus from the external world in order to look within. Here, the finger pressure on your ears enables you to deepen your listening and to hear the internal sound of your breath alone.

Garbha Pindasana B and Kukkutasana

WOMB EMBRYO POSTURE B AND ROOSTER POSTURE

garbha = womb
pinda = embryo
kukkuta = rooster

In Garbha Pindasana B, each roll of the soothing, rocking motion represents one of the nine months of gestation within the human womb. The lift of Kukkutasana develops strength in the upper body and especially in the wrists, arms and shoulders.

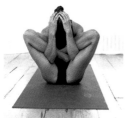 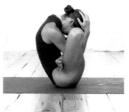 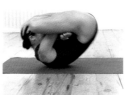 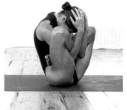

1a and b *Exhale* and move your chin in towards your chest, lowering your head and softly curling your body around like a ball. Place your palms on top of your head to seal yourself into this rounded shape.

2 As you continue to *exhale*, maintain the curve through your spine and softly roll back over on to your shoulders and swing your hips upwards.

3 *Inhale* and, as you begin to roll up, sway your hips slightly to the right side so that, as you arrive up on to your buttocks, you've rotated a little clockwise. *Exhale* and roll backwards again over your curved spine, and, as you begin to roll up with an *inhalation*, again sway your hips to the right so you rotate further clockwise. Repeat this rolling backwards and forwards in Garbha Pindasana another seven times (nine times in all) to complete a full circle.

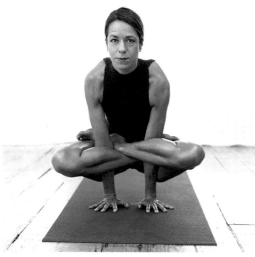

4 As you *inhale* into your ninth roll up, release your hands from your head and press your palms flat on to the floor with your fingers spreading open and pointing forwards. As your hands go down, press your chest strongly forwards and up. Lift the top of your head and firmly straighten your arms. As your arms straighten, raise your buttocks off the floor, connecting mula and uddiyana bandha deeper into your body. (Bandha control is exceptionally important here.) Balance on your broad, open hands and take *five to ten full, even breaths* here in Kukkutasana, looking towards your nose tip, <u>dristi</u>: **nasagrai.**

• *Exhale*, lower your seat to the floor and stretch into Dandasana. *Inhale*, draw your knees in and move into a **full vinyasa**.

Easing into the pose

As in the previous asana, you may wish to begin to practise this posture by wrapping your arms around the outside of your legs as you roll back and up. You can also build your strength towards the full balance by placing your hands on the ground by the sides of your hips to lift up

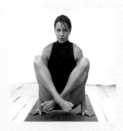

until you are able to slip your hands through your lotus legs.

Deepening the pose

Flow with the momentum of your breath to enhance a smooth, even, rolling motion and to connect yourself to the movement of your prana – the exhalation releasing your body down into the earth and the inhalation raising the energy of your body upwards.

Baddha Konasana A/B | BOUND ANGLE POSTURE A/B

baddha = bound or caught
kona = angle

These postures free up energy within the pelvic region and allow it to flow down to the feet to improve blood circulation and power in the legs. The stretch forwards of the back refreshes and rejuvenates the kidneys, helping to allieviate urinary disorders.

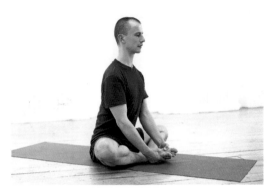

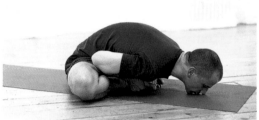

1 From Dandasana, *inhale*, bend your knees out to the sides and draw your feet together, bringing your heels close in towards your perineum and placing your hands on your feet. Now soften your hips and allow the soles of your feet to open upwards and the tops of your feet to roll down into the floor. Open your inner thighs wide and draw your knees down evenly to the floor. Breathe length into your spine, lifting your chest up and lowering your chin down so that the back of your neck feels long. Gently slide your shoulders down and broaden through your collarbones as you *take five to ten slow, deep breaths*, looking towards your nose tip, **dristi**: **nasagrai**. On your last *inhalation*, lengthen still further through your back.

2 As you *exhale*, softly lengthen your back out and over the soles of your feet, hinging deeply in your hip sockets and sending your pubic bone backwards and down into the floor. Lengthen through the front of your spine, torso and throat to bring your chin on to the ground in front of your toes. Look towards your nose tip, **dristi**: **nasagrai**, and *breathe slowly and deeply* in Baddha Konasana A for *five to ten breaths*.

Easing into the pose
Sitting on a yoga block or firm cushion will help to give your spine a lift up and out of your hips. This can be especially helpful if you have tightness in your pelvis and it will help to prevent your lower back collapsing or rounding.

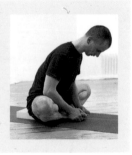

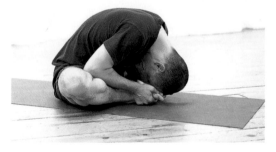

3 With an *inhalation*, return your torso upright and extend long through your back. On your *next exhalation*, deepen your engagement of uddiyana bandha to contract the abdomen in, softly curve your spine over and lower the top of your head down into the soles of your feet. Roll your chin inwards and release any tension in your shoulders by drawing your shoulder blades wide and down on either side of your spine. *Take five to ten deep, fluid breaths* in Baddha Konasana B while retaining your focus at the tip of your nose, **dristi**: **nasagrai**.

• *Inhale*, draw your back up straight, and flow into a **full vinyasa**.

Deepening the pose
Tuck your elbows inwards on to your inner thighs, and, with each exhalation, gently apply pressure down on to your legs to encourage your hips to open, your inner thighs to release and your knees to descend.

upavista = seated
kona = angle

This asana complements Baddha Konasana perfectly, as now the legs are stretched out, furthering the flow of energy from the pelvis to the feet. By releasing the legs wide and extending the torso forwards, flexibility in the hips and legs is developed.

SEATED ASANAS

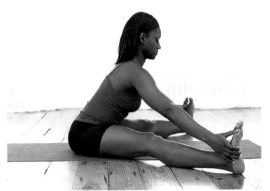

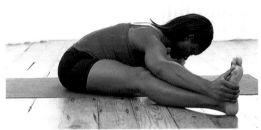

1 From landing in Dandasana from your **full vinyasa** continue to *inhale*, and stretch your legs open and wide out to the sides. Extend your back and lengthen through the front of your torso, stretching the abdominal wall long to tilt your pelvis forwards. Reach your hands on to your feet, placing each thumb in between the big toe and second toe joint and wrapping your fingers around the outer edges of your feet. Open your collarbones wide and press the centre of your chest forwards as you root your buttocks down into the floor, stretching both sides of your waist long.

2 On your *exhalation*, deepen the fold within your hips and pivot your pelvis forwards, sending your pubis and tailbone back and down behind you. Anchor your buttocks and backs of your legs firmly down into the floor. Open the centre of your chest forwards and out, lowering your torso towards the floor. Maintain uddiyana bandha and a long stretch through the front of your spine and throat to extend your chin towards the ground. Relax your shoulders and gently draw them back and down away from your ears. Focus awareness towards your third eye centre, <u>dristi</u>: **bru madhya**, and *take five to ten full, even breaths* here. As you breathe in this asana, with each *exhalation* soften in your hips and deepen uddiyana bandha as you release your torso long and further forwards and down. Now flow directly into Upavista Konasana B.

Easing into the pose
This posture develops flexibility in your hips, lower back and inner thighs. If these areas are tight, you may experience difficulty in reaching your hands to your feet. Rather than forcing the pose by rounding your back or bending your knees to catch hold of your feet, focus on creating full length and extension in both your

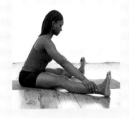

spine and legs, and place your hands on your ankles, or wherever you can manage, instead.

Deepening the pose
Engaging your bandhas in all postures is central to gaining internal support. In this asana, to extend deeper into the stretch without risk of groin strain, make sure you fully engage uddiyana and mula bandha to support the extension of your torso and the deep opening in your hips and thighs.

Be careful not to allow the fronts of your legs to roll inwards. Control this tendency by moving the outer edges of your thighs and knees backwards and down to direct your kneecaps and toes directly up. Keep your legs and feet active by extending your heels outwards and spreading your toes.

Upavista Konasana B | SEATED ANGLE POSTURE B

upavista = seated
kona = angle

Bandha control is essential here for providing support for the back when the torso is inclined and the legs extended up. As the body finds the balance point, the back and abdominal muscles are strengthened, helping to sustain alignment through the spine.

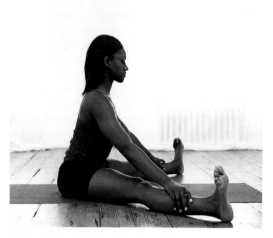

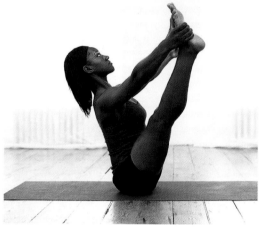

1 From Upavista Konasana A, *inhale* and lift your torso up while maintaining full length in your back and openness in your chest. Release the handhold of your feet and slide your hands on to your shins.

2 As you continue to *inhale*, lift from uddiyana bandha and rock back on to your sitting bones while reclining your torso backwards. At the same time, lever your straight legs up and off the floor. As your feet float up, extend your hands to catch hold of the outer edge of your feet again (as in Upavista Konasana A). Now, lift and press your chest high and roll your shoulders softly back and down. Extend up and out of your lower back and stretch the sides of your waist long, raising your lower abdomen. Once balanced, send the fold in the front of your hips down into your sitting bones to stabilize yourself. As you *breathe five to ten full, steady breaths*, extend your legs longer with each breath and root your sitting bones into the floor to balance high upon them. Lift your face skywards and take your focus up to the third eye centre, <u>dristi</u>: **bru madhya**.

• After five to ten breaths, *exhale* and let go of your feet without allowing them to crash down. *Inhale*, bend your knees to cross your ankles, and press your hands into the floor to swing back into Chaturanga Dandasana and continue into a **full vinyasa**.

Easing into the pose
Keeping your back strong and straight is fundamental to achieving this asana. At first, therefore, it is more beneficial to bend your knees rather than risk collapsing in your spine and hunching your back.
From a strong lifted spine and back, you can then work at gradually

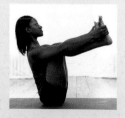

straightening your legs in this posture without shortening your torso.

Deepening the pose
Balancing high up on the tops of your sitting bones is the key to establishing a secure and open asana. Lifting from your lower back and bandhas while raising your chest strongly will help to shift your base forwards up on to your buttocks, rather then dropping back down on to your tailbone. It is a fine point of balance, and, once you're on it, you should continue to accentuate the lift through your chest by releasing your shoulders and stretching your legs like arrows.

supta = sleeping
kona = angle

As with all inverted postures the heart is placed on a higher level than the head. This stimulates the blood flow and oxygen supply to the brain. Sleeping angle posture introduces the first elements of inversion.

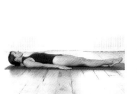

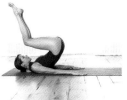

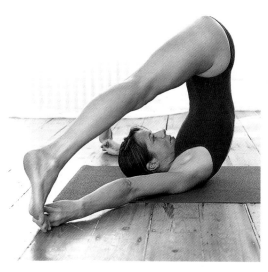

1 From Dandasana, *exhale* and softly roll your spine sequentially down on to the floor behind you, so that you are lying with your arms at the sides of your body, as if in a horizontal form of Tadasana.

2 *Inhale* and draw your knees up, pressing your arms and palms downwards as you swing your hips up and off the floor and roll over on to the back of your shoulders.

3 As you *exhale*, continue to roll completely over on to the back of your neck and head. Take your feet overhead and part them wide, stretching your inner thighs open. Catch hold of your right big toe with your right index and middle fingers and your left big toe with your left index and middle fingers. Press your sitting bones and pubis upwards to draw length into the front and back of your spine, and lock your chest up and into your chin. Extend your heels away, with your toes tucked under, and feel the stretch through the entire length of the back of your legs. *Take five to ten deep, long breaths*, focusing towards your nose tip, **dristi: nasagrai**, and deeply engage your bandhas to prepare for Supta Konasana B, which flows directly on from here.

Benefits of the pose

Rolling on to the back of the neck releases the cervical vertebrae, stretching the muscles in this area to relieve stiffness and tension. The lifting of the pelvis intensifies the action and toning benefits of uddiyana bandha.

Easing into the pose

If this posture causes strain in your back, bend your knees slightly to get hold of your toes. Alternatively, if you experience difficulty holding your toes at first, hold your ankles while maintaining the stretch through your legs, then gradually move towards your toes.

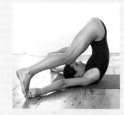

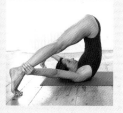

Deepening the pose

To enter this asana from step 1, as your back and abdominal muscles develop strength, try lifting your legs up straight and together and then rolling over on to the back of your shoulders. While in this posture, focus on opening the back of your neck and shoulders wide into the floor, at the same time as raising your pelvis higher to feel the polarity of energy directions through your body.

Supta Konasana B | SLEEPING ANGLE POSTURE B

supta = sleeping
kona = angle

The motion of rolling up through the spine helps to align the vertebrae and massages the back muscles along the floor. The head gently swinging up and down boosts the blood circulation from the brain to the heart, clearing the mind and refreshing the body.

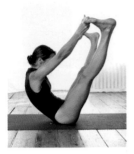
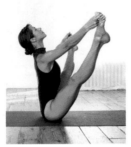
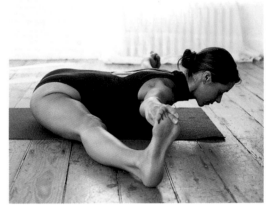

1 From Supta Konasana A, *inhale* and press from your tucked-under toes, gently rounding your back like a ball to roll up sequentially through your spine. Maintain your finger hold of your big toes, and send the top of your head forwards in order to roll smoothly upwards.

2 At the top of your *inhalation*, and just as you roll up on to your buttocks, strongly lift your chest forwards and up. Softly throw your shoulders back and extend through your spine to move your back from a curved to a straight position. Send the fold in the front of your hips down into your sitting bones to stabilize yourself here, and take a moment to suspend yourself in this fine point of balance, lifting your face and heart skywards as you look to your third eye centre, **dristi: bru madhya**.

3 As you *exhale*, drop forwards into Upavista Konasana, flexing your legs and feet fully and strongly with your fingers still securely holding your toes. This will carry the whole shape of the previous suspended position down on to the floor. Slide your shoulder blades down your back and lengthen the front of your torso along the floor, moving your chest forwards and your chin down towards the ground. On your next *inhalation*, and while still holding your toes, lift your body upwards, drawing more openness into your chest. With an *exhalation*, release your hands from your feet and bring your torso completely upright.

• *Inhale*, cross your ankles and press your hands into the floor to lift your seat up. Swing your feet back into Chaturanga Dandasana and continue to flow into a **full vinyasa** to softly land into Dandasana.

Easing into the pose
This flowing, rolling motion up and then down takes practice to achieve, and careful attention to how you roll through your back and drop forwards is essential. Keeping your back and spine consciously rounded will help you to roll like a ball, and, if keeping your legs totally straight impedes your sense of momentum at first, try bending them slightly as you roll upwards. However, once you reach your point of balance, stretch your legs long and your back straight. As you drop forwards, be careful not to crash land on your heels, though this may prove difficult, especially if, in the beginning, your tendency is to bend your knees. If this is the case, place your feet down one at a time until your flexibility and strength have developed sufficiently for you to progress on to the straight-leg drop forwards, as discussed in the "Deepening the pose" box (right).

Deepening the pose
Focus on completely flexing your feet and stretching your legs straight, so that as you drop forwards your heels do not touch the floor. This will not only develop both strength and flexibility in your legs but will also ensure that your calf muscles cushion your landing into Upavista Konasana B, rather than letting your heels crash down. Your bandhas, too, will greatly help a soft landing, so consciously engage them into your body and allow your body to flow and roll with the natural momentum of your breath.

supta = sleeping
pada = foot or leg
angustha = big toe

The preceding postures have prepared the muscles of the legs for the deep stretch of this pose. As one leg is lengthened up and over into the torso to increase flexibility, the other presses down and along the floor in the opposite direction to develop strength.

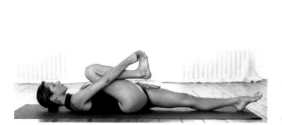

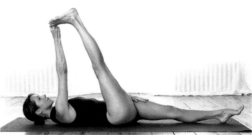

1 *Exhale* from Dandasana and softly roll your back sequentially on to the floor to lay your body long and straight. In this supine position, *inhale*, draw your right thigh and knee up, folding deeply within your right hip socket, and catch hold of your right big toe with your right index and middle fingers. Extend your left leg long, pressing the left sole of your foot out and away from your hips.

2 At the end of your *inhalation*, straighten your right leg completely by extending your right foot up and anchoring down through the back of your right hip to maintain even alignment through your pelvis. Lengthen through your back and broaden your shoulders and sacrum into the floor. Press your left palm firmly down on to your left thigh to encourage the full extension of your left leg.

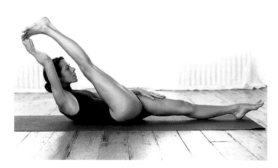

3 As you *exhale*, deepen the connection of uddiyana bandha into your body and raise your head, shoulders and upper back off the floor, moving your right leg up and in towards your face. Stretch out through your left leg, pressing your left heel and ball of the foot away and opening the entire length of the back of your left leg down into the floor. This creates a strong base for the stretching of your right leg. Be careful not to hunch your shoulders; instead, let them open wide and bend your right elbow sideways as your head draws higher towards your right leg. *Take five to ten steady, deep breaths* in this asana, looking towards the toes of your right foot, <u>dristi</u>: **padhayoragrai**. After a minimum of five breaths, *inhale* and, with control, softly lower your head, shoulders and upper back down on to the floor, as in step 2. From here, move directly into the next asana.

Easing into the pose
If you are unable to hold your big toe with your leg straight, take a strap and wrap it around the ball of your lifted foot. Work in this way until you are flexible enough to catch hold of your toe. If you have suffered from a back injury or any back pain, practise by bending your lifted leg and hugging your knee in with both hands as you lift your head and shoulders. This will help to develop abdominal strength and realign your spine. As you get stronger, work the full asana.

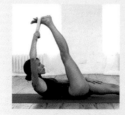 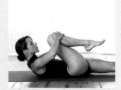

Deepening the pose
Keep both legs and torso evenly active – not overstretching or overworking one side of your body while the other side is underactive. Stretch the back of your lifted leg long and press the back of both hips evenly into the floor. Deeply activate uddiyana bandha by flattening the abdominal wall down as you move your chin to your shin.

Supta Parsvasahita A | SLEEPING SIDE ACCOMPANIED POSTURE A

supta = sleeping
parsva = side or lateral
sahita = accompanied

As the lifted leg is opened out to the side, the stretch through the leg muscles is intensified and a balance between flexibility and strength is developed. The lifting and rotation of the leg also promotes full blood circulation through the legs into the feet.

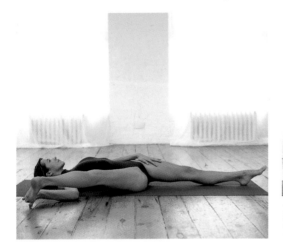

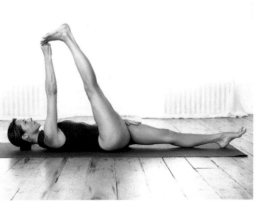

1 From Supta Padangusthasana, maintaining your finger hold of your right big toe, *slowly exhale* and rotate your right leg, deep within its hip socket, outwards to the right side. Fully engage uddiyana bandha to stabilize the pelvis into the floor. Open and stretch both your right arm and leg wide, lengthening through your right inner thigh until your right toes make contact with the floor. Press your left shoulder, left side of your ribcage, left buttock and the back of your left leg firmly down into the floor to create a strong, secure foundation from which to release and open your right leg out. This gives balance and stability to the stretch of your body in this asana. *Breathe five to ten full, even breaths*, turn your head to the left, as if your left ear were listening into the ground, <u>dristi</u>: **parsva**.

2 *Inhale*, draw your right leg up from the right side and anchor down through the back of your right hip while extending your right foot high and your leg long. Spread your back wide and open into the floor before continuing directly into Supta Parsvasahita B.

Easing into the pose
If you have been working with a strap in the previous posture, continue to do so for this asana. Alternatively, if you practised the previous pose with your knee bent, continue to do so, and open your bent leg out to the side with your hand cupping and supporting your knee.

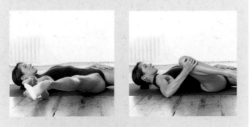

Deepening the pose
As in all of our asanas, both sides of the body need to work equally for strength and flexibility. Particularly in this posture, any imbalances of strength and flexibility through the right and left side become very apparent. It is therefore important to feel that both sides of your body are consciously involved and aware. Focus to open the left side of your body deeply into the floor away from your right side, as your right leg opens out and away from your left side.

If you find the left side of your body losing contact with the floor as your right leg opens to the side, this is an indication of imbalance between your strength and flexibility. To address this imbalance, move your right leg up to reanchor your left side down, and stabilize the pose here. From this centred place, focus on slowly releasing your right leg out and your left side down while maintaining full contact with the floor through the left side of your back. In this way, balance is created and flexibility and strength developed together, rather than one at the expense of the other.

supta = sleeping
parsva = side or lateral
sahita = accompanied

This posture is an intensified form of Supta Padangusthasana and is considered a purifying asana, as the deep and dynamic articulation of the legs focuses and stills the mind, helping to harness sexual energy.

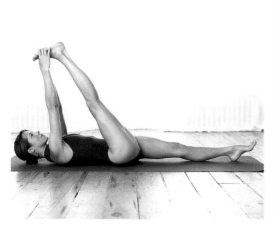

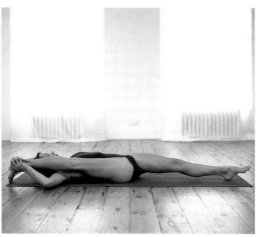

1 From Supta Parsvasahita A, with an *exhalation* take both your hands to catch hold of your right foot. Level your shoulders and draw the whole surface of your back and the back of your pelvis open and down into the floor. Press the heel and ball of your left foot away.

2 Continue to *exhale* and bend your elbows wide, keeping your chest open and both shoulders releasing down into the floor, and draw your right leg straight over to the right side of your head. Extend your right toes to touch the floor. Holding your foot with both hands still, bring your right inner calf to touch softly against your right ear and engage uddiyana bandha. *Breathe five to ten deep, even breaths*, looking to your nose tip, **dristi**: **nasagrai**. Focus on softening deeply in your right hip and through the back of your right thigh to extend and release into the posture fully. *Inhale* and return your leg to upright (at a right angle to your left leg), remaining open in your shoulders and centred in your back. *Exhale* and let go of your right foot, slowly releasing your right leg straight down to the floor by the side of your left leg to lie in a supine Tadasana. Without a vinyasa, repeat Supta Padangusthasana and Supta Parsvasahita A and B on the left side, then move into Chakrasana, as overleaf.

Easing into the pose
If you have been using a strap in the two previous postures, you will need to continue to do so. Do not, however, attempt to draw your leg beyond 90 degrees to the floor until you are able to catch hold of your foot while maintaining full length and straightness in both legs. A softer option

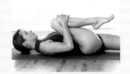

would be to hug your thigh in towards your front torso as you bend your knee.

Deepening the pose
As with Supta Padangusthasana and Supta Parsvasahita A, working evenly in this asana is essential for establishing balance in your body. In this pose it is easy to forget about engaging your bandhas and stretching your left leg while overfocusing on the lifting of your right leg in the ambition to deepen the stretch of this asana. Instead, draw your awareness into your left leg, opening the back of your knee down into the ground and extending your foot away from your hips. Engaging your bandhas will help to support your back, keep your torso long and your chest open as your body releases into this deep and demanding posture.

Chakrasana | CIRCLING WHEEL POSTURE

chakra = circle or wheel

The circular wheeling momentum of the body in this transitional posture boosts the circulation through the spine to the brain, as the back muscles are rolled and massaged into the floor to refresh and awaken the complete body.

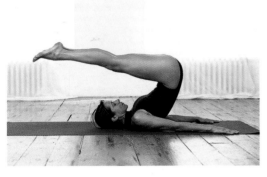

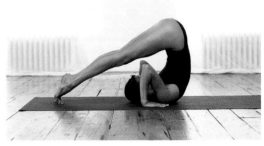

1 *Inhale*, draw your knees up, and press your arms and palms down by the sides of your body to help swing your hips and pelvis gently up off the floor. As your hips rise, soften your spine round, rolling further up and over your back on to your shoulders, like a ball rolling backwards. Let your pelvis float and the back of your neck and shoulders release wide and down into the floor.

2 Continue to *inhale*. Lengthen your legs, reaching your feet overhead, on to the floor. Take your hands on to the floor by the sides of your head. Your fingertips must be just under your shoulders with your elbows bent and pointing directly upwards.

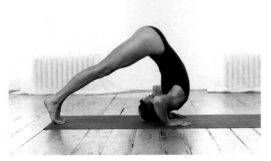

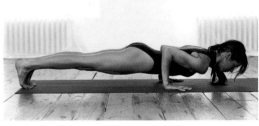

3 Towards the *end of your inhalation*, roll over on to the back of your head, allowing your neck to stretch gently with the rest of your spine rolling up off the floor. Press firmly down through your palms and stretch your legs strongly, with your toes tucked under. Transfer your weight now fully on to your hands and feet to roll further over on to the back and top of your head.

4 *Exhale* as you deepen uddiyana bandha, feeling dynamic energy pouring into your arms and legs. Release your head forwards and out to complete this full circular motion of Chakrasana and softly pounce out into Chaturanga Dandasana.

• From here, flow through a **full vinyasa**.

Easing into the pose
Go slowly, practising just up to step 2, gradually building your confidence to go further each time. Resist the tendency to roll over on to one shoulder more than the other by pressing evenly into both hands. Keep your mind relaxed and let it flow with the roll.

Deepening the pose
At all times it is of prime importance to keep your neck relaxed and your bandhas engaged, as this will enable you to roll with ease and without panic over your shoulders and neck. Be aware here of jalandhara bandha and allow your throat to yield.

ubhaya = both
pada = foot or leg
angustha = big toe

The soft, rolling motion of the preceding postures continues in the next two asanas, stimulating the spine and back muscles and helping to prepare for the back bends that follow. Ubhaya Padangusthasana also strengthens the back and tones the legs.

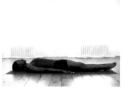 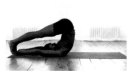

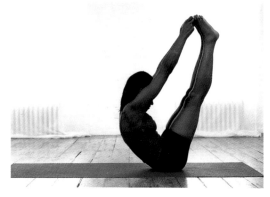

1 From Dandasana, *exhale* and roll your back down sequentially to lie supine on the floor.

2 *Inhale*, drawing your knees up and press your arms and hands down by the sides of your body. Roll your hips up, softly curling through your back to roll over on to the back of your shoulders. Extend your feet overhead, stretching your legs long with your inner thighs and feet together. Reach your hands to your feet to catch hold of your big toes with your index and middle fingers. *Exhale* here and soften the back of your neck. Release your shoulders wide into the floor as you draw your hips further over your shoulders and press your heels away.

3 As you begin to *inhale*, push off from your tucked-under toes. Deepen uddiyana bandha. Softly round your back, keeping your chin resting on your chest, and roll up through the curl of your spine. Lengthen the backs of your legs and lead the crown of your head forwards.

Easing into the pose
To gain a sense of momentum in this posture, practise rolling backwards and forwards with a curved spine and the knees slightly bent. Once you find a balance on your buttocks, work your back straight first and then your legs. If your back rounds as your legs straighten, rebend your knees to re-establish length through your spine, then try again to lengthen your legs while maintaining the straightness of your spine. Do not straighten your legs at the expense of rounding your back.

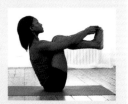

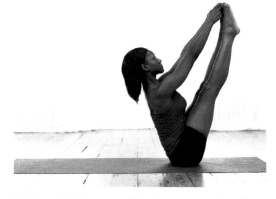

Deepening the pose
This posture is again a fine point of balance, and instead of passing through it, as in Supta Konasana, we maintain and breathe into it. To feel the correct placement up on your sitting bones and not collapse into your coccyx, send the fold at the front of your hips down into your sitting bones and lift strongly up from your lower back, pressing the sacrum and back of your waist forwards. Then release your neck and head back, stretching through the front of your throat.

4 Continue to *inhale* as your sitting bones make contact with the floor. Strongly project your chest open and upwards, lifting your heart high and face skywards. Release your shoulders back and lengthen your back out of its curve, balancing high up on your sitting bones. Deepen uddiyana bandha and stretch your legs as far as possible, looking towards your third eye centre, <u>dristi</u>: **bru madhya**, as you *take five full breaths*.

• *Exhale*, and release the clasp of your toes, placing your hands on the floor by your hips and bending your knees to cross your ankles. As you take your next *inhalation*, press down through your arms and raise your seat to enter into a **full vinyasa**.

Urdhva Mukha Paschimottanasana | UPWARD FACING INTENSE STRETCH OF THE WEST POSTURE

urdhva = upward
mukha = face
paschima = west
uttana = intense stretch

This is a progression from Ubhaya Padangusthasana, and the benefits are intensified by the pressure of the length of the front torso into the legs. This stretches and tones the abdominal wall, increasing the blood flow around and through the internal organs.

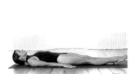 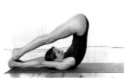 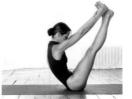 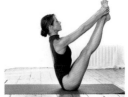

1 Landing in Dandasana from a full vinyasa, continue to *inhale* and roll your back sequentially down to lie supine on the floor. Keep *inhaling* now as you roll your hips up, softly curling through your back to roll over on to the back of your shoulders.

2 Complete your *inhalation* and extend your feet overhead, stretching your legs long with your inner thighs and feet together. Reach your hands to your feet to catch hold of their outer edge. *Exhale*, maintaining the hold of your feet, soften the back of your neck and release your shoulders wide as you draw your hips further up and press your heels away.

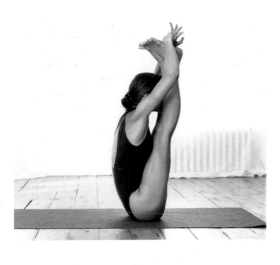

3 Push from your tucked-under toes and, as you *inhale*, softly round your back by deepening uddiyana bandha. Keep your chin resting into your chest to roll up through the curve of your spine like a ball rolling forwards. Lengthen the backs of your legs as you send the top of your head forwards.

4 Continue to *inhale* and, as your sitting bones make contact with the floor, strongly project your chest open and up, lift your head, aligning your neck with your spine, and extend your focus up to your toes, <u>dristi</u>: **padhayoragrai**. Release your shoulders back and lengthen your back out of its curve, securing your balance high up on your sitting bones. Deepen uddiyana bandha and stretch your legs as far as possible.

5 *Exhale* and release the hold of your feet, then recatch them, interlacing your fingers around the balls of your feet, or taking your right hand to hold your left wrist. Lengthen up through the front of your spine and torso, raising your chest and sending your pubic bone downwards. Lift out of your sacrum and stretch your back, bending your elbows to draw your legs and torso together. Draw your legs in towards your front torso and your torso in towards your legs. *Take five to ten long, steady breaths*, focusing energy up to your toes, <u>dristi</u>: **padhayoragrai**. *Inhale* and draw your torso and legs away from one another, still holding your feet. *Exhale* and release your feet. Bend your knees to cross your ankles, with your hands on the floor by your hips.

• *Inhale*, press down through your palms and lift your hips, then move into a **full vinyasa**, to jump through into Dandasana.

Easing into the pose
If drawing your legs and torso together causes your back to round or collapse, practise only up to step 4.

Deepening the pose
As you become stronger and more supple, focus on moving your chin and forehead up along your shinbones as you slide your shoulder blades down your back. Fold deeply in your hips to draw your legs and torso together like the pages of a book shutting.

setu = bridge
bandha = bondage or fetter

In this posture, an arching bridge shape is created through the body, producing spinal flexibility and preparing the back muscles for the back bend of Urdhva Dhanurasana. This pose strengthens the neck, dorsal, lumbar, sacral and back thigh muscles.

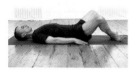 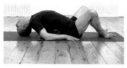

1 From Dandasana, *exhale* and roll sequentially down your spine to lie on your back. Now bend your knees, allowing them to part wide while turning your feet out and placing your heels together but your big toes apart. Open the soles of your feet face down towards the floor and place your arms by the sides of your body with your palms pressing down.

2 As you begin to *inhale*, arch through your spine, lifting your chest up and stretching through the front of your neck. Draw the very top of your head on to the floor. Tilt your pelvis, pressing your sitting bones down and raising the back of your waist and your ribs up. Spread your feet and toes while relaxing your face as you look towards your nose tip, <u>dristi</u>: **nasagrai**.

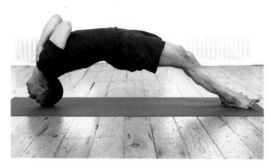

3 Continue to *inhale*, rooting down through your feet, and send your hips up, raising your seat off the floor. As your hips lift higher, press your feet into the floor to straighten your legs and arch more deeply through your upper spine, opening up your chest. Be careful not to grip your buttocks, as they will automatically engage and, if you overclench them, this will block the lift of your pelvis and lower spine. Release your hands from the floor and cross your arms over your chest. *Take five deep, smooth breaths* and look towards your nose tip, <u>dristi</u>: **nasagrai**. *Exhale* to lower your buttocks down. Release off the top of your head and lay your back flat on the floor, placing your arms at your sides.

• From here, lift your legs and roll back into Chakrasana and move into a **full vinyasa**. Jump through to land in Dandasana.

Benefits of the pose
Setu Bandha is a wonderful tonic for the entire body. The expansion of the chest and front ribs opens the heart to stimulate circulation and increases lung capacity.

Easing into the pose
If this posture is too strong on your neck and creates pressure, take your hands back on to the floor by the sides of your head with your fingertips pointing towards your feet. Press your palms down and roll your shoulders back to draw your chest open and high. Alternatively,

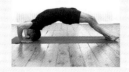

if you find this too intense, practise the back bend moderation of Urdhva Dhanurasana overleaf.

Deepening the pose
In this asana in order not to compress your neck vertebrae the legs must be fully active and the bandhas deeply engaged. As you practise this asana, concentrate on standing your feet firmly on the floor as you lift your kneecaps, thighs and abdominal muscles upwards. Draw your spine, especially your upper spine, up and in, pressing it through into the front of your torso to help raise your chest and ease pressure out of your neck.

Urdhva Dhanurasana | UPWARD BOW POSTURE

urdhva = upward
dhanu = bow

This strong back bend provides the body with a counter-stretch to the earlier forward bending postures. The front of the abdomen, hips and thighs are fully stretched and lengthened, and the hands and wrists are strengthened.

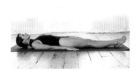

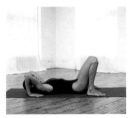

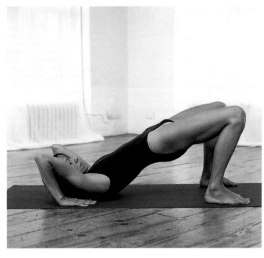

1 From Dandasana, begin to *exhale* and softly roll your back down to lie straight and flat on the floor, arms by your sides.

2 Continue to *exhale*, bending your knees and stepping your feet parallel and in line with the outer edges of your hips. Move your heels in so they touch the outer edges of your buttocks. Place your palms down on the floor on either side of your head, in line with your shoulders. Open your hands and extend your fingers underneath the tops of your shoulders, and direct your elbows upwards.

3 As you begin to *inhale*, press the soles of your feet into the floor, move your hips upwards and fully engage uddiyana bandha to support your lower back. Maintain the parallel alignment of your feet and legs as you move on to the next step.

Easing into the pose
Back bends are known for invigorating the nervous system and relieving nervousness, anxiety and fear. However, if a full back bend feels too intense, refer to the Urdhva Dhanurasana moderations.

Deepening the pose
As you gain in strength, suppleness and stamina, instead of lowering your whole body down to the floor, just bend your elbows to lower the top of your head to touch the ground as you exhale. From here, with your head still on the floor, take a step with each hand in towards your feet. Then, with a full inhalation, press firmly and evenly into your hands and feet to straighten your arms and energize your legs, raising your

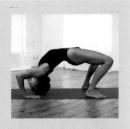

chest, torso and pelvis into a higher arch still. Take five steady breaths and repeat the lowering down on to your head and stretching back up twice more before releasing out of the asana.

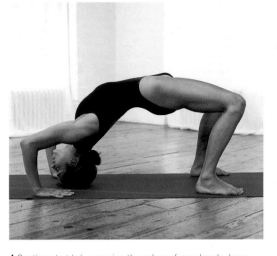

4 Continue to *inhale*, pressing the palms of your hands down and lifting your shoulders up off the floor. Open your chest to place the top of your head on the ground, and begin to arch in your upper back. Transfer all your weight evenly through your arms and legs. Engage uddiyana bandha to lengthen through the abdominal wall and give support to your lower back.

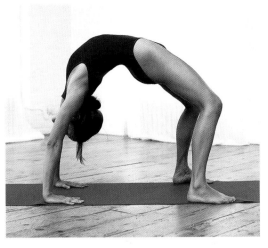

5 As you complete your *inhalation*, send energy down through your arms and legs into your hands and feet and press them firmly and evenly into the floor. Stretch your arms straight and roll your shoulders back, away from your ears, sending your shoulder blades into your back ribs. Do not tense your buttocks, as this will block movement in your lower spine. Draw your thigh muscles up to raise your hips, torso and chest higher. Slide your tailbone in towards your pubis. Feel the front of your pelvis opening: this will help you to arch evenly through the entire length of your spine. *Take five to ten deep breaths*, looking towards your nose tip, **dristi: nasagrai**. Then *exhale* and bend your elbows and knees, softly lowering your back on to the floor to the position shown in step 2. Repeat steps 3–5 twice more, so that you practise this asana three times in all, taking your body a little deeper into the posture with each repetition.

• Then, with an *inhalation*, roll over into Chakrasana to move into a **full vinyasa** landing on your feet into Tadasana.

Urdhva Dhanurasana Moderated | UPWARD BOW POSTURE MODERATED

This moderated posture can be practised initially to build the strength and flexibility necessary for the back bends of Setu Bandha and Urdhva Dhanurasana. It is a gentler asana than the full postures, with extra support provided from the base of the neck, head and arms as they press and root downwards, helping to arch the spine upwards.

1 Follow steps 1 and 2 of Urdhva Dhanurasana, but instead of putting your hands beside your head, keep your arms at the side of your body with your palms facing down.

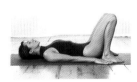

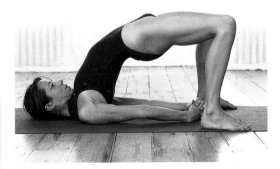

Easing into the pose
If you are unable to interlace your fingers while maintaining contact with your little fingers into the floor, leave your arms straight by your sides and press the entire length of them down, rolling your elbows in towards each other.

Deepening the pose
As the arch develops through your back and your legs grow stronger, try stepping your feet inwards so that you can clasp your ankles securely. Extend your heels down to send your hips higher, and draw your knees

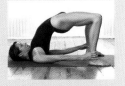

completely over and in line with your ankles.

2 *Inhale*, press firmly down through the soles of your feet into the floor, and raise your pelvis high without clenching your buttock muscles. Interlace your fingers on the floor behind your back, rolling your shoulders down and away from your ears and lengthening your arms. Extend your elbows, wrists and little fingers into the floor, moving your spine and back ribs in and up. Open up your chest, lifting it in towards your chin, and relax your throat and jaw. *Take five to ten even breaths*, gently drawing your tailbone in towards your pubis, still without clenching your buttocks. Focus on developing the support from the strength in your legs by extending your feet down and lifting your thigh muscles up, helping to raise your pelvis higher and to arch deeply through your spine.

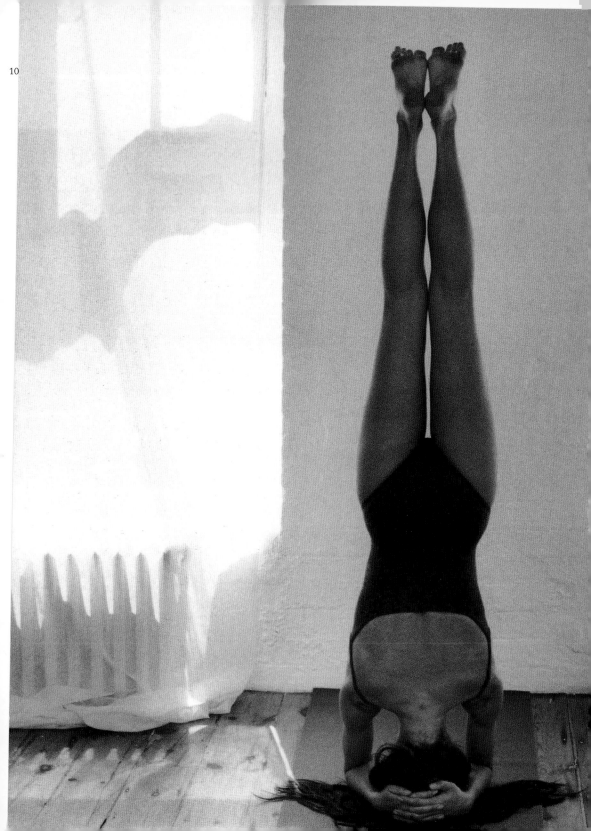

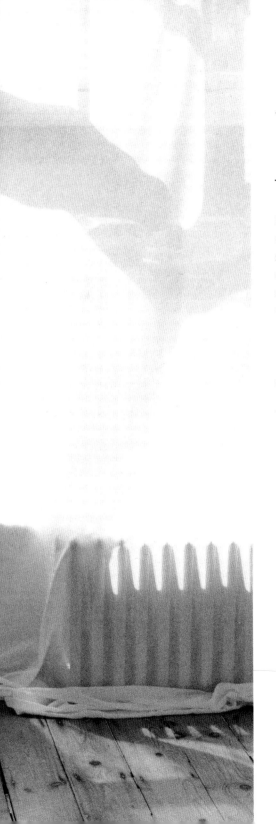

Finishing
Asanas

In the finishing postures we turn upside down to practise the shoulder and headstand sequences. Turning upside down can induce a sense of disorientation, insecurity, fear and anxiety, so challenging our comfortable view of the world. But if we practise with gentle patience and calmness, these inverted postures help us to clear our mind of negativity and find our own internal balance, security and stability.

The feet, which have been so firmly rooted into the earth, are now released skywards and root into the heavens instead, symbolically removing our standing in the physical and material world to seek inspiration from above. Bringing the head on to the floor to balance on it helps to focus the mind, surrendering our thoughts to the earth and ground.

Just as Surya Namaskara reflects the energy of the sun, warming the body and awakening the mind, this finishing sequence is reflective of the moon's energy. It balances the body and harmonizes the mind, preparing the way for the meditative posture of Padmasana (lotus posture) and the deep relaxation of Savasana (corpse posture), which is the final pose of the primary series.

Salamba Sarvangasana | SUPPORTED WHOLE BODY POSTURE

salamba = supported
sarva = entire or whole
anga = limb or body

Sarvangasana is the mother posture, creating harmony and balance throughout the human system. The inversion of the body boosts the circulatory and respiratory systems, and so nourishes and revitalizes the entire body on a cellular level.

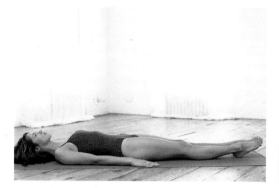

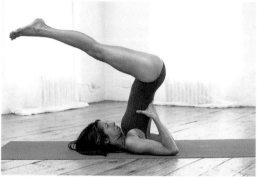

1 From a full vinyasa, *inhale* and jump through to land in Dandasana. *Exhale* and softly roll sequentially down through your spine to lie supine and straight on the floor, with your arms close by your sides. Feel the back surface of your body long against the floor and soften your shoulders down into the ground as you *take five full breaths.*

2 *Inhale*, pressing the backs of your shoulders, arms and palms down into the floor, then draw your legs up and roll over on to the backs of your shoulders and neck. Engage uddiyana bandha to create a lift through your pelvis and torso as you raise your hips directly over and in line with your shoulders. Move your chest up and into your chin, bending your elbows inwards no further than the width of your shoulders, and place your palms firmly on your back.

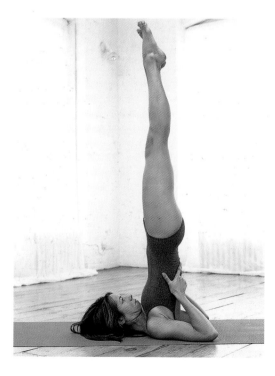

3 Continue to *inhale*, and stretch your legs up straight, coming into the full posture of Salamba Sarvangasana, balancing your entire body up and over on to the very top of your shoulders and back of your neck and head. Lift up out of your neck and shoulders by taking your hands lower down and pressing your palms on to your back ribs to help draw your upper spine away from your neck. Lengthen through your legs, opening the soles of your feet skywards, and align your heels together, directly up and over your hips. Move your tailbone in towards your pubic bone and draw your thigh muscles up and on to their thighbones. Draw in your lower abdomen to deepen uddiyana bandha. *Breathe here for 20–30 deep, steady breaths*, gently gazing towards your nose tip, <u>dristi</u>: **nasagrai**. Allow your face to relax, softening around your eyes and jaw muscles. From Salamba Sarvangasana, move directly into the next asana.

Warning
Do not practise this asana if you have high blood pressure, heart problems, a neck injury, a prolapsed disc, a hernia or glaucoma, or during menstruation (see the moderated posture opposite).

salamba = supported
sarva = entire or whole
anga = limb or body

Using the wall to support the legs in the shoulder stand helps to lift the torso up into vertical alignment. The benefits are the same as in the full pose, but this is a good way to acclimatize oneself to inversions of the body and is wonderfully rejuvenating.

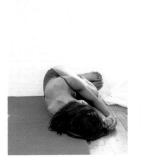

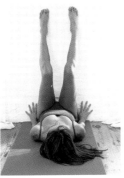

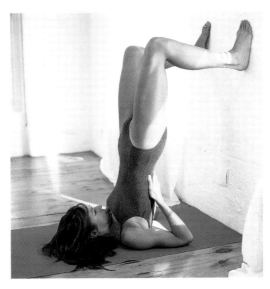

1 Place your yoga mat against the wall and lie on your side, with your knees drawn up, placing your right shoulder and hip along the edge of your mat with your buttocks touching the wall.

2 *Exhale* and roll over on to your back, levelling your buttocks against the wall, and keeping your spine straight. Step your feet up the wall, with your knees bent and your arms by your sides.

3 *Inhale* and press your feet firmly into the wall. Engage uddiyana bandha and raise your pelvis off the floor, lifting up through your back to open your chest up against your chin. Move your whole pelvis up and over your shoulders and draw your elbows in towards one another. Now press your elbows down into the floor and place your palms on your back. *Breathe here for 20–30 full, even breaths*, and then move into the next asana, or release your hands on to the floor and softly roll your back and hips down. Bend your knees and roll on to your right side to come out of this moderated posture.

Benefits of the pose
The action of lifting and pressing the chest up against the chin deepens jalandhara bandha and regulates the thyroid and parathyroid glands situated at the front of the throat. When these glands are balanced, this helps to maintain the health of the digestive, nervous, circulatory and endocrine systems, so ensuring the regeneration of cells, bones and bodily energy.

Easing into the pose
If you have health problems (see warning box), instead of raising your pelvis off the floor, simply extend your legs straight up the wall and soften your back, releasing it into the floor with arms outstretched.

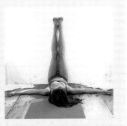

Deepening the pose
Focus on breathing steadily and slowly. Lift your sternum (breastbone) right up and into your chin to deepen the throat lock, which will stimulate and balance your thyroid gland. If you feel tension building up in your shoulders, softly roll them down into the floor and direct energy from your shoulders through your upper arms and into your elbows. Gently root your elbows down and send the energy from your elbows up into your palms to give support into your back and raise your pelvis higher. In this way, we can transform tension into positive energy.

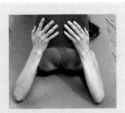

Halasana | PLOUGH POSTURE

hala = plough

Just as the plough drives through into the darkness of the earth to loosen the soil and uproot the old growth, so, in this asana, the blood is sent through the brain to clear and lighten the mind. It also stretches the arms and back and opens the shoulders.

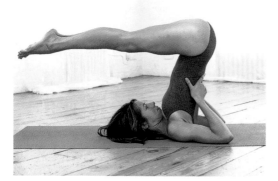

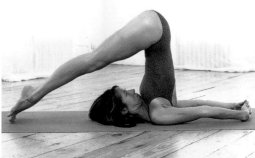

1 After *taking 20–30 breaths* in Salamba Sarvangasana, *exhale* and, while maintaining a strong lift through your abdomen, pubis and buttock bones, hinge your legs out from your hips, lowering your feet towards the floor. Keep your legs lengthening straight and support your back with your hands. Strongly lift your hips and allow the back of your pelvis to move very slightly back towards your hands in order to counter the weight of your legs as they lower down.

2 Continue to *exhale* as you keep lowering your legs with control, bringing your toe tips down on to the floor beyond the top of your head. Raise your buttock bones and pubic bone high, and lengthen through the front of your torso, stretching your front spine long. Release your hands from your back and interlace your fingers deeply, extending your arms straight out behind you. Roll your shoulders down away from your ears, and press your elbows, wrists and little fingers softly into the floor. Draw your collarbones wide, and open your chest up and into your chin to deepen jalandhara bandha. *Take 10–20 full, slow breaths* here before flowing into the next asana. Look towards your nose tip, <u>dristi</u>: **nasagrai**, relaxing your face and softening your jaw.

Easing into the pose
Lowering your feet on to a pre-positioned chair is a soft alternative to Halasana that is exceptionally soothing on your entire nervous system and is particularly beneficial to those who suffer from extreme neck tension and tightness. Bending your knees on to your forehead is another helpful way of easing into the posture of Halasana.

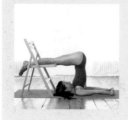

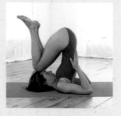

Deepening the pose
Do not stub your toes into the floor. Instead, place the very tops of your toes down and extend your legs long, drawing your kneecaps and thigh muscles up towards your hips, to help the pelvis remain lifted.

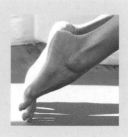

karna = ear
pida = pressure

Drawing the knees on to the ears deepens the stretch through the back, which tones and balances the nervous system. It also closes out external sound, making it possible to listen inwardly to the beat of the heart and the rhythm of breathing.

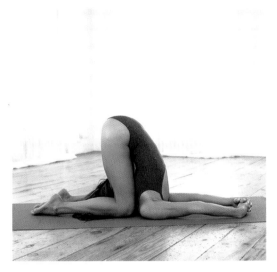

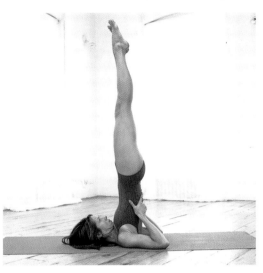

1 From Halasana, *exhale* and bend your knees, allowing them to part. Draw them in towards your ears, while projecting your buttock bones upwards to create length and space in the front of your spine and torso. Softly press your inner knees against your ears and extend your shinbones down on to the floor, stretching through the front of your ankles and feet. Bring your toes and heels together and release mula bandha, while maintaining uddiyana and jalandhara bandha. Lift and open your sternum up against your chin, and extend your arms backwards, gently pressing your elbows and little fingers down into the floor as your hands remain interlaced. *Take 10–20 even breaths*, quietly listening to the sound of your breathing as your knees close out the external sounds, which helps to induce pratyahara (sensory withdrawal). Look towards your nose tip, <u>dristi</u>: **nasagrai**, and relax behind your eyes.

2 *Inhale*, release your hands from their interlace, and bring your palms on to your back. Draw your knees away from your ears by lengthening your legs straight and together into Halasana. Extend your pelvis upwards and then lift your legs up to return into Salamba Sarvangasana. Re-engage mula bandha, then move directly into the next posture.

Benefits of the pose
This pose intensely stretches the entire length of the spine. It is particularly helpful in alleviating compression around the neck and upper back. Be mindful to distribute your weight evenly through both shoulders to help align the cervical vertebrae.

Easing into the pose
At first, you may find that your shinbones do not reach the floor. Do not try to force them, as this may cause injury to your neck. Instead, tuck your toes under as you draw your knees in, and, as your spine becomes more supple, slowly extend your toes

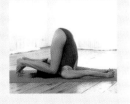

back until your shinbones can gently release down on to the floor.

Deepening the pose
It is also possible to practise this posture by wrapping your arms around the backs of your legs. The weight of your arms will help to send your shinbones further down into the floor.

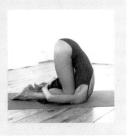

Urdhva Padmasana | UPWARD LOTUS POSTURE

urdhva = upward
padma = lotus

In this inverted position the posture of Padmasana may be a little easier to achieve, as the legs are made lighter by being lifted. This promotes full mobility and flexibility within the hips and energy circulation through the pelvic region.

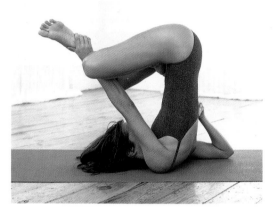

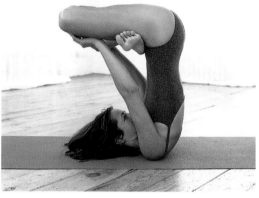

1 While in Salamba Sarvangasana, *exhale*, bend your right knee without dropping your hips, and bring your right foot across to your left upper thigh, as in half lotus. Now draw your left foot across to the top of your right upper thigh to create a full lotus posture in your legs. Use your hands at first to help move your feet across into Padmasana. With practice, you will be able to do this without the help of your hands.

2 Once your legs are securely and comfortably placed in Padmasana, take your hands just under your knees. Lengthen through the front and back of your spine and extend your back straight, with your pelvis balancing directly over and in line with your shoulders. Feel the connection between your palms and your knees and widen your shoulders evenly down into the floor as you straighten your arms, evenly pressing your palms upwards and your knees downwards. This will create a steady balance with your thighs aligned parallel to the floor and your torso and spine completely perpendicular. *Breathe here for 10–20 full breaths*, softly gazing towards your nose tip, <u>dristi</u>: <u>nasagrai</u>, then move smoothly into the next asana.

Easing into the pose
If full Padmasana causes knee pain, work into half lotus (Ardha Padmasana), and if half lotus also aggravates your knee joints, cross your ankles and align your feet to float over your buttocks. You may also at first place your hands on your back to help maintain a balance here until you

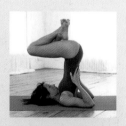

gain greater control to balance with your hands beneath your knees.

Deepening the pose
This is a wonderful asana to deepen your awareness and engagement of all your bandhas. As your arms straighten and your pelvis lifts, space is created in your front torso, allowing for the complete drawing in of your abdomen into uddiyana bandha. The openness of your chest presses into your chin to strengthen jalandhara bandha. Your pelvic floor and perineum in this

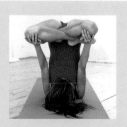

posture have no weight bearing down on them, so the energy of mula bandha can be fully harnessed within. Keep your buttocks level, as this will help you to balance in this pose.

pinda = embryo

In Pindasana the body is drawn into a foetus-like shape, softly curling in upon itself to resemble an embryo within the womb. Further suppleness is developed because the legs remain in Padmasana, creating an inverted forward bend action through the pelvis.

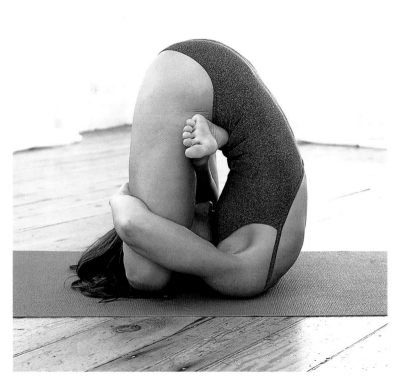

1 Maintaining Padmasana and full engagement of your bandhas, *inhale* and release your hands from your knees, balancing still over your shoulders and neck. With a *slow exhalation*, draw your lotus legs down and in towards your chest, wrapping your arms around your legs to clasp your hands together. Open the backs of your shoulders evenly and release your neck long into the floor to create a broad base on which to balance. Gently move your knees down on either side of your head and feel your body softly curling inwards into an embryo shape, as if resting inside the womb. *Take 10–20 full, even, deep breaths*, looking towards your nose tip, <u>dristi</u>: nasagrai, and relaxing the space in between your eyebrows to open up your third eye centre. From this asana, move smoothly and directly into the next.

Easing into the pose

As with the previous posture, care must be taken of your knees to prevent injury, so practise this posture with your legs in half lotus, or crossed if knee pain is felt. If, once in lotus, your balance feels unsteady or the stretch through your neck is too extreme at first, place your hands on your back to give your body extra support.

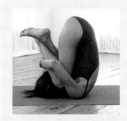
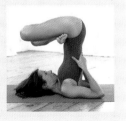

Deepening the pose

As you begin to feel more secure and comfortable in Pindasana, draw your knees closer together and lower your shins or ankles on to your forehead, taking hold of your wrist with your other hand.

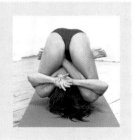

Matsyasana | FISH POSTURE

matsya = the fish incarnation of Visnu (preserver of the universe and second deity of the Hindu trinity)

This posture provides a complete counter-stretch to the four previous asanas. From the closed curling in of the body into the embryo shape, the back now reverses its position to arch open and stretch through to the front of the throat.

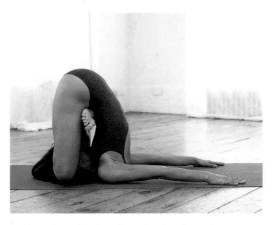

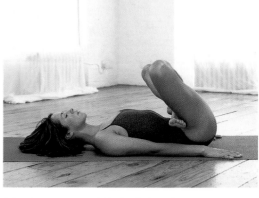

1 *Exhale*, release the clasp of your hands and stretch your arms out behind you, pressing your palms down and extending your fingertips away from your body. Feel your legs securely in the posture of Padmasana (or half lotus or crossed at the ankles, if lotus is not yet possible).

2 Continue to *exhale* and slowly roll down through your spine, sequentially lowering your back vertebra by vertebra on to the floor. Keep the back of your head down and use the pressure of your arms against the ground and the suction of uddiyana bandha to create a fluid roll of your back down on to the floor.

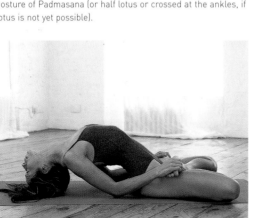

3 As the back of your pelvis touches down, press your knees down on to the floor and arch up through your spine, opening your collarbones wide and lifting your heart skywards. *Complete your exhalation* to release your head back so that the crown of your skull rests on the floor and the front of your throat lengthens long. Take your hands to your feet and roll your elbows in, without them pushing on to the floor. *Breathe here for 10–20 full, deep breaths*, feeling the expansion of your chest and the release of your throat. Softly gaze towards your third eye centre, **dristi: bru madhya**, and relax your facial muscles while drawing your lower jaw up to your upper jaw to stretch your underchin. The next asana, Uttana Padasana, flows on directly from this one.

Easing into the pose
If you practised the last two postures in half lotus or with crossed ankles, you can continue to do so here, but instead of catching hold of your feet, press your palms and forearms down on to the floor by your sides.

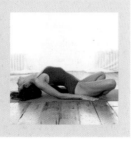

Deepening the pose
Deepen the arch through your back by taking your hands further over your feet and gently pulling on them to raise your chest. As you do so, draw your spine in and up into your body, moving it through into the front of your torso.

uttana = extended or intense stretch
pada = foot or leg

Muscular tone and strength are built through the legs and arms as they stretch up from the floor. The spine arches up, raising and expanding the chest and opening the front of the ribs and lungs to invigorate the heart and enhance deep respiration.

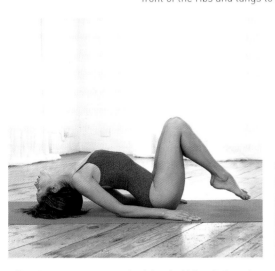

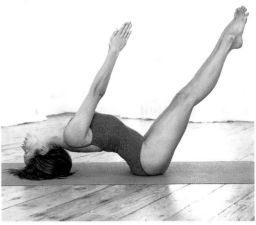

1 From Matsyasana, *inhale*, maintaining the high arch through your spine, and release your feet and legs out of lotus. Draw your inner knees tightly together to activate your inner thighs after their opening in the lotus posture. Stretch long through your shinbones into your feet, not allowing your toes to touch down on to the floor.

2 Continue to *inhale*, and stretch your legs straight, raising them sharply off the floor at a 45–50-degree angle. Extend your arms to follow the same alignment as your legs, and arrow your toe tips and fingertips outwards, lifting through your upper back and pressing your chest high. Draw your kneecaps and thigh muscles up and in towards your hips to stretch your legs fully. Take your focus towards your nose tip, <u>dristi</u>: **nasagrai**, as you *take 10–20 steady breaths*, then release your back on to the floor, keeping your legs lifted, and place your palms by the side of your head with your fingertips pointing towards your shoulders.

• With an *inhalation*, roll over your back to complete Chakrasana and move through a **full vinyasa**, but, instead of taking a **jump through** into Dandasana, lower your knees on to the floor to prepare for Sirsasana.

Easing into the pose
If you have back pain or weakness, practise this posture at first by pressing your forearms and hands down on to the floor by the sides of your body. If you have recently suffered a back injury, keep your feet and legs on the floor and press out through your heels to keep your legs active.

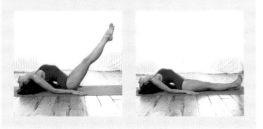

Deepening the pose
Press the back of your waist upwards, tilting your pelvis forwards to balance high up on your sitting bones. Draw your lower abdomen muscles upwards and in towards your navel in order to engage uddiyana bandha deeply. This will give support to your back and the lift of your legs in this asana. Stretch through to your fingertips to energize your arms.

Sirsasana | HEADSTAND POSTURE

sirsa = head

This is the father posture, which harmonizes the effects of Sarvangasana and creates a balance of energies within the body and mind. Here the body stands on the head in an upside down Tadasana, stimulating *sahasrara chakra*, the seat of enlightenment.

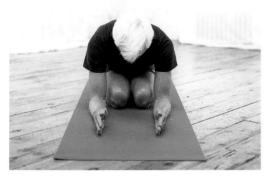

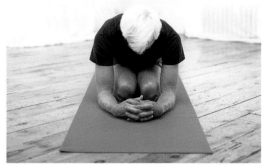

1 From Adho Mukha Svanasana, *inhale* and lower your knees on to the floor. Kneel down with your knees together and bring your hips back over your heels. Place your elbows on either side of your knees, aligned under your shoulders, and stretch your forearms and fingers forwards.

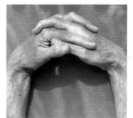

2 Continue to *inhale*, and deeply interlace your fingers, creating a semicircle through the palms (see left). Extend your forearms and elbows down into the floor and draw your shoulders back to open your chest and feel strong through your arms.

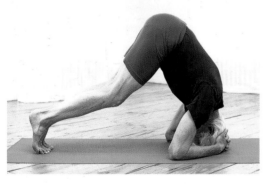

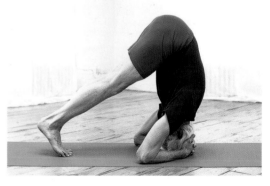

3 As you begin to *exhale*, lengthen through the back of your neck and extend the back of your head into your palms, cupping your head. Lightly place the top of your head on the floor and lift your shoulders up and away from your ears to create space and length in your neck. Engage uddiyana bandha as you tuck your toes under and raise your hips. Press your elbows down and begin to shift your weight evenly on to your forearms and clasped hands to create a tripod-like base for the headstand.

4 Continue to *exhale* as you walk your feet in towards your face and lift your hips further up, drawing them directly over your shoulders. Consciously press down through your arms and slide your shoulder blades upwards to release any compression in your neck.

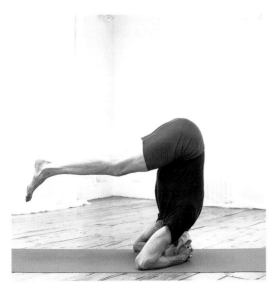

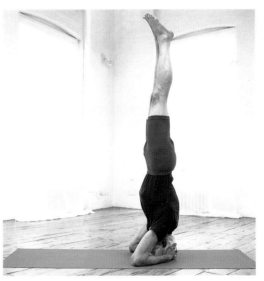

5 When your pelvis is aligned over your shoulders, sway your hips a little further back (this will help you to lever your legs up straight) but keep your toes on the floor for a little longer. Now, *inhale* and deepen your engagement of uddiyana bandha, energize your legs by drawing your kneecaps and thigh muscles up, and then float your feet up off the floor, transferring all your weight on to your arms, and just a little on to your head, and lift your legs to a right angle.

6 Continue to *inhale*, and raise your legs together, stretching them vertically up into the full head balance of Sirsasana. *Take 20–30 steady, deep breaths*, and gaze towards your nose tip, <u>dristi: nasagrai</u>, focusing on the support of your forearms and the open evenness through your shoulders. Breathe length into your spine and extend your legs from your hips, as the soles of your feet reach skywards and your elbows and the top of your head root down into earth. From here either go on to step 7 or on to Sirsasana Urdhva Dandasana (page 123).

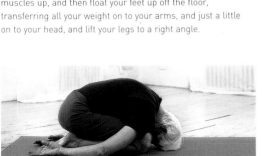

7 Keeping the lift of your pelvis and uddiyana bandha, lower your feet to the floor. Bend your knees and sit on your heels into Balasana (child's pose). Lay your forehead on the floor and take your arms back, with your elbows dropped, and rest here for a full 2 minutes. *Inhale* and place your hands underneath your shoulders, lifting your head and chest up. With your next *exhalation*, jump back into Chaturanga Dandasana and move through a **full vinyasa**.

Warning
Do not practise this headstand if you have high blood pressure, heart problems, a neck injury, a prolapsed disc, a hernia or glaucoma, or during menstruation.

Easing into the pose
If you are still building your confidence with the head balance, you may wish to spring your feet up softly one at a time, gradually working towards springing them up together, until your abdominal strength and confidence develop enough for you to float 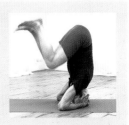 your legs up and straighten them together.

Deepening the pose
As your strength and confidence build, try moving your elbows and forearms deeper into the floor. Raise your shoulders and lift the top of your head 2.5cm/1in off the ground while maintaining full length through the back of your neck. This is a good test to check that your arms are active and that you are not dropping all your weight into your head and compressing the vertebrae in your neck.

Sirsasana Moderations | HEADSTAND POSTURE MODERATIONS

These two moderations, which use a wall for support, assist in the learning of Sirsasana for those who do not feel confident enough to attempt the free-standing form.

As with all asanas, learning from a teacher is always recommended, but for those who are unable to attend classes regularly, these two techniques are helpful.

Moderation A

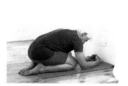
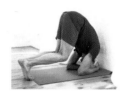
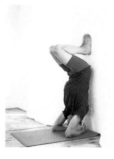
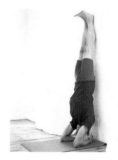

1 Position one end of your folded yoga mat along a wall and kneel down with your knees together. Align your elbows to your outer knees, and deeply interlace your fingers, with your knuckles touching against the wall.

2 Cup the back of your head into your palms and place the top of your head on the mat. Press your forearms down to strengthen the foundations of this posture, and draw your shoulders up. Tuck your toes under, and walk your feet in towards you. Raise your hips, drawing them up and over your shoulders while strongly engaging uddiyana bandha.

3 With an *inhalation*, spring your feet on to the wall.

4 Stretch your legs straight up along the wall. Start with *taking just a few breaths* in the headstand here, and then, with each practice, *add another breath*. As you develop your strength and confidence, begin to move one foot and then the other 2.5cm/1in away from the wall, so you start to find your balance, free-standing on your elbows, forearms and head without the support of the wall. It is very important that you do not become reliant on the wall: it is intended as a temporary aid, not as a permanent fixture of Sirsasana. Rest for a full 2 minutes in Balasana (child's pose).

Moderation B

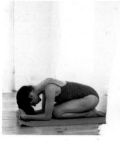
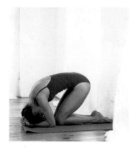
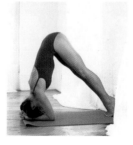
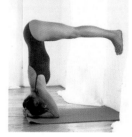

1 Bring yourself into Balasana with the tips of your toes touching the wall, interlacing your fingers ready to cup the back of your head in your palms.

2 Place the top of your head on the mat and extend the back of your head in to your hands. Press your forearms down to secure your base for this posture, then lift your shoulders upwards away from your ears and raise your hips.

3 Tuck your toes under and straighten your legs, keeping your toes still on the floor. Strongly engage uddiyana bandha and lift your hips up.

4 Walk your feet up the wall until your legs are parallel to the ground. Press your hips up and over your shoulders and stretch out through your legs, opening the soles of your feet into the wall. *Breathe steadily here for five breaths,* drawing your shoulders upwards and pressing your elbows down. On the final *exhalation,* walk your feet back down on to the floor and rest in Balasana for a full 2 minutes.

Sirsasana Urdhva Dandasana | HEADSTAND UPWARD STAFF POSTURE

sirsa = head
urdhva = upward
danda = staff, rod or stick

Once a stable headstand has been achieved, this posture, in which the legs are drawn downwards and then sent back up into the full inverted balance, may be tried. This movement stimulates the blood circulation, removing fatigue and tiredness in legs.

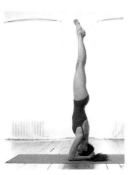 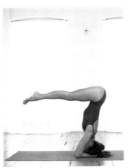

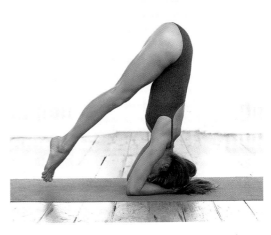

1 After breathing in Sirsasana for *20 breaths*, re-energize your legs by opening the soles of your feet upwards. Refresh the engagement of your bandhas, strongly lift your shoulders up and connect your forearms firmly into the floor to re-establish a sound base for your headstand and the following variation.

2 With a *slow exhalation*, lower your legs to a right angle, strongly projecting your sitting bones up and extending energy down through your arms, while actively sliding your shoulder blades upwards so as not to shorten your neck. Lengthen your legs, feeling the extension through the backs of your thighs, and stretch the backs of your knees straight.

3 Continue to *exhale*, and lower your legs straight down almost to the ground, so that your toe tips hover just 2.5cm/1in or so above the floor. Maintain the lift of uddiyana bandha and the alignment of your pelvis over your shoulders to control the lowering of your legs. Stretch up through your back and open your shoulders, rooting firmly down through your elbows and forearms. With a *full, slow inhalation*, lift your legs up straight again through a right angle and then into the vertical alignment of Sirsasana. Be careful not to tense your shoulders up in the effort to return your legs upright. Uddiyana bandha, along with the *inhalation* and the rooting down into the base created by your arms, needs to be the driving force that floats your legs up.

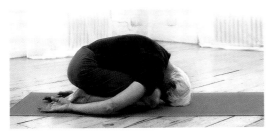

4 Repeat this lowering and lifting of your legs another four times, moving your legs down with an *exhalation* and floating your legs up with an *inhalation*. When you have performed this motion five times in all, lower your feet on to the floor, bend your knees and sit your buttocks back on to your heels. Lower your forehead on to the floor and take your arms back by the sides of your legs, allowing your elbows to drop to the floor. Rest here for a full 2 minutes in Balasana (child's pose).

• *Inhale* and place your hands under your shoulders, lifting your head and chest up. With your next *exhalation*, jump your feet back into Chaturanga Dandasana and move into a **full vinyasa**.

Easing into the pose

Once you feel secure in Sirsasana and can hold it for a full 30 breaths, then you may progress on to this variation. To begin with, move your legs downwards in slow motion so as not to lose control of your balance. As your legs extend forwards, focus on deepening uddiyana bandha and draw your pelvis back very slightly to counter the movement and weight of your legs as they stretch out and down.

Deepening the pose

As you become confident with this variation, you may wish to take five breaths with your legs extending out parallel to the floor before lowering them to let your toe tips hover just 2.5cm/1in or so above the floor.

Baddha Padmasana | BOUND LOTUS POSTURE

baddha = bound or caught
padma = lotus

In this asana, the arms extend backwards, expanding the chest and lungs and releasing tension and stiffness from the shoulders. The hips and knees are opened, improving flexibility, and the vertebrae of the spine align as the back is drawn straight.

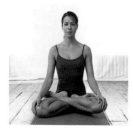 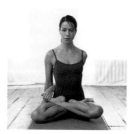

1 From Dandasana, *exhale* and bend your right knee, drawing your right foot up across on to the top of your left upper thigh into half lotus. Continue to *exhale* and bend your left knee, placing your left foot over on to your right upper thigh to come into the full lotus posture of Padmasana. Press your knees in towards one another to ensure your feet are sufficiently placed across your thighs, and fully engage uddiyana bandha. Draw length into your spine and consciously relax your shoulders.

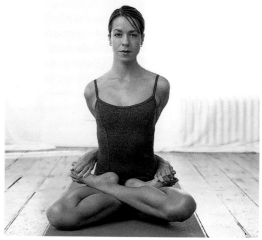

2 With an *inhalation*, softly sweep your left arm back, reaching your hand to your right hip and catching hold of your left big toe with your middle and index fingers.

3 Continue to *inhale* and now extend your right arm behind your back, taking your hand towards your left side to catch hold of your right big toe with your index and middle fingers. *Breathe steadily and fully here for 10–20 breaths,* and gaze softly towards your nose tip, <u>dristi</u>: **nasagrai**. Yield your weight down through your pelvis into the floor, and consciously feel any tension in your body draining down and releasing out on each *exhalation*. As you *inhale* feel energy rebounding up through your back, bringing lightness into your chest and openness across your collarbones. This in turn will help you to release your arms from your shoulders to secure the binding of your hands to your feet. As you complete your *10–20 breaths*, move into Yoga Mudrasana without taking a vinyasa.

Easing into the pose
If you are able to take your legs into full lotus, but not able initially to hold your big toes, use a strap to link your hands to your feet. If pain or strain is felt in your knees, proceed with caution and alternate the full lotus with a half lotus or with Sukhasana (cross-legged), and catch hold of your elbows behind your back.

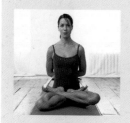 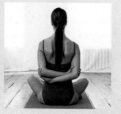

Deepening the pose
As you approach the closing of your practice, the deepening of the yoga postures takes place not only on a physical level but also, more importantly, on a spiritual and mental level. As you breathe here in Baddha Padmasana, cultivate your awareness of sitting in stillness as the internal motion of your breath washes through you.

yoga = union
mudra = seal or gesture

Mudras are subtle physical gestures that help to deepen awareness and connect individual energy to the universal energy within. Here, the head bows low to the earth, and the bound hands and feet allow unbroken energy to stream through the body.

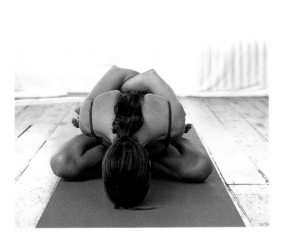

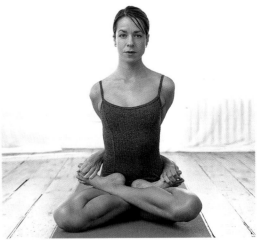

1 From Baddha Padmasana, maintaining an even anchor down through each sitting bone on to the ground, *exhale slowly* and fold your torso forwards, with the top of your head leading your back out and over your feet and legs to bring your face towards the floor. Lengthen long through the front and back of your spine and through into your neck to bring your face down towards the ground. *Take 10–20 deep breaths* here, and focus towards your third eye centre, <u>dristi</u>: **bru madhya**.

2 *Inhale*, drawing your spine upright and straight while keeping hold of your feet. The next posture, Padmasana, follows on directly from here, linked through the *inhalation*.

Easing into the pose
Do not be tempted to roll forwards off your buttocks in an attempt to reach your head all the way down on to the floor, as you will lose your foundation as well as the stretch of this posture. Go only as far as you can with both your sitting bones firmly rooted down into the floor. If you used a strap in Baddha Padmasana to enable you to catch hold of your big toes, continue to work with it here as you extend your torso forwards. If you held your elbows, also continue to do so as you extend your torso forwards.

Deepening the pose
Here, again, deepening of the asana is concerned with developing spiritual and mental, as well as physical, awareness. In Yoga Mudrasana, these three elements are intrinsically linked: while practising this asana, deeply engaging your bandhas will increase the benefits of the posture, as the action of the bandhas harnesses the energy of your breath, while the binding gesture of your hands on to your feet seals this harnessed energy within your body, raising your prana to awaken spiritual consciousness. As you breathe in this posture, tune into the flow of your breath washing through your body and mind, removing any blockages as it travels through you.

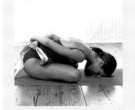

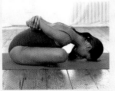

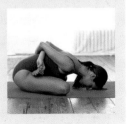

Padmasana | LOTUS POSTURE

padma = lotus

The lotus posture is often referred to as the royal pose, as energy rises up through the spine to lift the back majestically, directing the flow of prana from the first chakra (muladhara) through to the highest chakra of sahasrara at the crown of the head.

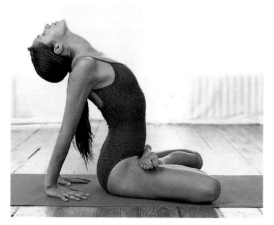

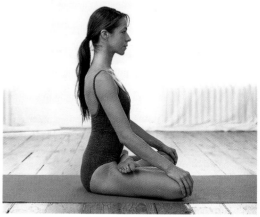

1 Continuing to *inhale*, release your hands from your feet and place your palms face down on to the floor behind your hips with your fingers pointing inwards. Draw up through your lower spine at the same time as pressing down through your sitting bones, hands and knees to send energy up to arch through your back. Lift your chest and open your heart as you release the breath. *Take a full 10–20 breaths*, focusing on expanding your chest with each inhalation, and with each exhalation softly roll your shoulders back and down while relaxing your neck muscles so that your head can gently fall as your heart lifts. Gaze towards your third eye centre, <u>dristi</u>: **bru madhya**.

2 With an *inhalation*, return your head and body to vertical and place your hands to rest on top of your knees. Softly lower your chin and focus to your nose tip, <u>dristi</u>: **nasagrai**. *Take 20–30 full, even breaths here*, yielding weight through into your pelvis to connect to the earth, and feel energy softly rippling up through your spine. Keep your gaze steady and your face relaxed.

• From Padmasana move straight into Tolasana.

Easing into the pose
All the previous asanas have helped you to tune into your body, so if you feel any discomfort or strain in your knees, listen to that warning and place your legs into half lotus, or Sukhasana (cross-legged) instead. If dropping your head back creates tension in your neck, draw your chin down and lift your chest up. Take 20 breaths here, softening the back of the neck while keeping it long.

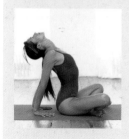

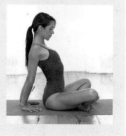

Deepening the pose
Breathe energy and space into your body, mind and heart as you free yourself from physical, mental and emotional restlessness. Allow yourself to drop into the stillness of Padmasana. This is known as practising *kaya sthairyam*, or complete body stillness. When your mind begins to wander and you feel the temptation to fidget, bring your awareness back to the sound and sensation of your breath. Let your pelvis and legs take root, and see your breath streaming up through your spine like a ray of sunlight, bringing illumination and lightness into your mind ... clearing the veils of darkness and obscurations.

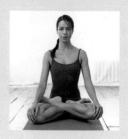

Tolasana | SCALES POSTURE

tola = a pair of scales

This asana is both demanding and challenging, allowing full appreciation of the relaxation of the closing posture of the sequence, Savasana. The strength of the bandhas is harnessed as Padmasana is raised up through the power of the arms.

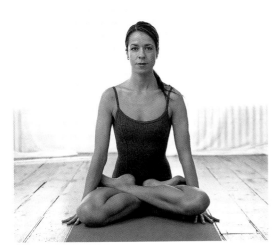

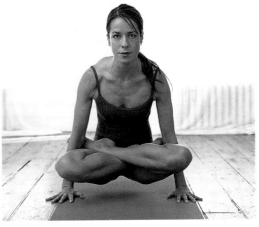

1 *Exhale*, releasing your hands from your knees and placing your palms on the floor by the sides of your hips. Draw your shoulders back and down, maintaining openness across your chest and deeply engaging uddiyana and mula bandha.

2 As you *inhale*, press down through your arms into your palms, and pick your knees up. Now, with full energy, straighten your arms to raise your seat off the floor. *Breathe here for 20–30 full, steady breaths*, focusing towards your nose tip, <u>dristi</u>: **nasagrai**, while maintaining uddiyana bandha. As this is a demanding asana, deepen your ujjayi breathing, feeling energy rising to help float your hips up with each *inhalation*. With each *exhalation* feel energy surging down through your arms and palms to help create a strong connection into the earth.

• *Inhale* and lower yourself back down on to the floor, then release your legs from lotus into Dandasana. Softly flow through your last **full vinyasa** of the practice. The total relaxation of Savasana follows.

Benefits of the pose

This finishing posture helps to cultivate the core strength of your bandhas while strengthening the arms, wrists and hands. As relaxation follows, direct all your energy into mastering this challenging pose.

Easing into the pose

Work this pose with your ankles crossed in Sukhasana if Padmasana is not yet possible. Refer to Lolasana (tremulous posture) on page 86 to remind yourself of the details.

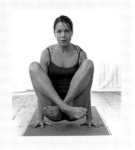

Deepening the pose

Do not rely on the tension of your shoulders to lift your torso and pelvis up. The key to raising your buttocks off the floor is uddiyana bandha. Keep shoulders level and release your shoulder blades down.

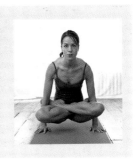

Savasana/Mrtasana | CORPSE POSTURE

sava and mrta = corpse

True, deep relaxation is the secret to health and happiness. Throughout our lives we accumulate tension, which can inhibit our growth, health, happiness and creativity. To fulfil our potential, therefore, it is necessary to relax fully and drop the tensions away.

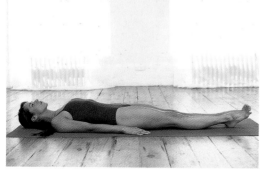

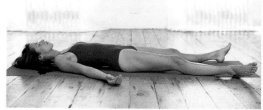

1 From your last vinyasa, jump through into Dandasana and softly roll your back sequentially down on to the floor, to lie in a straight line as you *exhale*.

2 Move your feet apart a little wider than your hips. Allow your breath to flow naturally and release your arms out to the sides of your body, turning your palms to face upwards. With a *deep exhalation*, sink your whole body into the ground, feeling the ground beneath you softening to receive the weight and shape of your body. As you lie here, slowly rotate your consciousness through your entire body, relaxing and allowing each and every part in turn to melt as it makes contact with the ground.

Deepening the pose

Savasana is one of the most important of all postures, and the way in which to deepen this asana is to carry it into the context of our everyday lives, practising not to hold on, allowing ourselves truly to let go in our body, mind and heart. In this way we can open up our lives to newness.

Benefits of the pose

The relaxation induced by Savasana allows your body and mind to absorb the harmonizing benefits and energy that have been generated through all the postures that have come before this point of your practice.

Breath by breath in Savasana, let tension flow out from your skin, muscles, organs, bones and cells, consciously relaxing your mind by consciously relaxing your body.

The series has cleansed, unblocked and released your body and mind from stagnant energy, tensions and toxins. Now the purified body may rest unburdened in this clear open space.

Listen within to the sound of your breath, the sensation of your body, the consciousness of your mind and the awareness of your heart.

As you relax in Savasana, the parasympathetic (relaxatory) and sympathetic (excitatory) nervous systems balance, inducing a state of yogic sleep (*yoganidra*). This enables you to discover an internal sanctuary of deep relaxation with inner awareness. This is a form of pratyahara, which leads the way to a higher realization.

Through the sensory withdrawal of yoganidra, your breath flows, saturating your body with the vital life energy of prana. This brings healing and rejuvenation into your entire being on every level – from cellular to intellectual – and allows the release of tensions, dramas, old habits and patterns (*samskaras*) from your life. This posture of the corpse drops and surrenders your bones into the ground.

In yogic thought, death is seen not as the end but rather as the route to rebirth. It is the stillness of the sea that pours in between the rising ripples of two waves.

...to make an end is to make a beginning...
the end is where we start from...
with the drawing of this love and the voice of this call
we shall not cease from exploration
and the end of all our exploring
will be to arrive where we started
and know that place for the first time.

T. S. Eliot

Once you are in Savasana

Starting at your head, move your awareness through your body, relaxing and softening each area as you go.

- Feel your skull heavy on the floor, relaxing all your neck muscles and softening your jaw.
- Feel your shoulders falling into the ground, and your elbows, wrists and hands heavy.
- Soften your chest and feel your ribs and stomach fall and rise with each breath.
- Relax your buttocks, feeling your thighs heavily releasing down and out from your hips.
- Soften your knees, relaxing all the way through to your calves and shins.
- Relax in your ankles, feeling your heels sinking into the floor as your toes relax.

- Return your awareness to your head and soften the skin over your face, relaxing your lips.
- Soften your cheeks and melt your eyes into the pools of their sockets.
- Relax the space in between your eyebrows and feel your brain softening gently within its skull.
- Keep warm and spread a blanket over you so that you can spend time here totally relaxing.
- Breathe, soften and release, sinking the landscape of your body into the floor. Feel tension melting away, breath by breath.
- As you lie here, free your body from the perpetual motion of doing and your mind from the wandering of listless thoughts, allowing yourself to rest in stillness, between the waves of your breath.

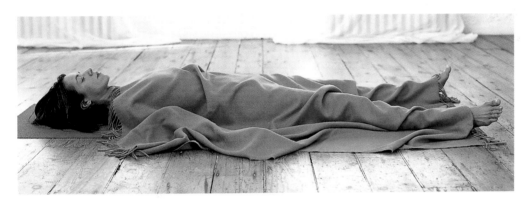

Variations to the pose

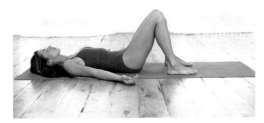

If your lower back feels tense and tends to arch off the floor, rest in Savasana with your knees bent and softly release the small of your back down into the ground with each exhalation.

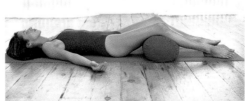

Alternatively, you may also wish to place cushions or a bolster under your knees, releasing the pressure on your lower back.

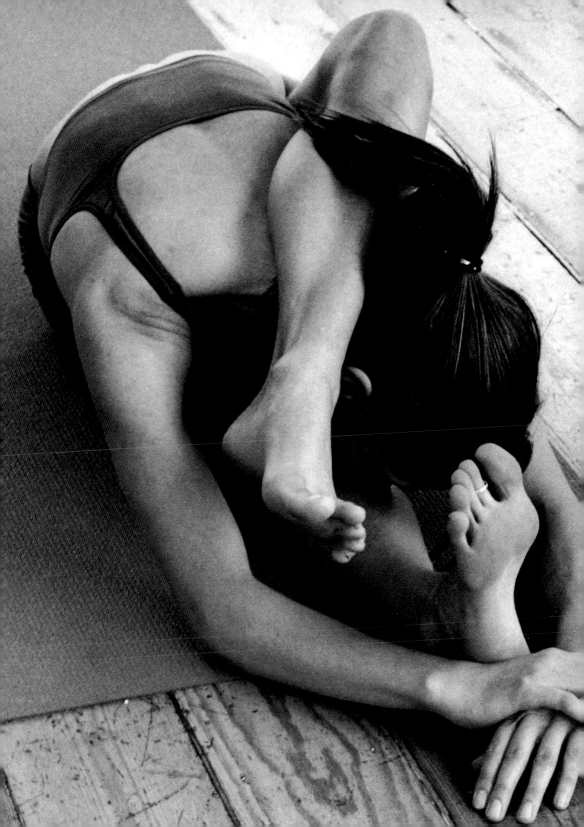

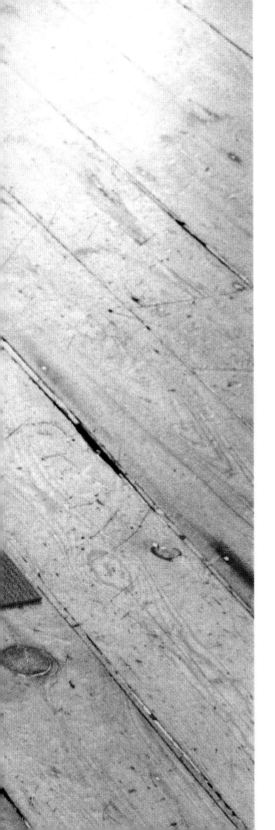

Abridged Sequences

The following sequences are designed for those occasions when we simply do not have enough hours in the day to practise the full primary series. Even though your time may be limited, do not be tempted to race through these postures. Take at least five full, deep breaths in each asana and practise the postures on both the right and left sides to work the body evenly.

Practising yoga a little and often is far more beneficial and balanced than doing a two-hour session once a week or every other week. Regular practice is the key, even if you only have 15 minutes to spare. It is better to practise fewer postures slowly and calmly than to rush more postures. Rather than feeling stressed about practice, do what you can and enjoy your time practising the postures.

15-minute Practice

The 15-minute sequence is composed entirely of moderated postures for those who are tired or recovering from injury, or who need a gentle route into the primary series. This gentle sequence of postures has a soothing effect on the nervous system, so it is ideal to practise after a hard day's work or even later on in the evening to help induce sleep. Start by practising Surya Namaskara A twice, and Surya Namaskara B twice, stepping rather than jumping back into Chaturanga Dandasana. Take a minimum of five breaths in each of the standing and sitting postures and be sure to practise the asanas on the both the right and the left side. Props may be used to ease into the postures.

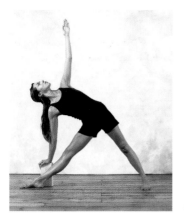

1 Utthita Trikonasana Extended triangle posture moderated p52

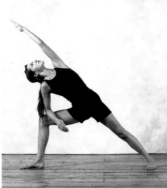

2 Utthita Parsvakonasana Extended lateral angle posture moderated p54

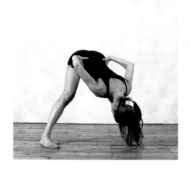

3 Prasarita Padottanasana B Expanded leg stretch posture moderated p57

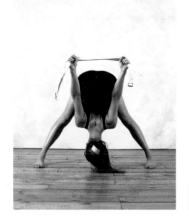

4 Prasarita Padottanasana C Expanded leg stretch posture moderated p58

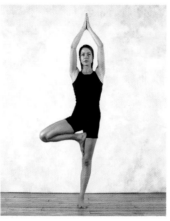

5 Ardha Baddha Padmottanasana Half bound lotus intense stretch posture moderated/Tree pose p64

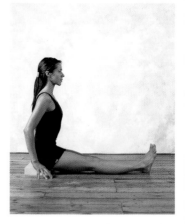

6 Dandasana Staff Posture moderated p72

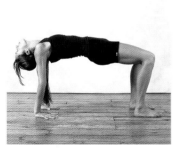

7 Purvottanasana Stretch of the East posture moderated p76

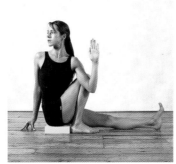

8 Marichyasana C Posture C dedicated to the great sage Marichi moderated p84

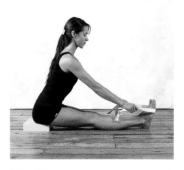

9 Paschimottanasana Intense stretch of the West posture moderated p72

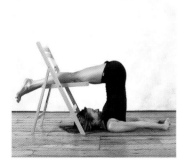

10 Halasana Plough posture moderated p114

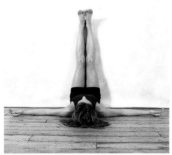

11 Salamba Sarvangasana Supported whole body posture moderated p113

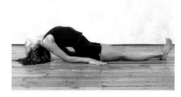

12 Matsyasana moderated Fish posture with legs out-stretched p118

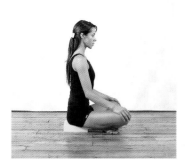

13 Sukhasana Easy happy posture moderated p134

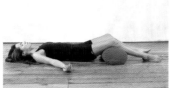

14 Savasana Corpse posture moderated p129

30-minute Practice

This 30-minute yoga session includes the basic key postures and so provides a good intermediate practice in order to begin to build the strength, stamina and concentration needed for the full series. It is an energizing sequence, so you may wish to make some time for this practice in the morning, as it is a great way to start your day. It will awaken your body and clear your mind of sleepiness while boosting your metabolism. In the mornings, the body may not feel as supple as it does later on in the day, but a couple of extra breaths in each asana will help you to ease a little deeper into the postures without straining. Start this sequence by flowing through Surya Namaskara A three times, and through Surya Namaskara B twice. If you are pressed for time, practise half rather than full vinyasas between asanas.

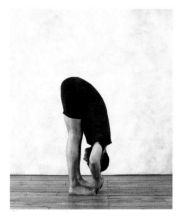

1 Padangusthasana Foot big toe posture p50

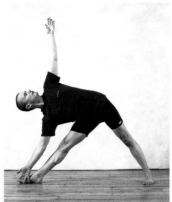

2 Utthita Trikonasana Extended triangle posture p52

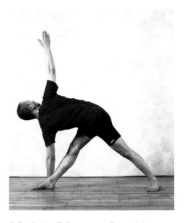

3 Parivrtta Trikonasana Revolved triangle posture p53

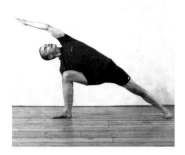

4 Utthita Parsvakonasana Extended lateral angle posture p54

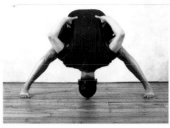

5 Prasarita Padottanasana B Expanded leg stretch posture B p57

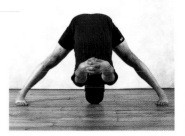

6 Prasarita Padottanasana C Expanded leg stretch posture C p58

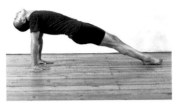

7 Paschimottanasana D Intense stretch
of the West posture D p72

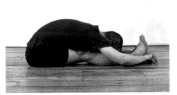

8 Purvottasana Stretch of the East
p76

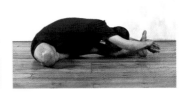

9 Janu Sirsasana A Knee head
posture A p79

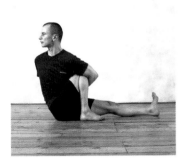

10 Marichyasana C Posture C dedicated
to the great sage Marichi p84

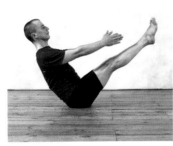

11 Navasana Boat posture p86

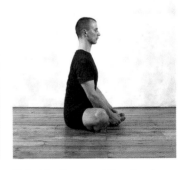

12 Baddha Konasana A Bound angle
posture A p94

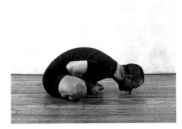

13 Baddha Konasana B Bound angle
posture B p94

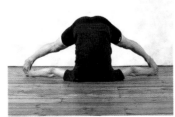

14 Supta Konasana A Sleeping angle
posture A p97

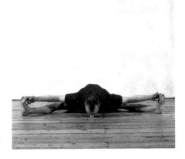

15 Supta Konasana B Sleeping angle
posture B p98

▷

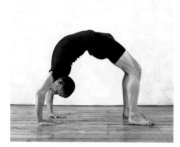

16 Urdhva Dhanurasana Upward bow posture p106

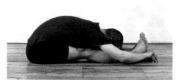

17 Paschimottanasana D Stretch of the West posture D p73

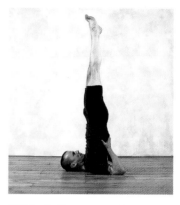

18 Salamba Sarvangasana Supported whole body posture p112

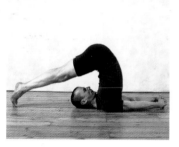

19 Halasana Plough posture p114

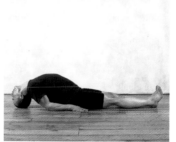

20 Matsyasana moderated Fish posture with legs out-stretched p118

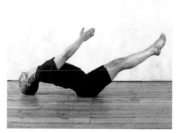

21 Uttana Padasana Extended feet posture p119

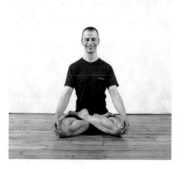

22 Padmasana Lotus posture p126

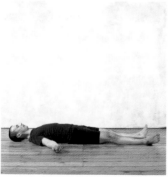

23 Savasana Corpse posture p128

45-minute Practice

This 45-minute routine creates a dynamic practice and is a definite step up from the previous 30-minute sequence. Before moving on to this sequence, therefore, make sure you are familiar with all the postures from the previous one, as the key asanas are now incorporated and developed with the inclusion of some of the more challenging postures.

The full finishing series of asanas included at the end will calm the mind and bodily system from the practice. This sequence may be practised at any time of the day, although it is generally considered to be most beneficial to practise in the morning at sunrise or in the evening at sunset.

Begin this 45-minute session by practising Surya Namaskara A and B three times each. As previously, replace full vinyasas with half vinyasas in between each asana if short of time. Practise mindful breathing throughout all of your postures, and five breaths on each side of a pose.

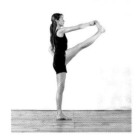

1 Pada Hastasana Foot hand posture p51

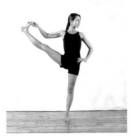

2 Utthita Trikonasana Extended triangle posture p52

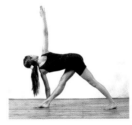

3 Parivrtta Trikonasana Revolved triangle posture p53

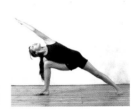

4 Utthita Parsvakonasana Extended lateral angle p54

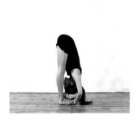

5 Parivrtta Parsvakonasana Revolved lateral angle p55

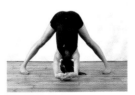

6 Prasarita Padottanasana C Expanded leg stretch C p58

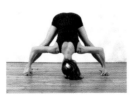

7 Prasarita Padottanasana D Expanded leg stretch D p59

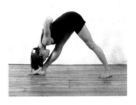

8 Parsvottanasana Side intense stretch posture p60

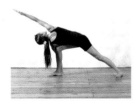

9 Utthita Hasta Padangusthasana Extended hand big toe posture p61

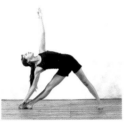

10 Utthita Parsvasahita Extended side posture p63

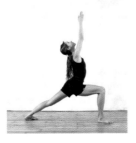

11 Virabhadrasana I Warrior posture I p66

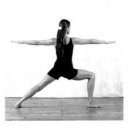

12 Virabhadrasana II Warrior posture II p67

▷

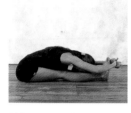

13 Paschimottanasana D
Stretch of the West D p73

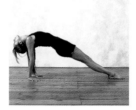

14 Purvottanasana Stretch
of the East posture p76

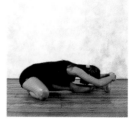

15 Janu Sirsasana B
Knee head posture B p80

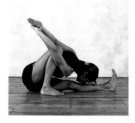

16 Marichyasana A
Sage Marichi posture A p82

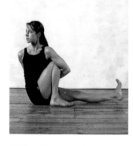

17 Marichyasana C
Sage Marichi posture C p84

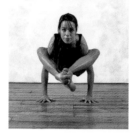

18 Bhujapidasana
Arm pressure posture p87

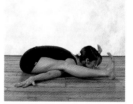

19 Kurmasana Tortoise
posture p89

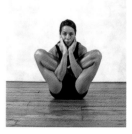

20 Garbha Pindasana A
Womb embryo posture A p92

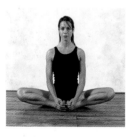

21 Baddha Konasana A
Bound angle posture A p94

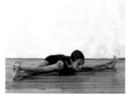

22 Upavista Konasana A
Seated angle posture A p95

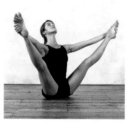

23 Upavista Konasana B
Seated angle posture B p96

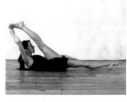

24 Supta Padangusthasana
Sleeping foot big toe p99

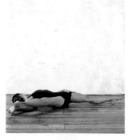

25 Supta Parsvasahita A
Sleeping side posture A p100

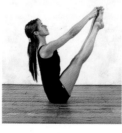

26 Ubhaya Padangusthasana B
Both feet big toe posture B p103

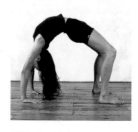

27 Urdhva Dhanurasana
Upward bow posture p106

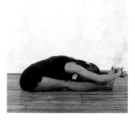

28 Paschimottanasana D
Stretch of the West D p73

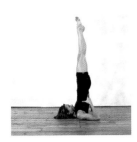

29 Salamba Sarvangasana
Supported body posture p112

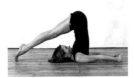

30 Halasana Plough
posture p114

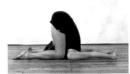

31 Karnapidasana Ear
pressure posture p115

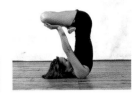

32 Urdhva Padmasana
Upward lotus posture p116

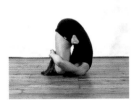

33 Pindasana Embryo
posture p117

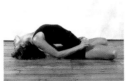

34 Matsyasana Fish
posture p118

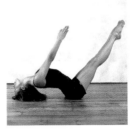

35 Uttana Padasana
Extended feet posture p119

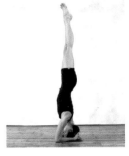

36 Sirsasana Headstand
posture p120

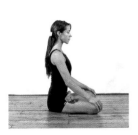

37 Padmasana Lotus
posture p126

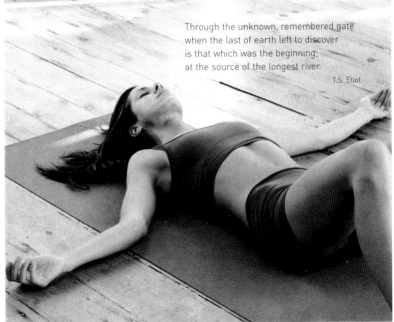

Through the unknown, remembered gate
when the last of earth left to discover
is that which was the beginning;
at the source of the longest river.

T.S. Eliot

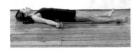

38 Savasana Corpse
posture p128

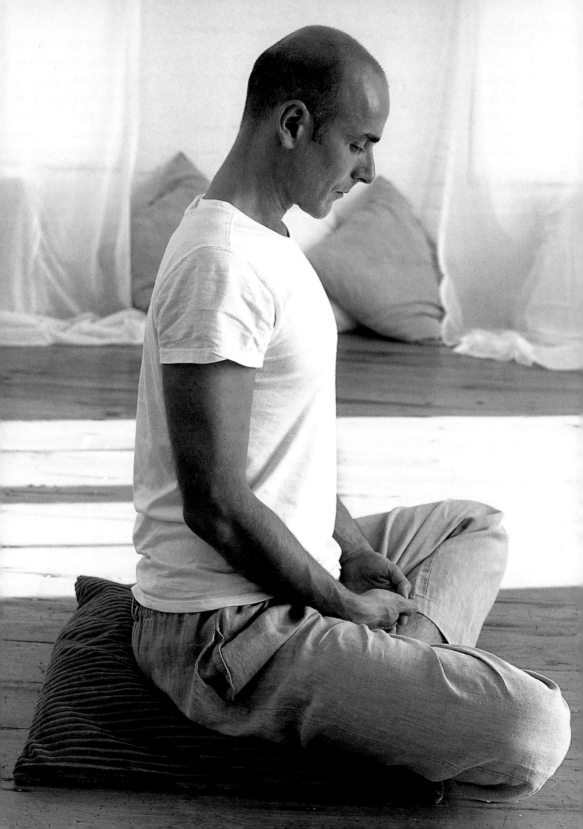

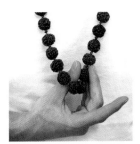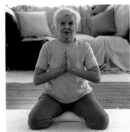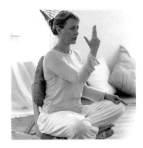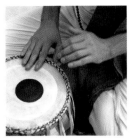

Meditation

Meditation is a way of focusing the mind, stilling the endless mental chatter that saps our energy and creates stress. In the yogic tradition it is dhyana, the seventh of the rishi Patanjali's eight limbs of yoga, and is the practice through which we are able to connect with universal consciousness. There are many routes to the meditative state: it can be reached in stillness or movement, with sound or in silence. With regular practice it can become a natural part of daily life, as essential as sleeping and eating.

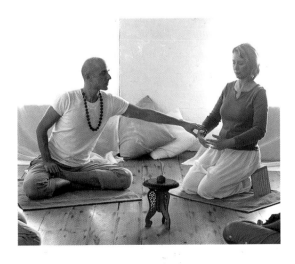

Finding Your Inner Self

Human beings have many levels: our physical bodies, energy flow, instinctive responses, thinking processes and wisdom each play a vital part in our overall functioning, and all need to be in balance to ensure health and wellbeing. All too often, however, a hectic modern lifestyle can unbalance these levels, making us feel jaded in body, mind and spirit. The regular practice of meditation helps us to rebalance ourselves so that all the levels are able to work together in harmony.

Meditation has three aspects: the regular practice of techniques that enable us to reach the meditative state, the experience of the state of meditation, and recreating this state in daily life. There are traditional meditation techniques appropriate to all temperaments and levels of attainment. They all involve symbolically "going up into the solitude of the mountains" so that we can then "return to the bustle of the marketplace" and live a changed life as a result of our experience.

We practise meditation because we believe (with Robert Browning) that:

There is an inmost centre in us all,
Where Truth abides in fullness…and to know
Rather consists in opening out a way
Whence the imprisoned splendour may escape.

Meditation allows us to experience that splendour for ourselves and live our lives in the glow of our own inner radiance.

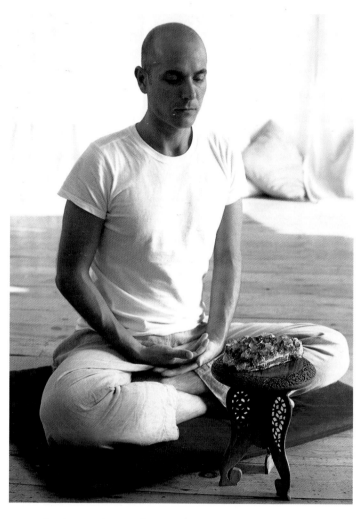

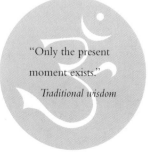

"Only the present moment exists."
Traditional wisdom

removing inner obstructions

The path to and from our "inmost centre" may be obstructed by lack of awareness, self-obsession, the stress of an unbalanced lifestyle, or by negative attitudes and thought patterns.

Most of us try to crowd too much activity into our lives, and lack the stillness and silence that are necessary to rebalance the nervous system. Regular meditation

△ Meditation is practised with the spine erect and the body motionless. The mind is still but alert, vibrant and focused inward.

practice establishes a healthy rhythm of activity and rest for both mind and body. Our minds are constantly active, mulling over current problems, planning anxiously for a future we cannot control, regretting past actions or creating personal doctrines

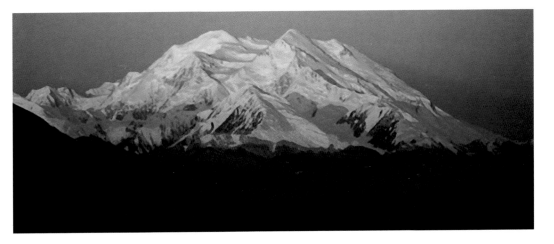

△ Symbolically compared with the solitude of the mountains, meditation involves a withdrawal from the bustle of human activity.

▷ These traditional clay figures in a circle of friendship represent the unity nurtured by the meditative way of life.

and dogmas, opinions and prejudices. These mental "games" draw us, like magnets, away from the present moment. Meditation teaches us to live in the moment, and grow through the experiences of here and now. When we are inclined to wallow in negative emotions such as anger or resentment, and to see insults and dangers where none exist, meditation helps us to replace defensive energy-sapping reactions with open and trusting responses that enable us to build loving relationships.

reducing stress

If you practise the meditation techniques outlined in this section regularly and with enthusiasm, you will soon start to feel the benefits, as both the causes and the effects of stress diminish.

Stress is a normal part of life, and a certain amount is essential to motivate and develop humans, but the pace and complexity of life in modern Western society can overburden our systems and block our natural ability to manage stress. Human beings are (as far as we know) the only animals with brains that are constantly

thinking – but the result may be that we allow ourselves to remain stuck in negative thought patterns, squandering our precious energy and unbalancing the nervous system.

Like that of any other animal, the human nervous system operates instinctively and is programmed to deal physically with threats to survival. Stress is a natural reaction that enables us to respond to danger, either by fighting or running away. Once the threatening episode is over the nervous system should rebalance itself as we return peacefully to our normal activities. Unlike other animals, however, humans are apt to remain in a state of arousal, because we go on feeling anxious about past and future events, as well as preferring to be continuously active and stimulated in the present.

Because stress hormones make us feel excited, it is easy to become addicted to activities and challenges that trigger their release. This is why we want to watch exciting programmes on television and take part in testing activities. But if we remain in a constant state of arousal, we deny our bodily systems the chance to rest and renew themselves. Stress accumulates until the system reaches breaking point – and the result is illness and malfunctioning of the body or mind. By practising the techniques of meditation, we can reverse this build-up of stress by learning to stop and consciously clear the mind and emotions of negative attitudes the moment we become aware of them.

STRESS AND YOUR HEALTH
Meditation practice can help to reduce the unpleasant effects of prolonged stress, protecting you from symptoms such as:
- muscle tension and pain in the joints
- tension and migraine headaches
- the inability to concentrate or think clearly
- digestive problems, which may include diabetes
- interrupted sleep patterns
- breathing difficulties
- cardiovascular problems
- allergic reactions
- physical fatigue
- nervous exhaustion
- weakness of the immune system
- other auto-immune problems

▽ Regular meditation gives you the energy and clarity you need to deal with the multiple demands of daily life.

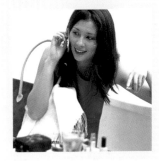

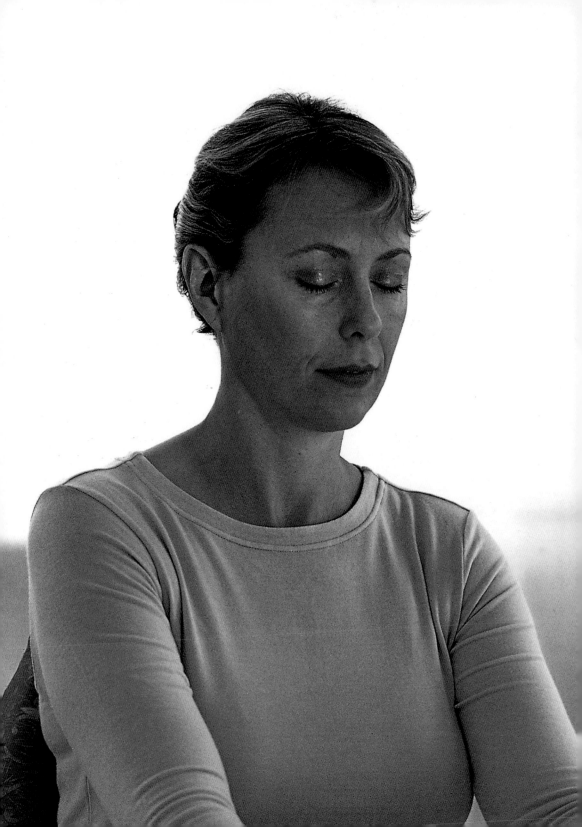

What is Meditation?

During an experience of meditation we are calm, focused, happy and loving. We let go of the burden of ourselves and enter into a wider state of consciousness, awakening ourselves through practices such as yoga asanas and pranayama.

Having achieved this wonderful state, we can then learn to transfer the attitudes and awareness it fosters to all our interactions, and to maintain them in everyday situations, regardless of what is happening around us. The practice of meditation increases our awareness of ourselves and of how we relate to the rest of creation, and enables us to live fully in each moment with contentment, serenity and love.

It is possible, through the regular practice of meditation, to transform the quality of our lives totally. Many of us live constantly with the stress that arises from an overload of negativity. Meditation can free us from this, to find peace we never thought possible.

Treading the Path of the Ancients

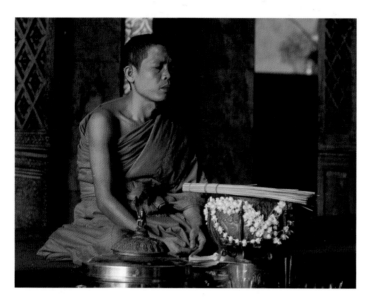

△ **In the Buddhist tradition, the energy and insight gained from meditation are dedicated to the enlightenment of all living beings.**

The practice of meditation may be as old as humanity itself, and its origins certainly predate written records. When we look at the most ancient civilizations that still exist today, such as the aborigines of Australia or the native peoples of North and South America, we find that meditation, and spiritual practices generally, have always been the special preserve of those few who were chosen to undergo many years of training and tests before being considered fit to gain access to hidden wisdom and to be the spiritual leaders of their people.

In many cultures, spiritual mastery, and the techniques that led to it, were taught secretly to those destined to become spiritual leaders – either by being chosen at a very young age (like the Dalai Lama of Tibetan Buddhism) or by being born into a family chosen to fulfil this role for generations (such as the Brahmins of Hinduism). It is only recently, with the explosion of worldwide communications, that this secret wisdom has become widely available to all who are prepared to learn and practise the techniques.

meditation techniques and traditional lifestyles

When they are stripped of the symbolism and mystery that have traditionally concealed them from prying eyes, the secret meditation techniques of every culture are remarkably similar. These techniques all help the meditator to quieten body and mind and to let go of thoughts about the past, the future and daily life in order to turn attention inward. This switches the nervous system into the "all is well" state of serenity and changes the quality of the brain waves from active to reflective. In these conditions, an experience of the state of meditation can develop.

In many traditions, spiritual practices are learned while the meditator lives in a

▷ **The doctrine of love and trust preached by Jesus and other great spiritual leaders stemmed from their experience of the meditative state.**

community, such as an ashram or monastery, that is set apart from society as a whole. Regular solitary meditation is always balanced with activity performed as a service to that community. When the meditator is considered able to maintain a state of meditation "in the marketplace" as easily as "on the mountain top", he is sent out to preach and teach the wider community. Once back in the world, there is a danger of spiritual teachers being seduced by fame and the adulation of their followers and falling from grace, becoming "false gurus".

Only a very few are accepted for training. In the past, the majority of people were excluded – especially women (who were the property of their menfolk), serfs, peasants and labourers (who were virtually owned by rich and powerful landlords), and foreigners. Nevertheless, members of these excluded groups have produced some of the greatest practitioners, in spite of the obstacles they have faced. In today's world we are fortunate that almost everyone – regardless of nationality, class or gender – has the opportunity to practise the meditation techniques of the ancient spiritual traditions.

Buddhism and Christianity

The Buddha was a Hindu prince, born in India around 560BC. He left his life of luxury when he saw the sufferings endured

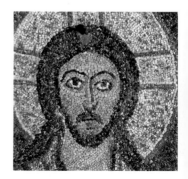

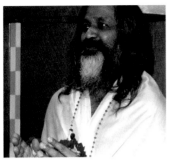

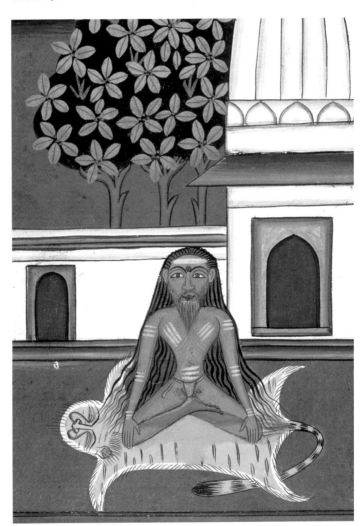

by the poor outside his palace gates. The Buddha practised the severest austerity in a vain attempt to become "enlightened", but through meditation came to realize that the "middle way" of moderation is the best spiritual path. To free ordinary people from the burden of the restraints and rituals imposed by the Hindu priests of his time, he preached a new religion based on love and respect for all beings.

There are parallels between the Buddha's teaching and that of Jesus, who also saw the lives of his fellow Jews being dominated by the harsh laws imposed on them by the religious hierarchy. It is likely that Jesus spent periods in a meditative state as he preached love and forgiveness. Both the Buddha and Jesus restored basic human freedoms, but after their deaths their followers built new religious institutions in their names that again suppressed this freedom. Today many of us are again free to choose our own path to the hidden splendour within, despite all the pressures of a greedy and secular world. We should take advantage of this opportunity.

▽ In North American and other shamanic traditions, rhythmic drumming is a powerful way of connecting with the world of spirit.

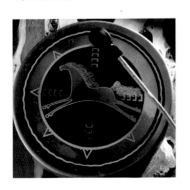

meditation and Hinduism

Hinduism is a vast melting pot of ideas based on the teachings of the Vedic scriptures, which are thought to date from about 2000BC. Two schools of meditation that are currently popular in the West have arisen out of Hinduism.

The first is that of the Indian sage Patanjali. His *raja yoga* – the "royal path" of meditation – was originally designed for Hindu monks. It teaches yoga posture, breathing and relaxation as preparations for meditation. Many yoga and exercise systems are based on these aspects of Patanjali's teaching. Another popular path is Transcendental Meditation (TM), which was introduced to the West by the Indian Maharishi Mahesh Yogi in the early 1960s. His system, which is designed to fit into everyday life, promotes mental relaxation – leading to the state of meditation – through sitting twice daily for silent repetition of a personal mantra, or sacred sound, specially chosen for each individual.

Universal Meditation Techniques

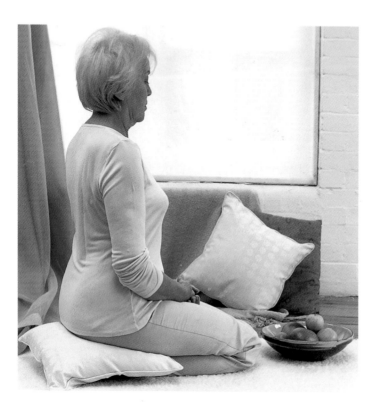

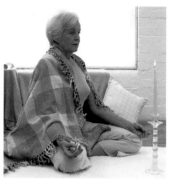

◁ The postures traditionally used for meditation allow the body to stay motionless while keeping the spine erect.

▽ Wrap a shawl or blanket around your shoulders so that you stay comfortably warm while sitting still to meditate.

Most classical meditation techniques are common to all the great spiritual traditions, although their forms may vary. Whatever the methods used, the meditation will follow a similar pattern.

For meditation practice to bear fruit in daily life there are four essential elements: detaching the attention from competing distractions outside and within; returning the mind to a single focus in order to enter a state of expanded awareness (the state of meditation); recalling and reflecting on the insights gained while in the meditative state; learning to apply these insights to daily life. The final stage of mastery is to live constantly in the meditative state, "enlightened while still embodied". It is said that the effects of meditation are cumulative and that "no effort is ever wasted".

stilling the body

Settling into a position that can be held without effort means that the body can cease to occupy our attention. Hindus, Buddhists, Zen Buddhists and yogis usually sit on their heels or cross-legged on the floor. Christians may kneel and many Westerners prefer to sit upright on a firm chair. Classical yoga postures are designed to hold the body upright and still for long periods. The eyes may be closed to avoid outside distractions or open to gaze upon a specific object.

breathing and chanting

Slowing and deepening the breath induces relaxation of the nervous system. Chanting aloud is a traditional way to lengthen each breath and the repetition of a mantra or prayer is soothing and uplifting. Buddhists, Christians, Hindus and yogis all practise chanting and repetition, either aloud or silently. A string of beads – such as the mala used by yogis or the Christian rosary – is often used for counting the repetitions of a mantra or prayer.

focusing on a single object

When the attention is focused, the incessant chattering of the mind quietens naturally, and we become oblivious to outer or inner distractions. Sound is a universal focus, and may take the form of music, the note of a Tibetan singing bowl, a mantra or *nada* (the mystical sounds of our inner vibration).

Gazing – often upon a flower or lighted candle – is another universal practice. Christians may choose to focus on a picture of Christ or a saint, Hindus and Buddhists on an image of a divine being or incarnation of God. If you prefer an impersonal image, you might choose the Sanskrit symbol of OM, the *sri yantra* or a *mandala* (both of which are pictorial

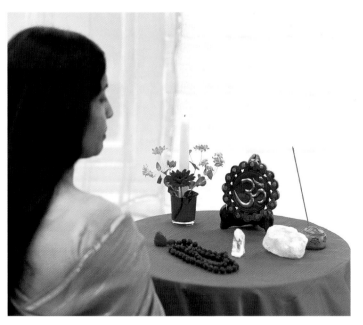

◁ You may wish to sit for meditation before a low table holding natural or symbolic objects on which to concentrate your gaze.

▽ One of the most basic focusing techniques involves gazing at a single object: focusing on a flower helps you to feel at one with creation.

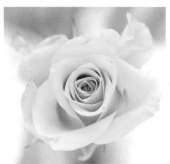

representations of universal energies). The focus may be something touched or felt, such as mala beads or the breath within the body. Even the senses of smell and taste may serve as focal points for meditation.

observation and acceptance

"Witnessing impartially" consists of relaxed observation and acceptance of what is, without any reaction of liking, disliking, criticism or judgment. After watching the contents of the mind in this way we can record them truthfully in a diary. Once we stop reacting instinctively we can start to respond from the heart and open ourselves to life as it is. This is the aim of both Western and Eastern psychotherapies.

mental visualization

Visualization is the intentional creation of a mental image or series of images, which may be of objects, feelings or symbols, as a focus for meditation practice. Informal visualizations are often used by Western psychotherapists and might, for instance, involve experiencing a walk by the sea or in the countryside using all five senses. Skill in visualization enhances the ability to create and maintain healthy and happy attitudes, thoughts and emotions, replacing former negative feelings.

healing through love

"Placing the mind in the heart" is an essential step, for love is an attribute of the heart – or feeling nature – and not of the mind. Love should serve our highest aspirations. When loving feelings and thoughts radiate outward from the heart like light from a lighthouse, both the meditator and those meditated upon receive healing.

living in loving kindness

When we live consciously from the highest we can glimpse in meditation, we are living from the heart. We feel strong, relaxed, focused, accepting, creative and joyful.

People in all ages and traditions have achieved this goal. The Hindu tradition has always perceived the divinity in everyone – hence the Indian greeting of "Namaste", meaning, "The divine in me greets the divine in you." Both Buddhists and yogis practise the meditation of loving kindness, in which love is beamed from the heart to all sentient beings, including those who cause pain and distress. Jesus said, "You shall love the Lord your God with all your heart and soul and mind and strength, and your

▷ The Buddha is represented in contemplation of a lotus, the symbol of enlightenment, with his right hand raised in a gesture of reassurance.

neighbour as yourself." St Francis of Assisi included all of nature in his love, and the 14th-century English monk who wrote *The Cloud of Unknowing* declared that "God can be known by thought never – only by love can he be known." This wisdom is available to us all: we can find it for ourselves through the practice of meditation.

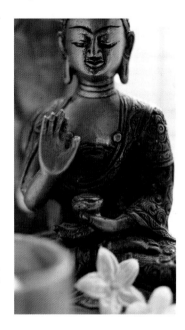

Patanjali's System

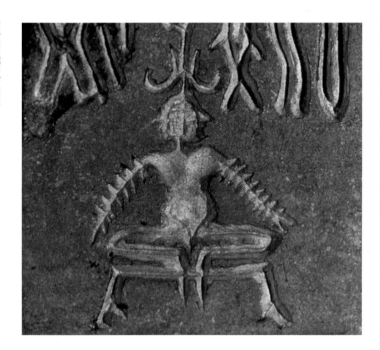

△ This stone seal showing a seated yogi belongs to the Harappa civilization of the Indus Valley, which worshipped a deity associated with meditation in the third millennium BC.

The Yoga Sutras of the ancient rishi Patanjali are a sequence of aphorisms on yoga meditation (raja yoga). They form the basis of most yoga taught today, and of the meditation techniques presented here. Western yoga teachers study the text as part of their training, even when the yoga they teach is predominantly physical yoga. The core hatha yoga text (*Hatha Yoga Pradipika*) agrees with Patanjali that "Hatha yoga is to be practised solely for the purpose of attaining raja yoga" – in other words, as a preparation for meditation. All the benefits of yoga for health and stress relief are incidental to its main purpose, which is "the settling of the mind into silence" to achieve the state of meditation.

who was Patanjali?

Yoga did not originate with Patanjali and he may not even have been a single person. All that is known about him is that he fused together the many yogic traditions that existed in his time – thought to be around 100BC–AD100 – into one coherent philosophical system. Some scholars consider that the section on the "eight limbs" of yoga (which includes the hatha yoga element) was added later, since the Sutras form a more consistent treatise on meditation without it. Whatever their origin, the Yoga Sutras are a masterpiece of conciseness and precision. They were handed down orally from teachers to students for generations, before being written down in Sanskrit and later translated for Western readers.

▷ The philosophy of yoga pervades Indian sacred texts, beginning with the Vedas, which are among the world's most ancient scriptures.

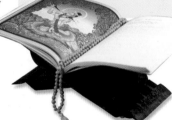

ASTANGA: EIGHT LIMBS

Patanjali defined eight intertwined aspects of yoga, of which the first five are "outer" or active practices. They prepare for the three "inner" limbs which together constitute the meditative state of *samyama*.

Yamas: social restraints reflecting an attitude of respect, consideration and love for others, as taught by all the great religions

Niyamas: inner purificatory practices reinforcing an attitude of respect for ourselves as embodiments of consciousness

Asanas: the perfection of seated postures for meditation, becoming impervious to the opposites (such as heat and cold) that disturb meditation practice

Pranayama: breath regulation to balance and increase vital energies, used to launch us into meditation

Pratyahara: turning the senses away from the outside world (relaxation) to the world within (witnessing and visualization)

Dharana: focusing techniques to make the mind "one-pointed" and shut out mental chatter

Dhyana: the state of meditation arrived at by maintaining relaxed one-pointedness, using the mind to go beyond the mind

Samadhi: the state of expansion of consciousness that lies beyond the thinking mind

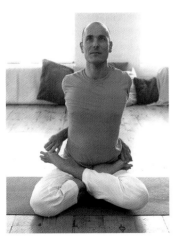

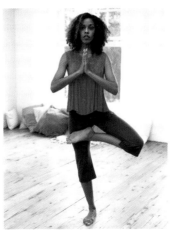

concentrated on a single object so that the meditator becomes one with the object and perception is transformed.

Finally, Patanjali describes the wonderful state of unclouded truth that is the pinnacle of human perception: "Now the process by which evolution unfolds through time is understood." (Quoted passages from Alistair Shearer's translation.)

△ Those who practise advanced poses such as Baddha Padmasana (bound lotus), a traditional pose for meditation, sometimes attain the meditative state as part of achieving the pose.

the teachings of Patanjali's Yoga Sutras

Patanjali follows an ancient Indian philosophy called *samkhya* (dualism). This sees *prakriti* (nature) and *purusa* (consciousness) as forever separate and distinct, and our perceived existence as embodied human beings as a result of the relationship – or "entanglement" – of consciousness with nature.

According to this belief system, the human mind is a part of the colourful, active and ever-changing mirage that is nature. Patanjali describes the human mind in detail, together with the obstacles and

suffering we have to contend with. He outlines the illusions that trip us up when we keep entangling consciousness, which is unchanging, within our natural and incessant mental activity: our hopes and fears for the future, and our memories of the past.

Patanjali sets out a wide range of meditation practices, shared by a number of traditions, to train the mind to relax in one-pointed stillness so as to reflect consciousness (the eternal self or spirit) "as a clear crystal". "Yoga is the settling of the mind into silence … [so that] pure unbounded consciousness remains, forever established in its own absolute nature. This is enlightenment" – and the goal of meditation.

There is a detailed section on the eight limbs before the Sutras describe at length the extraordinary powers of a mind trained in *samyama*, or meditation perfectly

PATANJALI'S MEDITATIONS
Meditative practices recommended by Patanjali include the following, quoted from Alistair Shearer's translation of Patanjali's Yoga Sutras (Ch 1, verses 23–39):

- "**surrender to the almighty Lord** who is the Teacher of even the most ancient tradition of teachers and who is expressed through the sound of the sacred syllable OM"
- "**bringing the mind repeatedly to a single focus**"
- "**cultivating the qualities of the heart:** friendliness towards the joyful, compassion towards the suffering, happiness towards the pure, and impartiality towards the impure"
- "**[practising] various breathing exercises**"
- "**experience of the inner radiance** which is free from sorrow"
- "**attuning to another mind** (such as a saint or guru) which is itself unperturbed by desire"
- "**the witnessing of dreams**" (learning how dreams can access our subconscious levels)
- "**any [type of] meditation held in high esteem**" (Patanjali recognizes that his way is not the only one)

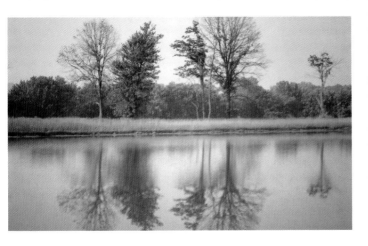

◁ The quality of stillness is central to Patanjali's belief system.

Peeling Away the Layers

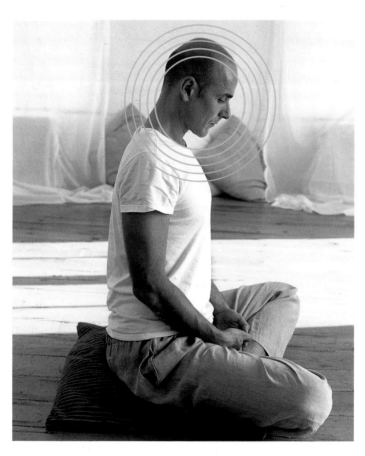

◁ The concept of the five koshas gives us a mental map to help us on the spiritual journey inward during meditation.

THE LINE OF COMMAND THROUGH THE KOSHAS

Through meditation we can influence the levels above, as well as the levels below, the one that is the focus of our meditation.

• At soul level (called *ananda maya kosha*, or sheath of bliss) we form our life's purpose and express this through our attitudes

• which influence our conscious choices (in *vijnana maya kosha*, or sheath of intellectual understanding)

• which influence our unconscious mental programming (in *mano maya kosha*, or sheath of mental activity)

• which directs our flow of vital energies (in *prana maya kosha*, or sheath of life force)

• which move our physical bodies (*anna maya kosha*, or sheath of food) to perform our actions and behaviour, such as thinking and communicating.

According to the ancient Hindu philosophy of Vedanta, a human being consists of five bodies, each contained within the next, which hide the immortal spirit as if with a series of veils of varying density. These bodies are known as the *koshas* (sheaths).

Our progress towards self-realization through meditation can be seen as a journey inward, through each of these five sheaths, from the outermost layer – the physical body – to the deepest "soul body" of unchanging consciousness, where we are in loving touch with all souls.

the five koshas

The further from the physical body they are, the finer the veils become. The most dense of the koshas is sthula-sarira, or the physical body, which can be weighed and measured by scientific instruments.

The next three koshas constitute suksma-sarira, the subtle body. The first is the energy body, perceptible to clairvoyants and detected by Kirlian photography (a technique that uses a high-voltage,

◁ The koshas can be visualized as the layers of an onion, forming a series of sheaths around the centre.

low-current electric charge to represent the body's energy in visual form). This is the level at which we are aware of the presence of someone entering our "space" before we see them. It contains a web of energy channels meeting at the chakra points, or energy centres, that correspond to the concentrations of nerves, or plexuses, of the brain and spinal cord. All physiological processes interact through these channels.

Next comes the "lower" or instinctive mental body. This contains the "mental computer" that is programmed to react

▷ Learning to understand your own nature and shedding negative feelings of fear through the practice of meditation puts you at ease with yourself and makes for trusting, open relationships with others.

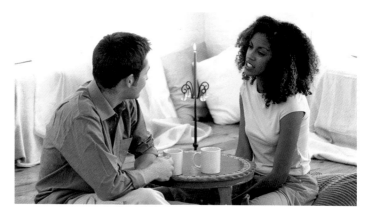

according to the input keyed in by our temperament and previous conditioning. The nervous system operates this computer, mostly at instinctive and tribal levels below conscious awareness.

The next level is the veil of the intellect, involved in thinking, discrimination and choice. It can choose to override mental programming, and to respond consciously rather than reacting instinctively.

The finest veil of all, often called the soul body, is linked with the spiritual dimension and survives death. If we can reach this level in meditation, we can change our whole attitude to life and the way we live. This is conscious evolution, opening up the dormant areas of the brain.

instinct, interaction and reasoning

It often seems that different forces co-exist within us, pulling us in opposing directions. This is because we have three distinct brains governing how we behave, feel and think. Our ancient reptilian brain is tiny but very powerful. Situated at the top of the spinal cord, it controls the primitive instincts and urges that ensure physical survival in animal bodies. It drives the basic needs that ensure

our physical and species survival – food, safety, shelter, sleep and procreation. The mammalian brain, above the reptilian brain at the back of the skull, evolved later and processes herd, tribal and social instincts. The rest of the skull contains the most recent development, the neo-cortex. This uniquely human brain enables us to think, reason and evolve spiritually.

The neo-cortex is so new that we use less than ten per cent of it, and it cannot easily override our older brains. However altruistic our intentions, we feel frightened and angry, and may indulge in self-centred behaviour, whenever we consider our basic needs are not being met. We actually need very little to survive, but modern society depends on inflaming our instinctive fear and addictive greed, so that we keep buying the products that keep the wheel turning – unsustainably in the long term.

trusting more, needing less

The practices of meditation help us to balance our evolved and primitive natures. The tradition of Vedanta claims that all creation arises from the desire of the one absolute reality to experience itself as life (nature) and light (consciousness or spirit) in relationship (love) with each other. This relationship is continuously enacted within us, and is seen as the purpose of human existence. The attributes of life, light and love (sat-chit-ananda) are immortal, and therefore so are we, as part of the one indivisible whole. Trusting in the divine process of life-light-love creates joy rather than fear and makes the accumulation of things seem less important than expressing our true nature. It is like being protected from negativity by a shield that beams out goodwill to all, while hiding a glory we cannot yet understand.

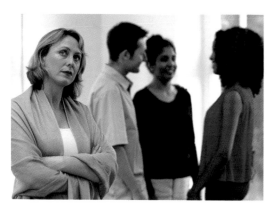

△ Fear of isolation and exclusion from the crowd can be a result of feeling unhappy with yourself at a fundamental level.

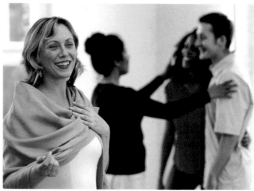

△ Reaching a state of inner content means that you can be happy and relaxed whether you are alone or part of a group.

Freeing Vital Energies

"It is just as unbalanced to be held fast by material concerns as to be too heavenly to be any earthly use."
Traditional wisdom

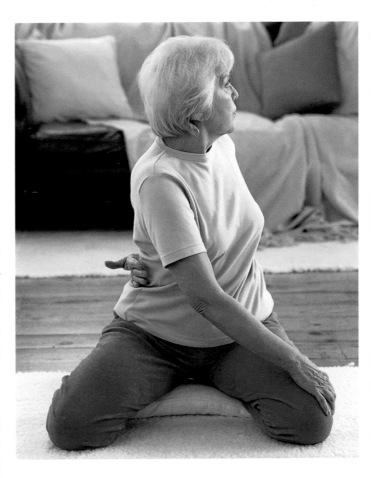

In the Eastern traditions (and also in many modern therapeutic systems) it is assumed that our vital energies – or "life force" – flow through the energy channels (nadis) of the subtle body. Techniques that operate at this level are aimed at healing, balancing and increasing our energies. Yoga asanas can get energies flowing when they are sluggish or blocked, while the practice of pranayama, or breathing with awareness, clears and balances the energy channels.

chakras and granthis

The subtle body's major energy channel, the susumna nadi, follows the spinal cord and links the seven main chakras, which can be thought of as spinning vortices of energy. Pranayama is practised to influence the energies in the chakras and to weaken the three *granthis* (knots of attachment) that bind us to our negative attitudes and prevent us from experiencing the fullness of life-light-love. Although the granthis are seen as obstacles on the path of spiritual awareness, they also act as safety valves, protecting us from surges of vital energy and misplaced enthusiasm for changes we are not ready for. We need to practise well-tried and tested methods (such as meditation) to open them slowly and naturally, rather than forcing them with drugs or stimulants.

△ Yoga postures use movement and stretches to tone the physical body and stimulate the chakras and the connecting energy channels.

▷ The chakras are often visualized as lotus flowers; meditation makes them bloom and perfume our lives with their positive attributes.

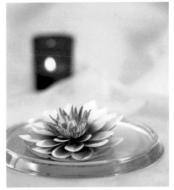

The energies of all the koshas are expressed in each chakra. We can behave spiritually in practical ways from the base chakra, or serve the divine efficiently from the crown chakra. However we behave, feel or think we cannot help bringing life and

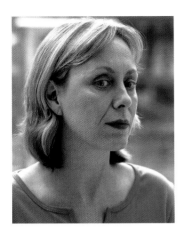

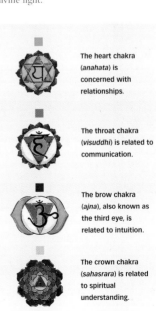

◁ The granthis are visualized as three knots that bind us to negative attitudes and material concerns, keeping our minds and spirits closed. The granthis constrict the free flow of energy that leads to true understanding and acceptance.

light together in the relationship of love – even if we can perceive only conflict and fear. Awareness is the key to all meditation practice, so we must first "switch on the light" in the brow (mind) chakra before doing anything else, through breathing techniques that quickly "light us up".

Life chakras and the life granthi

The life chakras correspond to the positions of the nerve plexuses attached to the spine behind the abdomen. Their energies are concerned with our survival in the physical human body (the base chakra, connected to the legs and feet), our role in human society (the sacral chakra) and our sense of self-esteem as a human personality (the navel chakra). The life granthi that binds us is our attachment to material wellbeing, physical comforts and luxuries, and the amassing of things. Patanjali teaches self-discipline for regulating the energy through the life chakras and life granthi.

Love chakras and the love granthi

The love chakras are situated in the chest (the heart chakra, connected to arms and hands) and neck (the throat chakra, connected to voice, mouth and hearing). In this area self-concern gives way to sharing with others. The heart chakra energies are concerned with relationship – especially unconditional love – and the throat chakra with expressing the truth and hearing what others are telling us. The love granthi that binds us is our attachment to emotional excitement and the desire to be the hero of every drama, so that we are not receptive to the needs of others. Patanjali teaches

self-surrender for increasing the energy through the love chakras and love granthi.

Light chakras and the light granthi

The light chakras are situated in the skull. They are the brow chakra (connected to the mind) and the crown chakra (connected to the spirit). "Taking the mind into the heart" is an essential element of meditation, bringing the realization that relating, not thinking, is the purpose of life. The light of divinity is received through the crown chakra and is present in us as "the eternal flame burning in the cave of the heart". The light granthi that binds us is our attachment to our own opinions, prejudices and fantasies. It is hard to relinquish treasured opinions and pride in our own intellect, yet it is not our minds but the light and love in our hearts that make us divine. We cannot claim ownership of universal life-light-love. Patanjali teaches self-awareness to dissolve pride and those mental habits that obscure divine light.

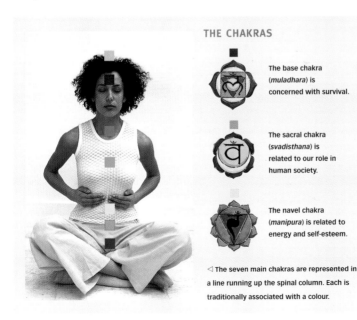

THE CHAKRAS

The base chakra (*muladhara*) is concerned with survival.

The sacral chakra (*svadisthana*) is related to our role in human society.

The navel chakra (*manipura*) is related to energy and self-esteem.

◁ The seven main chakras are represented in a line running up the spinal column. Each is traditionally associated with a colour.

The heart chakra (*anahata*) is concerned with relationships.

The throat chakra (*visuddhi*) is related to communication.

The brow chakra (*ajna*), also known as the third eye, is related to intuition.

The crown chakra (*sahasrara*) is related to spiritual understanding.

Achieving Balance and Harmony

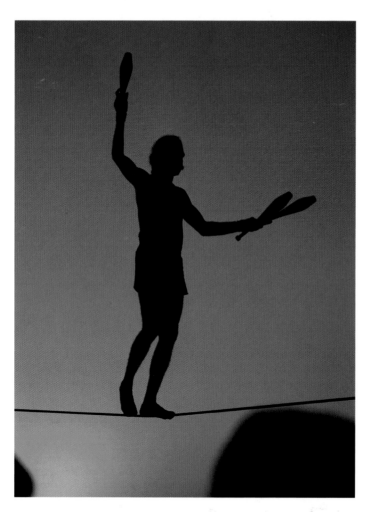

lacking in hope. A tamasic attitude among those in power – such as bureaucrats or those running businesses – will perpetuate laziness, procrastination, ignorance and lack of concern.

However, even though tamas is a "constipating" quality that can block progress in both individuals and institutions, it is also characterized by resilience and staying power. Inertia also has its positive side – we all need to take time out for rest, sleep and recuperation when our systems are depleted. Tamasic feelings of lethargy and dullness can be a sign of exhaustion or illness, and may be the body's warning to stop or suffer the consequences.

THE BALANCE OF OPPOSITES

There is a correspondence between the interaction of the three gunas, or qualities of nature, and the three attributes of the absolute or non-nature (light-life-love), in that when the two opposites merge in a balanced state a third quality arises that contains and transcends both the opposites. This principle seems to underlie the way the universe works at the deepest levels. Some examples are:

- Sat/existence (life) + chit/consciousness (light) = ananda/bliss (love)
- Tamas (inertia) + rajas (motion) = sattva (equilibrium)
- Patanjali's self-discipline + self-awareness = self-surrender
- Male + female = a new being
- Day + night = time

All aspects of nature possess inner properties called *gunas*, which are described at length in many of the ancient texts of India. There are three gunas, all of which are present in varying proportions in everything, from the human mind to the food we eat, but the dominance of one of them characterizes everything in the physical world. According to the dualistic philosophy of samkhya, this imbalance between the gunas is a result of the disturbance caused by Creation.

tamas

The first guna is *tamas*, the state of darkness, silence and ignorance, where nothing happens. In scientific terms, tamas is inertia. This quality receives much abuse in the texts because it blocks any attempt to change and therefore obstructs evolution.

The tamasic state of mind is lethargic, selfish and dull. When we are dominated by tamas we are lacking in energy, fearful and dependent on other people, regretful and

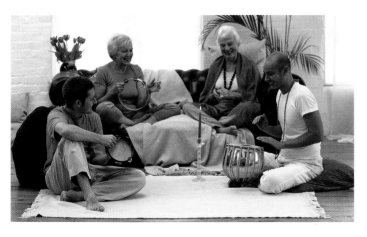

"The difference between the best and worst of us is nothing compared to that between what we are and what we will become."
Traditional wisdom

rajas

Opposed to the tamasic state is *rajas*, the quality of desire, arousal and passion – or motion. Rajas is an epidemic in modern society. We are urged to want more, to buy everything on credit and to work harder and longer to pay for the luxuries we think are necessities. Our nervous systems are whipped into a constant state of "red alert", so that we rush around ever faster to fight or flee imaginary threats. A rajasic attitude perpetuates fear, greed, delusion, desire and many other exhausting stimuli.

Although rajas causes addiction, obsession, dissipation of energy and burnout, it also has its positive aspects. Without zeal, ardour and drive nothing in life can be achieved. The spiritual path requires intense and ongoing commitment.

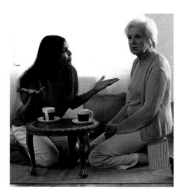

△ The rajasic character (left), prevalent in modern society, is turbulent and excitable and impatient, whereas dullness and indifference characterize the tamasic state (right).

△ Meditation practice helps us to achieve a balance in our lives between activity and rest, interaction and solitude, fostering inner peace and loving relationships.

sattva

When the two opposite qualities of tamas and rajas blend together, *sattva* is created, the state of balance and harmony – or equilibrium. This quality combines the best aspects of the other two, making us relaxed yet energetic, trusting and accepting yet innovative and creative, committed to goals yet unattached to outcomes. Needless to say, sattva is the quality we aim for as the preparation for meditation – for when we are lethargic it is hard to maintain focus and when we are obsessive it is hard to maintain non-attachment.

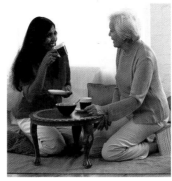

△ When the opposing qualities of rajas and tamas are in balance with each other, the result is the sattvic state: happy, alert, clear-thinking and compassionate.

PATANJALI'S THREE PRELIMINARY PRACTICES

Patanjali defines three qualities we need to develop before we can enter the meditative state. Each makes us more mindful of the dominance of tamas or rajas within us, and helps us to bring them into balance to achieve the inner harmony of sattva.

- *Tapas* **(self-discipline)** removes the inertia and procrastination that is typical of tamas, which can block us when we plan to do our practices. Nothing is achieved without disciplined commitment.
- *Swadhyaya* **(self-awareness)** enables us to discover patterns of rajas and tamas as we witness our thoughts, feelings, reactions and behaviour throughout the day without involvement or excuses. Patanjali also prescribes the study of uplifting texts, to learn from enlightened saints and sages.
- *Iswara pranidhana* **(self-surrender)** to a higher power than the drives and resistances of our own personalities. We may picture this power as a divine person or as an impersonal source, fullness or void.

Through self-discipline and self-awareness we let go of the attachments represented by the three granthis and free ourselves to reach our potential.

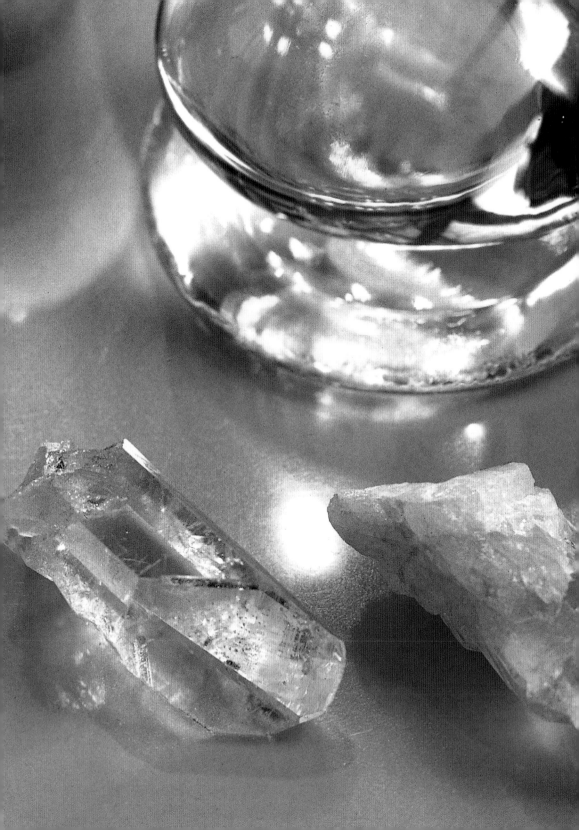

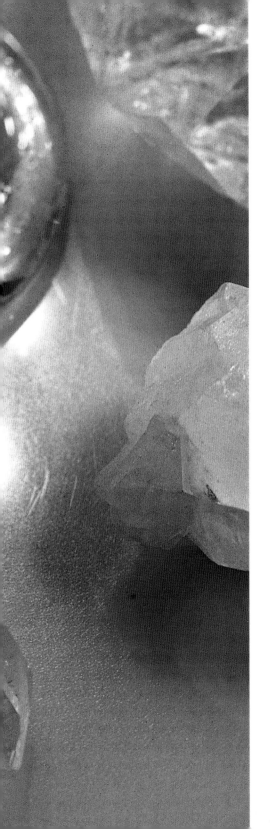

Preparing Body and Mind

The most external levels of our being are our physical body and our energy flow. Through a sequence of gentle movements and techniques that foster awareness of the breath, we can bring both these levels into a state of harmony, so that we can sit comfortably and peacefully for meditation practice.

Exercises that slow and deepen the breathing bring a "feel-good" factor to the body, while also relaxing and resting the mind. Yoga practice releases tensions in the physical body and also frees obstructions in the nadis, or energy channels. The easy movements described in this chapter can also be followed as a gentle preparation for meditation.

It is important to choose a posture that is comfortable and sustainable. The traditional postures for meditation, such as the yoga poses of Padmasana (lotus posture) or Virasana (hero posture), hold the body in stillness on a stable foundation, while allowing energy to flow freely along the spine as we start to turn our focus inward.

Basic Body and Breath Awareness

The traditional position for meditation practice is to sit with the knees out to each side. This creates a pyramid with a firm triangular base so that it is difficult to topple over and easy to keep the spine erect, even when you are totally engrossed in inner experiences. However, in Western society people seldom sit in this position.

Although the hips, like the shoulders, are ball-and-socket joints, designed to turn freely in all directions, we normally move through a very narrow range of standing and sitting positions. Imagine how restricted you would feel if you could move your elbows only up or down in front of you but

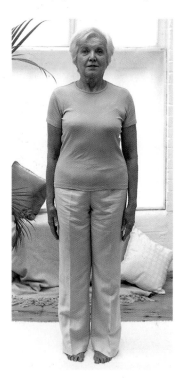

△ In Tadasana (mountain posture) the body extends upwards from a firm base, with the sides, front and back of the body aligned, creating a sense of equilibrium and repose.

not to the sides – yet this is what we do with our knees as we sit at a desk and in a car or armchair, while walking or running, and even when we are lying down. In traditional societies it is as natural and comfortable to sit cross-legged on the floor as sitting in an armchair is for us, and with gentle practice and suitable props you can enjoy the benefits of this pose and also regain a more natural range of movement in your hip joints.

breath with posture and movement

In exercise, moving with the breath brings a new mental awareness and a feeling of both relaxation and energy flow, so it is important to develop the habit of leading every movement with a conscious slow breath either in or out, as directed.

Do the exercises suggested for just a few moments, as frequently as possible during the day. Relax and enjoy them, and never force your body into any position. You will be amazed how quickly you begin to shed the tightness that has been restricting your body for years. A relaxed body and mind creates a wonderful sense of well-being and makes meditation practice very rewarding.

Start by standing in Tadasana (mountain posture) – feet parallel and rooted, ankles lifted, knees straight and springy (not locked), tailbone (coccyx) tucked under, waist pulled in and back, breastbone (sternum) lifted, chin parallel to the floor. The gaze is soft and straight ahead. Imagine a straight line down each side of your body. It should pass through your ankles, knees, hips, waist, shoulders and ears. Having located all these points, breathe in to stretch up, and out to bring them into line. You should feel as though you are hanging from the ceiling by a strong cord, with your limbs loose like a puppet. The same exercise – stretching up on the in-breath and aligning on the out-breath – can be practised while seated on a chair or on the floor.

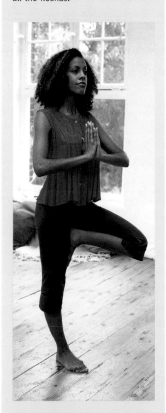

△ Vrksasana (tree posture) is one of the classic yoga postures used in preparation for meditation practice.

swing a leg

This exercise, repeated frequently at odd moments during the day, releases muscular tension, improves balance and develops body awareness. At the end of the sequence, quietly observe everything you can feel in your body.

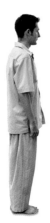

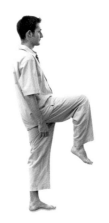

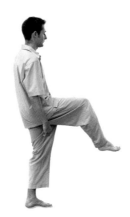

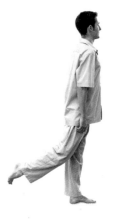

△ **1** Standing in Tadasana, become comfortable with your breath, awareness and posture, so that you can maintain them throughout the exercise. If your balance is shaky, stand where you can hold on to a table, the back of a chair, or a wall if you need to.

△ **2** Raise one leg, bending the knee, until the thigh is parallel to the floor. Balance on the other leg, using your breath to stretch up and align your body, and to hold the position. When you are balanced, shake your raised ankle gently and rhythmically.

△ **3** After a moment, change the movement so that you are swinging the lower part of the raised leg, from the knee, with the ankle relaxed. Continue to focus on the breath, and maintain the Tadasana pose.

△ **4** Now swing the whole of the raised leg from the hip, forward and back, keeping it relaxed and maintaining Tadasana. Take a deep breath in, then breathe out, as you lower your leg and stand on it. Breathe in to raise the other thigh parallel to the floor and repeat the sequence.

deep standing squat

This exercise brings awareness and strength to the legs and back. Loosen the muscles around the hip, knee and ankle joints by practising a few squats frequently.

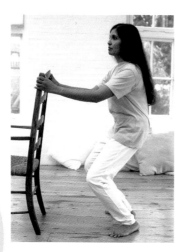

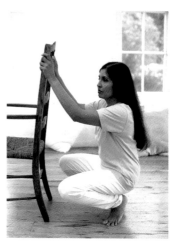

> "The physical postures should be steady and comfortable. They are mastered when all effort is relaxed and the mind is absorbed in the Infinite."
> *Patanjali's Yoga Sutras, Ch 2, translated by Alistair Shearer*

△ **1** Stand at arms' length in front of a stable object, such as a chair or table, and grasp it firmly for support as you squat. Your feet should be comfortably apart and turned out at 45 degrees, so that your ankles, knees and hips are in alignment when you sink down into the squat. Keep your spine erect and your gaze forward.

△ **2** Breathe in and stretch up through your spine and neck, then breathe out to squat down as low as you are able. Keep your heels on the floor if you can, or raise them until your lower back becomes more flexible. Breathe in to rise and out again to repeat the squat.

Opening up the Chakras

Gentle stretches and movements, working with the breath, help to release muscular tension in the physical body and also to free obstructions at the energy level. Breathing up through the body from the floor, and down from above the head, increases the energy in the susumna nadi, which flows through the chakras.

increasing vitality

The knees, hips and pelvis are all part of the "life" area of the body, where the centres that process vitality are located. The legs and the base of the spine are under the influence of the base chakra, and the hips and pelvis are under the influence of the sacral chakra. Seated stretches and bends energize these two chakras. If you add a twist to your movement you will be activating the navel chakra as well.

opening the chest

Exercises that open up the chest will foster improved breathing and better posture, and these can be done in a standing, kneeling or sitting position.

To start, the breath in is focused upon stretching up. If you are standing or kneeling, this stretch begins through the legs, then continues through the lower, middle and upper spine, and the neck. The upward stretch opens your chest to create space for deeper breathing and improves your posture by lengthening your spine to allow increased energy flow through the chakras, including the heart chakra in the chest and the throat chakra above. The breath out – done with the same relaxed attention – can be focused into movements involving the limbs, while still maintaining the strength and openness of the spine and neck.

By linking your breath with movement in these exercises, you are working from within, rather than making the correct "shapes" as seen from outside. In this way you can release physical tension and mental and emotional stress with every combined breath and movement. It is best to start with simple movements in order to focus on this co-ordination of mind and body with the rhythm of the breath.

Every nerve impulse that passes between the brain and the body has to travel through the neck, so it is very helpful to release any tension that has built up in this area. Continue the upward stretch of the spine through the neck and into the skull, and maintain the stretch during the movements to open the chest. At the same time, be aware of any tension in the throat and face and keep them relaxed.

wide-angled seated movements

The more you sit on the floor with your legs comfortably wide apart and practise these movements, the more quickly your hips, lower back and spine will release the muscular tension that is so restrictive and can also cause pain and malfunction.

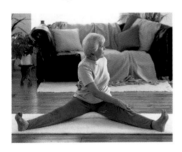

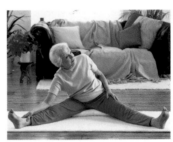

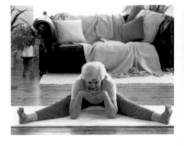

△ **1** Twist for navel chakra: sit on a cushion with your back straight and legs apart, toes pointing to the ceiling and the backs of your knees relaxed on the floor (though tight hamstring muscles may keep the legs bent to begin with). Breathe in and stretch the spine up. With your right hand on your left thigh, breathe out, twisting your trunk to the left and your left shoulder round behind you. Breathe in to return to the centre and stretch up. Breathe out to change sides. Repeat several times.

△ **2** Side bend for sacral chakra: breathe in and stretch up. Place one hand on each thigh. As you breathe out, slide your right hand down your right leg and look up to the left, bringing your left shoulder back to open the left side of the chest area. Breathe in to straighten up and repeat on the other side. Repeat several times.

△ **3** Forward bend for base and sacral chakras: place your fingertips on the floor in front of you and gently "walk" them forward, keeping your spine stretched. Avoid rounding your back and jutting your chin forward to reach further than is comfortable, as this causes tense muscles, whereas relaxation loosens them. Breathe in to stretch right through your spine. As you breathe out, sink forward a little more. As you relax deeply, you may want to rest your head in your hands with your elbows on the floor and smile. Come up again gently and slowly.

opening the book

This can be done standing, seated or kneeling. It is important to keep the chest open and the breastbone (sternum) lifted. The upper spine and neck are stretched up, strong and unmoving, and the elbows are at shoulder level as you move the arms.

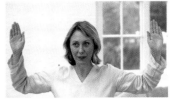

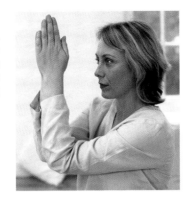

▷ **1** Stand "tall", stretching through the spine, with palms joined in front of your body and elbows at shoulder height. Breathe out for this "closing" position, stretching your ribcage at the back.

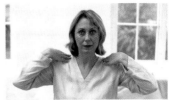

△ **2** Breathe in to "open the book", bringing your elbows (still at shoulder height) to the sides, palms facing forward. The spine and neck should not move at all as you press the elbows right back. Repeat the movement several times.

elbow rotations

As with all arm movements, the spine and neck are not involved and need to be held firmly in position throughout.

▷ **1** Place your fingertips on your shoulders and, keeping your breastbone lifted, bring your elbows in front of your body, as high as possible. Breathe out for this "closing" position, stretching your ribcage at the back.

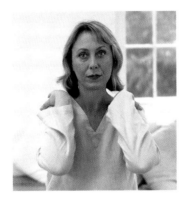

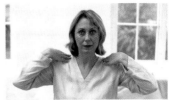

△ **2** Breathing in, rotate your elbows up, round and back, squeezing your shoulderblades together and stretching your ribs at the sides. Your spine and neck should remain stretched up and unmoving. Repeat several times, then circle your elbows the other way.

chest expansion

It is important to keep the spine and neck stretched up and unmoving as the arms are raised and lowered. This is an isometric exercise (developing muscle strength without moving) for the spine and neck and an isotonic exercise (stretching and moving) for the arms and the pectoral muscles in the chest.

"Open the window in the centre of your chest and let spirit move in and out."

Rumi, 13th century

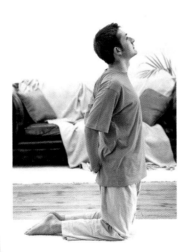

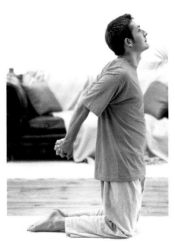

△ **1** Clasp your hands behind your back, keeping the palms firmly pressed together all the time. As you breathe in, push your clasped hands down toward the floor, squeezing your shoulderblades together.

△ **2** As you breathe out, raise your straight arms up behind you, keeping the palms firmly pressed together. Repeat several times. Even if only a little movement is possible at first, this is a powerful exercise, and you will find that your range of movement will increase with practice.

Learning to Let Go

The combination of relaxed stretching and deep, slow breathing is a quick and effective way to settle the "bodymind" in preparation for meditation. You can practise the following stretches and breathing techniques at any time of the day – preferably several times during each day. The resulting reduction in your stress levels will be gradual but cumulative. The practice leads to a calmer mind, clearer thinking, a more comfortable, relaxed body and a more open-hearted acceptance of the way things are – including the inadequacies of other people and of yourself.

active preparation

Of the eight limbs in Patanjali's system of raja yoga, the yoga of meditation, five are *bahir* (outer) or active limbs. All five physical aspects are to be practised together, and all are necessary to remove tensions from the body, emotions and mind, in order to experience the meditative state.

If we are angry with someone, or discontented with ourselves, or unable to sit still, or struggling with unhealthy breathing patterns and high stress levels, or if our minds are distracted by outer sensory stimuli and constant inner chatter, it is

impossible to give our full attention to meditation practice. Patanjali's first two limbs reinforce an attitude of respect and care for others through social restraint (yama) and for ourselves through purification (niyama). These are followed by a firm, comfortable seated position (asana) for meditation practice, breathing exercises (pranayama) to balance and increase energy, and finally relaxation and "switching off" (pratyahara). Only then are we ready to practise the three *antar* (inner) limbs that make up samyama (these are concentration, meditation and absorption/ecstasy).

skiing

This exercise stretches and flexes all the muscles that hold the spine, releasing tension and tightness that may be restricting blood flow, nerve communications and energy flow. It also opens the front of the chest and makes the breastbone more flexible, for better breathing.

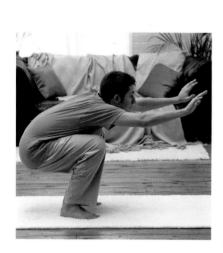 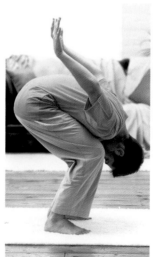 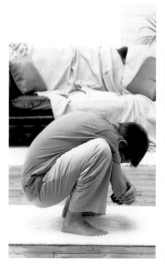

△ **1** Stand with your feet comfortably apart and parallel. Bend your knees and squat right down, stretching your arms out in front of you for balance. Lift your arms, opening your chest, as you breathe in. Imagine you are holding two ski poles and plant them firmly in the snow ahead of you.

△ **2** Breathing out, sweep your arms down and back, reaching as high behind you as you can to wave your imaginary ski poles in the air after they have propelled you forward. Repeat this movement several times. The visualization of the movement should make you feel flushed with exertion and enjoyment.

△ **3** When you feel you have done enough skiing, squat down with your arms and trunk between your knees and rest. Breathe naturally and feel the weight of your body stretching your lower back and legs.

easing the spine and neck

When you exercise lying down, gravity supports and cradles you, so these exercises are very soothing – especially if you feel stiff or have painful twinges in your lower back, hips or neck. You may feel more comfortable lying on your back if you place a small cushion under your head (not your neck) to lengthen your neck and bring your chin down toward your chest. Keep your neck area free, so that it can stretch.

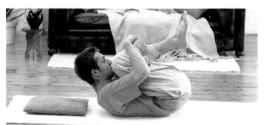

△ **1** Bend your knees on to your chest and clasp your hands around your shins (or the backs of your thighs). Breathing out, curl up your spine to bring your nose or forehead (not your chin, as this constricts your neck) to touch your knees. Breathe in to replace your head on the cushion, with your chin tucked in. Breathe out to begin the sequence again and repeat several times.

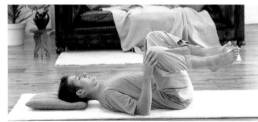

△ **2** To ease your lower back and hips, lie with your bent knees comfortably apart and one hand on each knee, with your elbows resting on the floor if possible. This is an open and relaxed pose that can ease pain from trapped nerves (such as sciatica). Breathing deeply and naturally, use your hands to circle your knees in toward each other then out to the sides in slow circles, really relaxing all your back and leg muscles.

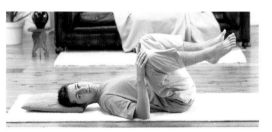

△ **3** Keeping your spine relaxed and knees wide and supported by your hands, with elbows resting on the floor, take your full attention to your neck. Breathing out slowly, turn your head to one side and turn your eyes to look at the floor.

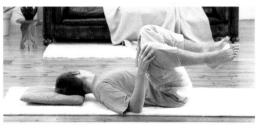

△ **4** Breathe in to raise your head and eyes to the centre and out to turn them to the other side. Repeat several times, focusing on awareness and relaxation of all your neck muscles. Keep your spine, legs, arms and jaw completely relaxed throughout.

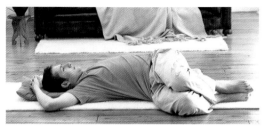

△ **5** Bring your arms overhead, clasping your hands loosely if you can, or simply bringing your bent arms as high as possible – your elbows should be relaxed on the floor. This position stretches the front of your body. Place your feet together on the floor close to your buttocks, and relax your upper body, neck and jaw. You will move only from the waist down. Breathe in and, as you breathe out, drop your knees (keeping them pressed together) to the floor on your right side. Breathe in to raise your knees and out to lower them to the left.

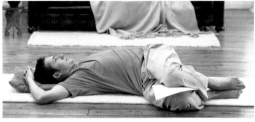

△ **6** For extra strengthening of the upper inner thighs – essential for good posture – press a sheet of paper between your knees and hold it there as you move your knees from side to side.

Breathing Techniques

Focusing on the breath is a universal technique for enlightenment and healing, and many traditions use breathing practices either as a way to prepare for meditation or as meditation techniques in themselves. Conscious control of the breath, or pranayama, is the fourth limb of Patanjali's system. The technique of holding the breath – either in or out – is beyond the scope of this book, as accomplishing it safely requires one-to-one teaching, but becoming aware of the breathing process and directing the flow of the breath is within the capacity of everyone.

Slowing down the breathing and lengthening the breath out (which is what happens when we sing or chant) switches the nervous system into its peaceful happy mode, allowing stress to be dissolved and rest, digestion, absorption and healing to take place at every level of the five koshas.

Patanjali's path to enlightenment

This use of the breath fits in perfectly with Patanjali's philosophy. He describes three vital steps (which have been called "preliminary purificatory practices") that

encapsulate his path to enlightenment. The steps are as follows (quotations are from the translation of Patanjali's Yoga Sutras by Alistair Shearer, Ch 2, verses 1–2):

"Purification" [through self-discipline]
"Refinement" [through self-awareness]
"Surrender" [through self-surrender and continual letting-go]
"These are the practical steps on the path of yoga." They nourish the state of samadhi [absorption/ecstasy/expansion]
"And weaken the causes of suffering."

The whole process of self-development starts with taking conscious control over our own nervous system, so that we experience more "expansion" and joy and less stress and unhappiness. Our circumstances influence the outcome of events far less than our own basic attitudes, and these can be changed from negative to positive by the simple act of changing our breathing pattern.

The breath forms part of the energy system and the physiological processes in the energy kosha, while nervous energy runs the mental computer in the kosha of

unconscious programming. All the koshas meet and blend in the chakra system in the energy kosha and all can therefore be consciously influenced through the practices of breathing and meditation.

Although some translations of the Yoga Sutras describe Patanjali's three "purificatory steps" as "preliminary", there is really no end to our need of them. We always have to maintain our discipline and keep our attention focused – and we never stop needing to let go of something or other.

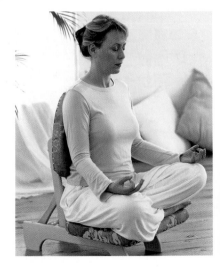

"Those who see a glass as half empty feel deprived, whereas those who see it as half full feel blessed."

Traditional wisdom

viloma: focusing on the breathing muscles

This useful focusing technique can be practised anywhere, sitting with the spine erect and the hands and eyes still.

▷ **1** Place your hands on your knees, palms either up or down, with thumb and index fingers touching to close the energy circuits. As you breathe in deeply, feel your ribs expand and your diaphragm contract downwards against your stomach. Notice how these movements cause air to flow into your lungs.

2 As you breathe out, count "One and two and ...", then stop your breath in mid-flow for the same count. Repeat until you have slowly and comfortably expelled enough air, then repeat this cycle four times more and rest. Then reverse the cycle, breathing in counting "One and two and ..." and out slowly for five breaths. Use the fractional breath in to start your day or whenever you need energy, and the fractional breath out to relax before meditation.

WATCHPOINTS FOR BREATHING PRACTICE

Regular practice will calm the mind and raise your energy levels. As the lungs strengthen, their capacity will be increased. Practise little and often – a few rounds of the breathing exercises now and then throughout the day will prepare you for longer sessions during meditation practice.

- Avoid any breathing practices after meals – when your stomach is full it presses against your diaphragm, constricting your lungs.
- Keep your spine stretched and as straight as possible (allowing for its natural curves) whether you are standing, sitting, kneeling or lying down to practise breathing. This allows maximum lung expansion and helps the free flow of both air and energy.
- Keep your breastbone lifted to open your chest and give your diaphragm room to move freely. Keep it lifted even when breathing out, letting your diaphragm and rib muscles do all the work.
- Always breathe in through your nose, as it is the filter that protects your lungs from cold, dust and infections from outside. Breathe out through your nose unless you are making sounds.
- Develop your focus on, and conscious awareness of, your breathing patterns, so that you constantly monitor their effects upon you. Develop the habit of watching yourself breathing.
- Slow your breathing down – especially your breath out – whenever you feel agitated or anxious, in order to gain conscious control over your autonomic nervous system.
- Stop your breathing practice and rest for a few natural breaths the instant you feel breathless. Start again when your nervous system has settled down and relaxed. It is not used to being watched and controlled, as breathing is usually an unconscious process.

alternate nostril breathing

This universally popular exercise quickly balances the nervous system, so that you feel calm and centred after just a few rounds – ready either for meditation practice or to get on with your day refreshed.

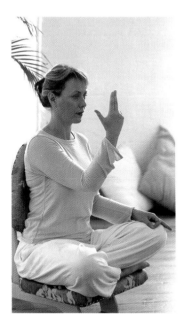

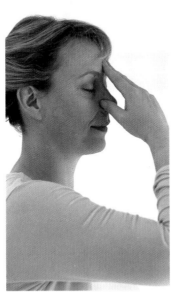

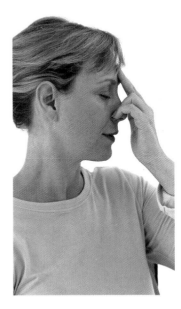

△ **1** Sit erect with your left hand on your knee or in your lap. Raise your right hand to place it against your face. Your thumb will close your right nostril, your index and middle fingers will rest aginst your forehead at the ajna (brow) chakra and your ring finger will close your left nostril.

△ **2** Your eyes may be closed, or open and gazing softly ahead. Keep your eyeballs still, as quiet eyes induce a quiet mind. Close your right nostril with your thumb. Breathe in through the left nostril.

△ **3** Release the right nostril and close the left with your ring finger. Breathe out slowly, and then in again, through your right nostril. Then open the left nostril, close the right and breathe out. This is one round. Do five rounds, breathe naturally to rest, then repeat a few times.

double breathing

This exercise fosters your self-awareness and observation. It also tones the muscles that give you "core strength" and support your spine, giving you increased energy and stamina for self-discipline, and improving posture and energy flow. Start each round by breathing in from your feet up (if you are standing), or from the base of your spine if you are sitting.

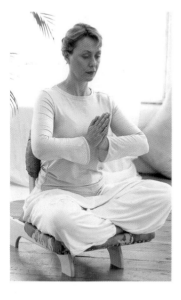 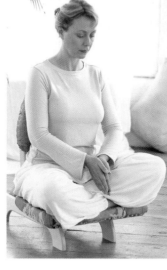 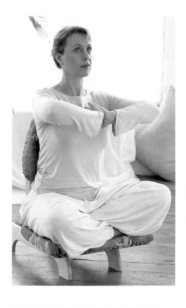

△ **1** Bring your palms together at chest level with elbows wide, lifting your breastbone and drawing your spine erect. Breathe slowly and deeply a few times to settle yourself.

△ **2** Point your fingers downwards and focus on the base of your body. As you breathe in, tighten the muscles of your upper inner thighs and pelvic floor, and at the same time draw your lower abdominal muscles back towards your spine. This movement lifts your life energy upwards.

△ **3** As you breathe out, turn your hands so your fingers point toward your collarbones, at the base of your throat, lifting your elbows to shoulder level. At the same time draw your energy up from the base, through the waist as you tighten your abdominal "corset muscles", and up to your head as you lift your chin. In this position breathe in, opening your ribs at the back of your chest by pressing your palms firmly together, as you bring spiritual energy down into your heart centre. Breathe out as you lower your fingertips and take your energy to the floor. Repeat the cycle twice more, then rest.

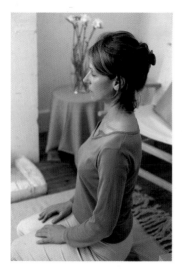

◁ Breathing practices can be done in a kneeling position if you find this comfortable. The pose creates a strong, stable base and helps to keep the spine erect to maximize the flow of energy. When you are kneeling or sitting, start the upward breath in from the base of your spine.

"We can keep only what we are prepared to surrender."

Traditional wisdom

grounding ritual

This is an essential step at the end of your meditation, so that you clear your mind of all you have experienced and go back to daily life refreshed and in "active mode", rather than "heady" and "spaced out". It is an exercise in self-surrender, as you give to the earth all the relaxation and joy you feel as a result of your meditation practice. This is one reason why we meditate – to share positive energy with those with whom we interact.

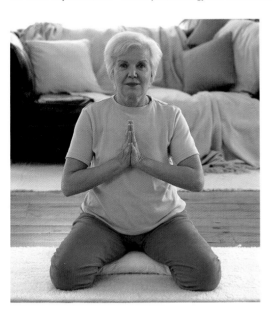

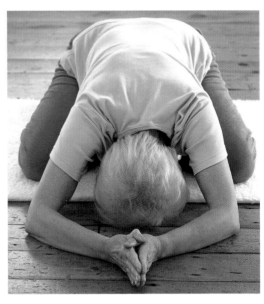

△ **1** At the end of your visualization or other meditation practice, bring your palms together and breathe in, mentally giving heartfelt thanks for the experience, whatever it was like for you.

△ **2** As you breathe out, fold forward to ground yourself by placing your hands on the floor – and your head also if you can reach – giving to the earth all the experience and benefit you have received.

bee buzzing breath

This technique uses sound to begin extending the length of the breath out. It induces instant relaxation and reduction of stress, and is an exercise in "letting go".

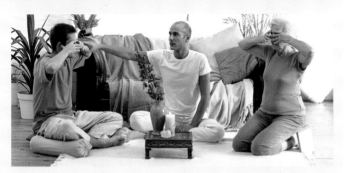

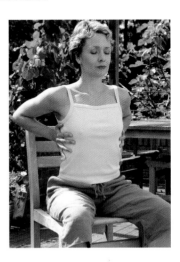

△ **1** Sit erect, placing your thumbs in position ready to close your ear flaps, and your fingers ready to close your eyelids and lips.

2 Breathe in deeply. As you breathe out, "close down" and make a humming sound like a bee. Feel this sound vibrating through your body, loosening tightness and tension. Before you run out of breath, open your eyes and ears to breathe in and repeat.

△ **Explore the physical effects of your breath on your abdominal organs by placing your hands on the sides of your ribs, then on the front and finally on your lower abdomen.**

Posture Principles

Meditation practices are traditionally performed sitting with the spine erect and vertical, so that energy flows between the "heaven" (light) and "earth" (life) poles of our being. Energy needs to flow smoothly up and down through the physical spine and the energy channels of the subtle body, so that the brain and breathing function optimally and the chakras are balanced and full of vitality. An erect spine is quite easy to maintain if the right props are used to begin with and the right exercises are performed regularly to strengthen the muscles that hold the spine erect and open the hip joints.

meditation and relaxation

Relaxation is quite different from meditation. It is part of the fifth limb of Patanjali's system – pratyahara, or withdrawal of the senses from outer stimuli. Relaxation practices are done lying down in as comfortable a position as possible. Western psychotherapists usually favour a reclining position because their techniques require the client to be relaxed as they follow a guided visualization or answer questions about their past. Meditation practice takes us deeper than this, with the mind quietly focused on a single object. Relaxation – like physical stretching and awareness of breathing – is very useful as a preparation for meditative practice but should not be confused with it.

sitting on a chair

When starting to practise meditation, most Westerners find it easiest to sit upright on a firm chair. Your thighs should be parallel to the floor – in order to achieve this you may need to raise your feet (without shoes) by resting them on a cushion. Sit erect with your hands, palms down, resting on your thighs, hands and feet parallel and pointing forward. This posture is known as the "Egyptian position". If you lean back at all you will quickly develop a backache, so sit

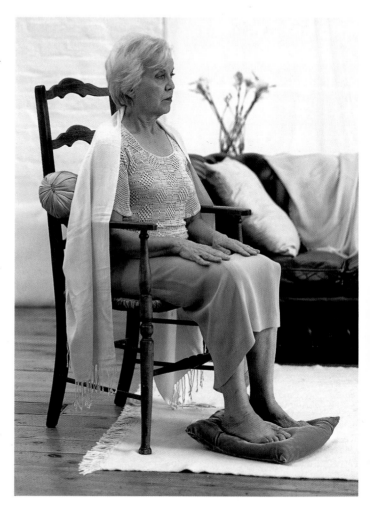

erect with the base of your spine pressed against the chair back or a firm cushion.

Once you are settled in this position you can gradually increase the time you can comfortably remain motionless. Spend up to ten minutes watching your natural breath or practising breathing exercises to centre your energies along the axis of the spine. You will feel energized and relaxed as a result. Later you may wish to sit motionless for half an hour or longer while you practise

△ **If you choose to sit in a chair for meditation practice, make sure it gives firm support and is a suitable height. Your spine should remain erect, with your head and neck aligned.**

your meditation techniques. If the seated position suits you, you may decide always to practise meditation seated on a particular chair, or you may want to try out a variety of positions as your hips become more flexible through regular stretching exercises.

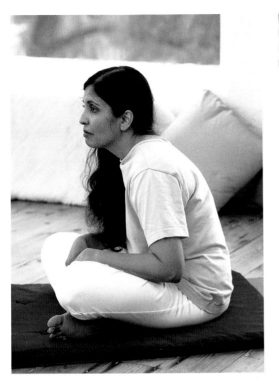

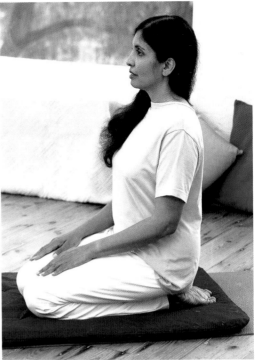

△ Lack of spinal strength and the right support result in poor posture, with the head jutting forward and the spine rounded. The neck automatically shortens and tenses when the back is humped in this way, constricting the flow of energy, and it is impossible to maintain the position comfortably for the whole period of meditation practice.

△ Good posture results from choosing the right position. The head and neck are aligned and erect, and the spine is vertical. To prevent strain and help with alignment, the base of the spine can be supported on a firm cushion or a folded blanket positioned between the feet.

sitting on the floor

This is the traditional Eastern way to meditate, since chairs were not used in homes until very recently. As a result, people had very flexible hips, so sitting cross-legged on a cushion on the floor was easy and natural. Most Westerners first need to loosen up their hip joints – which has the additional benefit that it reduces the risk of developing arthritic hips in old age. Meanwhile, it is better to sit on a chair, or on your heels in Vajrasana (thunderbolt posture) than with a slumped spine in an attempt to sit with crossed legs on the floor. Whatever position you adopt, do use support where it is needed until your muscles and joints have strengthened and loosened enough for you to be comfortable without support. Many excellent meditation stools and chairs are available, some of which are illustrated in this book.

WHERE SUPPORT MAY BE NEEDED

Your spine may need help in order to remain comfortably erect. You can sit supported by a cushion against a wall – if you are on the floor or in bed – or with a cushion against the back of a firm upright chair (not an armchair). Sitting on your heels may be the easiest way to learn to sit erect without support.

Your hips may not yet open freely enough to allow your knees to rest on the floor in a cross-legged pose. Cushions supporting your thighs will help you to stretch up through your lower back and a firm cushion under your tailbone will relieve pressure in the lower back by lowering your knees. Strategically placed cushions can make sitting on the floor the most comfortable option.

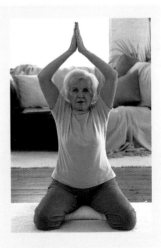

△ A cushion under the tailbone eases the lower back by lifting the hips.

Choosing a Posture

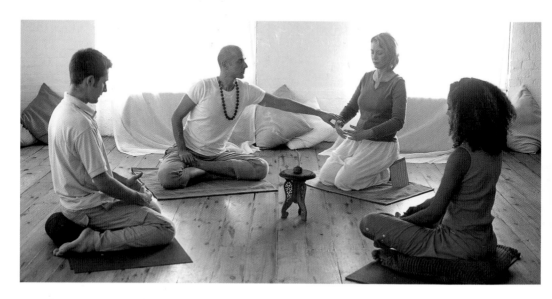

Regular practice is the best teacher, as your body quickly gets used to the new routine and settles into it more and more easily. When you find a position that is comfortable for you, practise sitting in it until you can remain motionless, relaxed yet alert, for half an hour or more. It is helpful to vary your position when you sit at home, or to change purposefully from one position to another without disturbing your inner focus whenever your muscles begin to ache. This is much better than focusing on the complaints coming from your body when you push it to sit too long without moving.

△ You may find it helpful to attend a meditation class, where you can be shown different ways to sit and try out the various props available before buying any of them for yourself.

easy cross-legged pose

This involves sitting erect with hips loose and knees wide. Each foot is tucked under the opposite thigh so that the weight of the legs rests on the feet rather than the knees. Place cushions under each thigh and/or under the buttocks if you feel pressure in the lower back. The tailbone (coccyx) should hang freely, letting the "sitting bones" take the weight of the trunk. Place your hands on your knees or rest them in your lap with palms facing up.

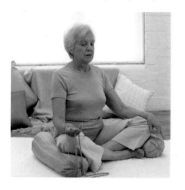

◁ If the hips are not sufficiently flexible for the knees to rest on the floor when sitting cross-legged, support them with a couple of cushions. Resting the hands palms up enables you to hold a mala or rosary.

▷ This low chair, which folds for easy carrying, is specially designed for meditation. It supports the back when sitting in the cross-legged pose. The hands are in *gyana mudra*, with the tips of thumb and forefinger joined to complete the energy circuit.

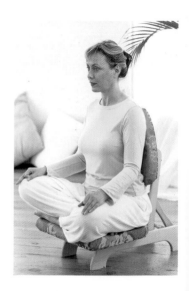

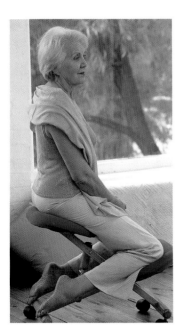

Buddhist position

The kneeling pose called Virasana (hero posture) is sometimes used for meditation. Buddhists often choose to sit on a very firm cushion that lifts the hips, with the knees resting on the floor on each side of the cushion and the shins and feet pointing back. Lifting the hips in this way helps to keep the spine correctly aligned, and this position can be very comfortable as long as your knees are fairly flexible.

◁ Using a "kneeling" chair helps to keep the spine straight and gives a good, well-supported position that is similar to the Buddhist kneeling pose.

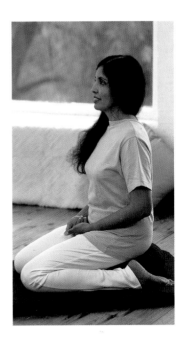

▷ While sitting on a firm cushion in Virasana, the knees and feet can also be supported on a larger cushion. The meditator sits between the feet, rather than on the heels. The hands are in the gesture called *bhairavi mudra*, to focus the energy for meditation.

early morning meditation

Many people like to meditate first thing every morning, while the mind is quiet and before the events of the day have a chance to distract it. If you meditate in bed, use a V-shaped pillow or ordinary pillows to support your back, so that you can sit erect in a cross-legged position. Wear a shawl round your shoulders and pull up the bedclothes so that you feel warm while you are doing your meditation practice. Choose a practice that energizes rather than relaxes you, such as chanting or repeating a mantra using a mala. You may prefer to keep your eyes open in a soft gaze.

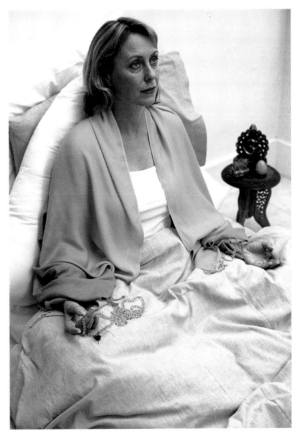

▷ Your bed can be a haven of peace and warmth if you prefer to meditate on waking in the morning.

▽ A V-shaped pillow helps you to maintain an erect posture while meditating in bed. A mala, used for counting the repetitions of a mantra, is traditionally kept concealed in its special bag when not in use.

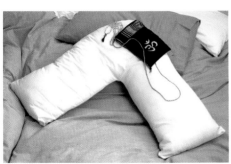

The Time, the Place

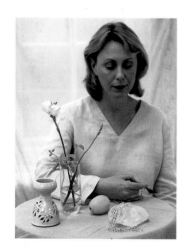

It takes determination to establish a new habit and to make room in your life for a new regular activity. It helps if you train your mind to meditate routinely at a specific time and place. You may still be tempted sometimes to skip your meditation slot and do something else instead, but you will begin to feel uncomfortable when you miss your practice. There will be days when you have to forgo your normal routine, but that will be a conscious decision rather than simply forgetting or procrastinating.

◁ Your "meditation corner" may contain a number of objects on which to focus: any object can act as a trigger to put you in the right frame of mind for your practice.

▷ A crescent-shaped "moon cushion" is often used as support when sitting for meditation.

meditating at a regular time

It is helpful to place your meditation practice in the context of long-established habits – such as before showering in the morning, or after cleaning your teeth, or before lunch or supper. Since you do all these things daily you will meditate daily as well. A good time is when you wake up or before a meal – after meals people are apt to feel sleepy – or in the evening after a brisk walk or listening to soothing music. You might read an uplifting book in bed and then meditate before going to sleep. Choose a time when you are normally alone and undisturbed – the fuller your day, the more rewarding and de-stressing your meditation session can be. Couples often meditate together at a mutually convenient time, or get up early before the household is awake. Whatever time you choose, stick to it to establish your meditation habit.

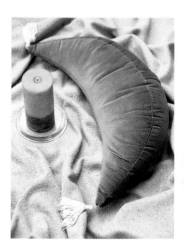

creating a meditation corner

If you always do your meditation in the same place this will also help to establish your meditation habit. Choose a quiet and uncluttered space so that the moment you sit there your mind becomes calm and focused. Make sure you will be warm enough, as body temperature drops when you relax and turn inward.

Your "meditation corner" might consist of a special chair in a peaceful part of your home, or perhaps you might sit on a

MEDITATION IN BED

If you practise meditation in the early morning, your bed (with a warm shawl around you and the covers pulled up) can become your "meditation corner". Have a wash, a drink and a good stretch to really wake you up first – and make sure you sit with your spine erect.

If you regularly meditate in bed in the morning, and this is the place where you are in the habit of turning your mind inward, it can also be very soothing to perform simple meditation techniques before you go to sleep at night.

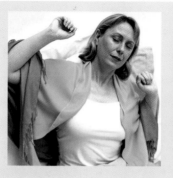

△ When you wake up, have a relaxed, "releasing" stretch before starting your early morning meditation.

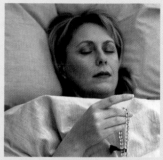

△ Last thing at night, relax with your mala and repeat a mantra or simple prayer before you go peacefully to sleep.

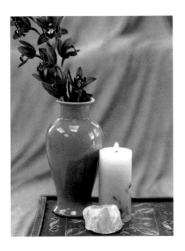

△ If you choose to meditate sitting on the floor, a low table is useful for holding objects on which you wish to focus your gaze.

favourite cushion, or spread out a lovely rug. The corner might contain a table holding a candle and flowers, or anything you find soothing and inspiring.

objects of devotion

The things you keep in your meditation corner can be used for the classic technique called *tratak* – or "gazing". This involves sitting erect and motionless while focusing your gaze upon an object.

The point of focus is often a lighted candle. If you practise this form of meditation, check that there are no draughts to move the candle flame, as this can give you a headache. (Epileptics and migraine sufferers should avoid gazing at a flame.) After gazing softly, without staring, for a while, close your eyes and keep the image in your mind's eye. When it fades, gaze at the candle again and repeat the visualization. Your mental image will gradually become firmer and your concentration deeper.

You may like to light a candle before starting meditation practice and blow it out with a "thank you" as a final gesture. A flame is a universal symbol for the presence of the divine, and you may like to develop a greater awareness of this presence dwelling within you and surrounding you.

There are different forms of tratak. A flower can be held and turned around in the hand, as you observe every detail of its

postural stretch

If you have been sitting all day in a car or at your desk, you may want to regain a strong upright posture before you start an evening meditation session. You could try standing with a weighty object on your head to strengthen the spinal column and improve your sense of balance. Previous generations learned "deportment" by walking around the room balancing piles of books on their heads, and porters the world over have strong straight backs, developed by carrying loads on their heads.

▷ Stretching your spine up against the weight of gravity makes your meditation pose "firm and comfortable", as Patanjali recommends.

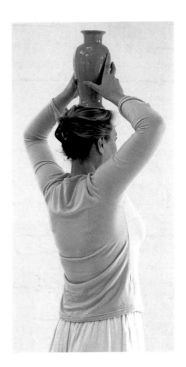

beauty and structure. Holding a crystal in your hands and feeling its contours and coolness is another form of tratak – in this case the eyes are closed throughout and the "gazing" is accomplished through the sense of touch. You could equally well choose to gaze at any object that inspires you.

relaxing horizontal stretch

Stretching out on your back is the perfect preparation for meditation. Ten minutes lying stretched out on the floor on your back, with your mind gently but firmly focused on the movement of your breath while your body relaxes, is an instant restorative.

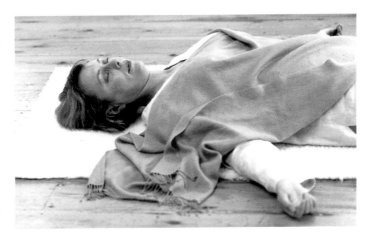

△ Keep alert and warm while you relax on your back. Stretching in this position prepares you for keeping your spine erect – the spine should always be as straight as possible when meditating. While you lie on your back and relax your body, many meditation techniques can be used to keep your mind alert and focused, such as counting your breaths from one to ten and back again, visualizing energy moving through the spine, repeating a mantra, or visualizing a tranquil scene in the country or by the sea. After your relaxation take a few deep breaths, move your fingers and toes, stretch and yawn and sit up very slowly. You are now ready for meditation practice.

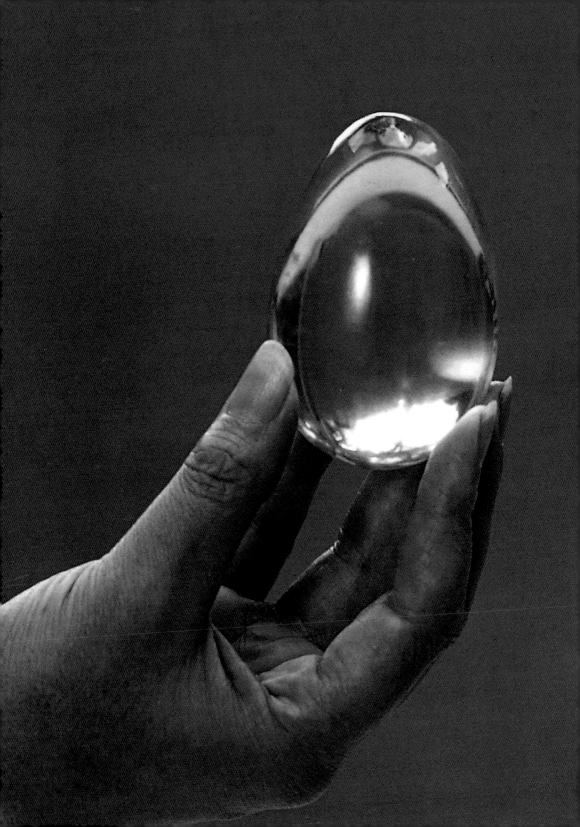

Using the Senses

We relate to the world around us by means of our five senses, and these same senses also tell us what we are thinking and how we are feeling. They are the link between the physical world outside us – which everyone else can also experience – and the world within us that only we can know.

By increasing our powers of observation, visualization and imagination, meditation practices help to sharpen our senses. By these means we can actually change how we feel inside ourselves.

Dharana, which is interpreted as concentration or "one-pointedness", is the sixth of Patanjali's eight limbs of yoga. If we focus on one sense and concentrate all our attention on the message it conveys, whether we are gazing at a candle flame, listening to a bell or the sound of a mantra, or smelling a flower, we can reflect that steady focus inwards to our inner life and thoughts, shutting out the sensory assault of the everyday world in preparation for the meditative state. We can also use the memory of sensory experience in visualizations that enrich our inner world.

Meditation and the Five Senses

Our senses are the antennae that our minds use to probe the world, both outside and within us, so that we can become aware of what is happening, and what we are doing and thinking. What we are unable to feel, see, hear, taste or smell we can neither conceive of nor describe. Without our five senses we could have no first-hand information about anything and would remain in ignorance, even of our own bodies. Yet their range can pick up only a tiny fraction of what is actually "out there" and "in here" – even when enhanced by modern technology.

We may claim to have a "sixth" sense – or intuition – but this arises from the five physical senses working together. Try thinking about anything without "hearing" yourself thinking about it or "seeing" it in your mind's eye. We can even "feel" in two minds about some issue and "hear" voices arguing the pros and cons in our heads.

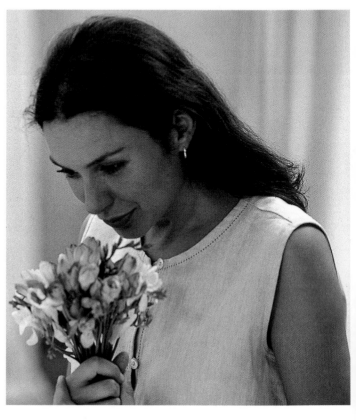

△ All that we know about the world – from the scent of a flower to the beating of our own hearts – is conveyed to us through our senses.

CHAKRAS AND THE SENSES

 1 Base (muladhara): earth element and sense of smell.

 2 Sacral (svadisthana): water element and sense of taste.

3 Navel (manipura): fire element and sense of sight.

 4 Heart (anahata): air element and sense of touch.

 5 Throat (visuddhi): ether or space element and sense of hearing.

pratyahara for focus and awareness

Meditation is a state of expanded awareness, and awareness is simply becoming conscious of specific sensory messages once the general sensory "noise" of everyday experience is switched off.

Pratyahara is the fifth of Patanjali's eight limbs. It is often translated as "withdrawing the senses from their objects", so that we are no longer distracted by what is going on around us. However, if we are fearful or anxious, the nervous system will not allow us to be off guard in this way, even for a moment. This state of anxiety is very stressful and eventually exhausts the body's systems, leading to illness.

Pratyahara is associated with deep relaxation, which is the opposite of being "on guard", and it is possible to relax like this when we feel completely safe and at ease in a protected environment, such as a personal meditation corner at home. In this situation we can let our guard down, but if we switch off all the senses we go to sleep. Instead, the answer is to focus on one sense, or turn the senses inward to practise visualization and witness thoughts as they arise. These techniques prepare us for the state of meditation.

prana mudra: gestures for moving energy through the spine

You can increase your awareness of the energy "highway" that corresponds to the central nervous system by visualizing energy moving up and down the spine and passing through the chakras. Eventually you will perceive these movements as actual rather than imaginary, and can start meditating on the qualities of the chakras. This will deepen your relationship with your senses.

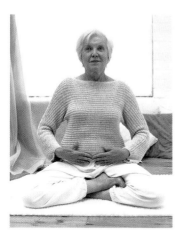

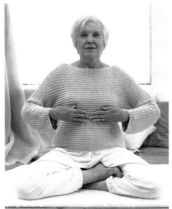

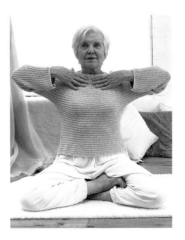

△ **1** Sitting erect and comfortable in a cross-legged position, bring your palms to face your lower abdomen with fingertips just touching. Start to breathe in, feeling that you are drawing vital energy up from the earth through the base of your body into the life chakras in the abdominal area.

△ **2** Continue breathing in as your raise your hands slowly up the front of your body, "drawing" the energy up through the spine and into the love chakras in the heart area.

△ **3** Continue, still breathing in, raising your hands and drawing the energy up through the throat area.

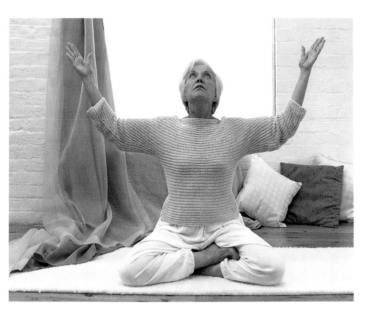

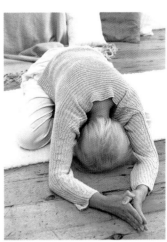

△ **5** Now breathe out slowly as you lean forward to bring your head and joined hands to the floor in an attitude of relaxed and trusting surrender. This is the basic grounding position. Repeat the sequence once or twice more.

△ **4** Finish the breath in by taking your hands up past your face (the area of the light chakras), spreading your arms wide and looking up. This is a joyful, exuberant movement.

Sight, Taste and Smell

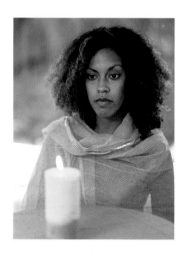

Many traditional meditation techniques are based on focusing with awareness upon one or more of the five senses through practising pratyahara. In Patanjali's system this is the last of the outer, or "active", limbs, before the mind turns "inward".

using sight for meditation

Tratak – gazing at an object such as a candle flame or a flower – is a favourite meditation technique that is common to many traditions. It is a simple but highly effective way to rest a busy mind.

1 Look softly upon your chosen object without staring, blinking or thinking. When you feel the need to close your eyes do so, but keep the image of the object motionless in your "mind's eye". The image will gradually fade and, when it does so, open your eyes and gaze again upon the object. Repeat for a total of about ten minutes.

2 You may find that tears will start to flow as you practise tratak, washing the eyeballs. In ancient India, where clean water was in short supply and the environment was very dusty, tratak was practised as a safe cleansing technique for the eyes. Sometimes tears bring emotions to the surface to "wash away" ancient sorrows – let them flow, as this process can be very healing.

◁ Bringing the full intensity of the sense of sight to bear on a candle flame is a popular meditative technique. Place the candle at about arm's length, with the flame at eye level. (You should avoid gazing at a candle flame if you are prone to migraines or epilepsy.)

the sense of sight

Sight is probably our most conscious and developed sense in modern western society. Our environment is constantly lit, so that we can move about and work at any hour, regardless of the natural rhythms of day and night, and we are bombarded by visual messages, ranging from traffic lights or advertising hoardings to television and computer screens. It is hard to find a place that is softly lit and visually soothing unless we create it for ourselves in our own home. Most of us find it easier to picture something with the "mind's eye" than to feel or hear it, so visualization is a popular pratyahara technique.

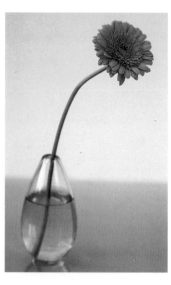

△ Gazing at a single flower, focus all your attention on every aspect of its appearance: its intricate form, colour and texture.

THE CHAKRAS IN COLOUR

In Western healing circles the chakras are often "seen" as the colours of the rainbow, rather than using the intricate traditional Eastern diagrams of energies, known as *yantras*:

- **Base chakra:** a deep fiery red like the embers of a coal fire; it is dull blackish red when unhealthy or stagnating.

- **Sacral chakra:** a glowing orange; drab and brownish when lacking energy

- **Navel chakra:** a bright sunny yellow; tinged green when resentful or envious

- **Heart chakra:** emerald green, or often its complementary colour, rose pink; faded when energy is blocked

- **Throat chakra:** brilliant sapphire blue, especially when inspired or defending the truth

- **Brow chakra:** royal purple or amethyst, sometimes indigo (containing the three primary colours of red, yellow and blue)

- **Crown chakra:** brilliant white or pale lilac, radiating as a beacon of light

As you breathe slowly up and down through your chakras, what colours do you "see" them? Remember to ground yourself in prana mudra after you finish this visualization.

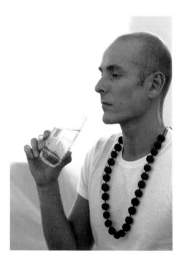

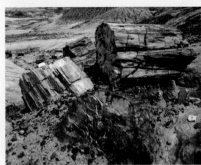

◁ Focus on your sense of taste by experiencing pure flavours, in this case lemon-flavoured water, with total attention.

the senses of taste and smell

Taste and smell are closely linked, each affecting the other extremely powerfully. They are also our most primitive senses, associated with the reptilian brain and the two lowest chakras, and they are essential for our survival. The most fleeting fragrances have the power to release emotions and memories, and in many religious traditions, aromatics such as incense are used to elevate the spirit or to induce altered states of consciousness. Taste and smell can be included in your meditation by burning incense or fragrant oils and by eating or drinking as an exercise in awareness.

VISUALIZING THE GUNAS
It is easy to understand nature's three "strands" in visual terms and to create our own imagery:

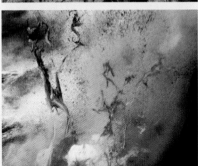

- **Tamas** (inertia, depression, obstruction) looks dull and dark, like an immovable rock or a stagnant murky pond. Everything appears gloomy when we are feeling unhappy.

- **Rajas** (movement, passion, obsession, anger) looks hot and fierce, like a devouring and uncontrolled fire. We say that we "see red" when in a fury.

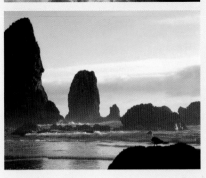

- **Sattva** (balance, harmony, peace) looks bright and light, like polished silver or gold. We can see love "shining" in someone's face and angels are often represented dressed in gleaming white robes.

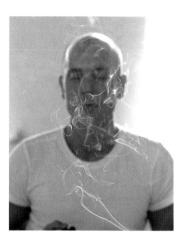

△ Incense is a traditional aid to meditation. Burn it in your meditation corner to purify the air and focus your sense of smell.

Do any of these images correspond to how you are feeling right now? The gunas are intermingled in every aspect of nature, like a plaited rope, but one of them usually predominates. The only guna suitable for meditation practice is sattva, as neither of the other two makes us feel safe and relaxed.

Hearing and Touch

Pratyahara involves a gathering in of the thoughts by consciously detaching the mind from all the fleeting sensations presented to it by the five senses, which are constantly bombarded by all the distractions of the outside world.

the sense of hearing

We are so beset by noise pollution in modern society that our sense of hearing often becomes blunted by the cacophony, yet this sense can take us more quickly and also deeper into meditation than any of the others once we have learned to really listen intently but in a completely relaxed manner. The Hatha Yoga Pradipika, one of the classical treatises on hatha yoga, leads the student through all the hatha practices – "for the sole purpose of attaining the yoga of meditation" – until the object of meditation can be heard within.

inner sound

What you can hear, once you know how to listen, is the inner vibration or sound, which is called *nada*. This sound is described as having several levels of subtlety. Moving from the grosser sounds to the most subtle,

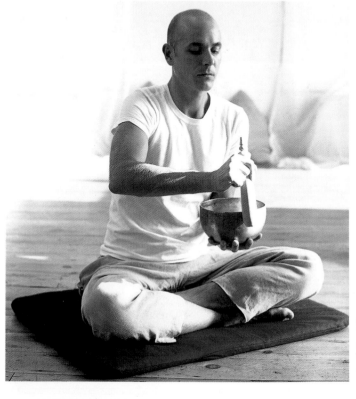

△ To draw the deep resonant sound from a Tibetan singing bowl, a wooden wand is held very firmly against the side of the bowl as it is stroked around the rim.

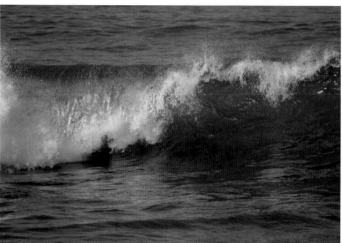

◁ At its most resonant level, the inner sound, or nada, is compared with the crashing of waves in the ocean.

the levels are likened to "the ocean ... [thunder]clouds, kettledrum ... conch [a seashell that can be blown into to create a sound], gong and horn ... tinkling of bells, flute, vina [a stringed instrument] and humming of bees".

Anyone who has learnt to relax, still the chattering mind and really listen will be able to hear nada. It is often heard at first as a

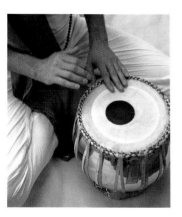

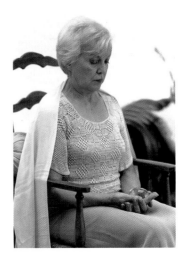

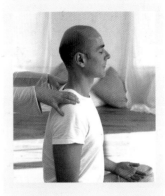

◁ Complicated rhythms can be created by a drummer, but keeping time can be as simple or as complex as you wish. Clapping is an excellent and simple way to sustain a rhythm, either alone or in a group.

△ Really feeling the shape, weight, coolness and texture of an object such as a crystal is a valuable meditative practice.

high-pitched vibrational hum, such as you might hear when standing beneath overhead power cables. Once you can hear nada you should listen for the more subtle levels of sound behind the one that is apparent.

the primordial sound

Many spiritual traditions claim that creation began with sound. St John's gospel opens with the statement: "In the beginning was the Word," and this primordial word is clearly a sound caused, like all sounds, by a vibration. The same claim is made in the *Mandukya Upanisad*, one of the philosophical and mystical treatises that form part of the Vedas: "Whatever has been, is or shall be is OM and whatever transcends time is also OM." OM is known as the *pranava* (primordial sound) and is placed at the beginning of most mantras, as well as being the source of every mantra. It is the sacred sound or vibration that gave rise to the universe as we know it. Therefore the reverent chanting of OM takes us back to our creator or source, God or Brahman. Nada is the sound of the divine within us.

developing your ability to listen

An effective pratyahara technique is to sit quietly and focus upon your sense of hearing without involving any movement of the mind. Start by picking up the most obvious sounds, such as a car in the street or a dog barking somewhere. Listen to these sounds, simply becoming aware of them without making any mental comment such as "That is a dog's bark," or framing any judgment or description of the sound, such

as "ugly" or "loud". Gradually listen for more subtle sounds, such as your own breathing, heartbeat or digestion – still without the addition of any mental comments. Hear your own thoughts without making any comment upon them. Eventually, when you have learned how to listen impartially to whatever sounds you are picking up, you will hear nada.

making your own sounds

Having learned to hear sounds impartially, you can learn to produce sounds without any of the "mental baggage" that usually accompanies attempts to create tuneful noises such as singing or playing musical instruments. You can chant a simple mantra, stroke a Tibetan singing bowl with a wooden wand, sing a scale up and down through an octave, create rhythm on a drum, all without embarrassment or stress, whether you are alone or in company. Both listening to and creating sounds are wonderfully relaxing practices that can quickly take you into the meditative state.

the sense of touch

Every emotional response is a matter of "feeling", involving some aspect of the physical sense of touch. Feeling safe is like being held by loving hands or feeling the presence of friends around you. Feeling inspired or uplifted creates a tangible feeling of inner lightness and expansion. You can also feel "in touch" with your body – whether you are hot or cold, comfortable or in pain, still or moving.

Most of these sensations remain below consciousness unless we need to notice them. In our daily lives, we are unaware of the muscles that keep us standing upright until we trip and are in danger of falling, or of our breathing cycles until we run too fast and feel out of breath. Learning to consciously feel safe and relaxed while becoming more focused and aware is a wonderful antidote to stress.

SHARING A SENSE OF TOUCH
Massage is an excellent way to explore and enhance your sense of touch – whether as "giver" or "receiver". You do not need to be an expert. Simply remember that your hands are extensions of your heart chakra, ask your partner how they feel and tune in to their responses. It helps communication to synchronize your breathing with your partner; press down as they breathe out and relax, lightening your touch on the breath in.

△ Giving or receiving massage allows both of you to focus on the sense of touch.

Combining the Senses

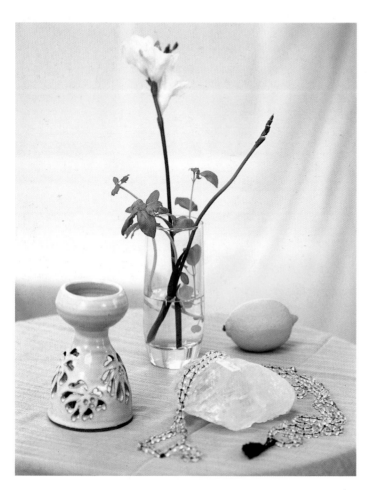

Sensory perception is a mental activity. The brain turns the constant input of nervous impulses from the body into touch, sight, hearing, taste and smell so as to make internal sense of the external world. We do not actually know what lies outside our brain, only what it tells us is there as it translates the impressions picked up by the sensory nerve endings.

Most of what our senses pick up is filtered out from our conscious awareness. For instance, while we are reading a book that is engrossing our interest, we may not

△ A meditation table can cater for all the senses: include a flower to look at; a lemon and some sprigs of an aromatic herb such as basil for smell and taste; essential oils in a burner to create fragrance conducive to meditation; a crystal to look at and touch; and a mala to handle as you hear yourself repeating a mantra.

notice other people moving about around us. All kinds of forces exist that we cannot sense, such as the cosmic rays called neutrinos that pass straight through our "solid" bodies and our planet.

the dominant sense

People often have a bias toward one of the five senses. The sense of sight is probably dominant for most people in modern Western society, though some people rely more upon hearing or touch than upon sight, and the other senses may be far more important to us than we realize.

It is impossible to write anything without hearing the words spoken in our own mind, or to move around without being aware through the sense of touch of the body's relationship with everything around it. The senses of taste and smell are far more active than we may imagine. Therefore combining the focusing of several senses in meditation practice is likely to be more effective than concentrating on just one.

combining sensory tools to deepen meditation

Start with simple techniques that use only one sense until you have learned to stay focused on it for several minutes at a time. Then gradually increase the complexity of the exercise and find what works best for you and holds your attention for longest.

Practise regularly a simple technique such as feeling the movement of your breath within your body (which relies on your sense of touch). This technique may eventually become so familiar that your mind can wander even while you are doing it, making focusing difficult. When this happens you can change to a different technique – perhaps alternate nostril breathing with counting (combining the senses of touch and sound). Then explore "seeing" or "feeling" prana, or energy, as light or warmth or tingling as you breathe. Direct this prana mentally as you breathe in and take it to a specific place within your body on the breath out (combining the senses of sight and touch).

These sensory tools are deceptively simple to use in order to reach the meditative state, yet they can have profound

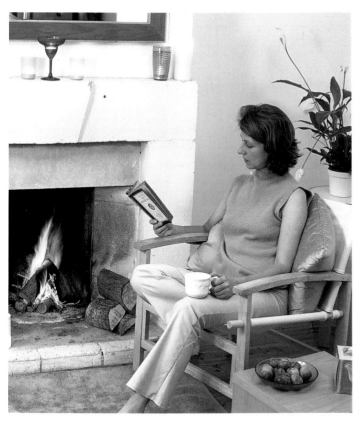

△ When you become absorbed in a book your brain is able to ignore outside distractions even though all your senses are still picking up all the signals from them.

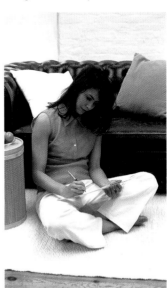

▽ While you are watching yourself writing, and feeling your hand steering the pen, you are also hearing the words inside your head.

effects over time. Just taking three deep breaths – if that has become your trigger – can immediately lift you out of a state of stress and into inner silence. The art is to combine several tools so as to maintain mental awareness and focus, and avoid slipping into daydreaming.

All meditation practices use the natural senses, usually touch, sight or sound and often a combination of these. You can learn to sharpen all your senses, one at a time, and then to switch off your perception of the outer world at will in order to create an inner world. Visualization is the technique of creating your own reality. "As we think, so we become", so think happy and relaxed thoughts, flowing with life–light–love. Your external world will reflect the attitudes that you project on to it from within.

MALA AND MANTRA

Fingering a mala (a string of traditional meditation beads) while chanting a mantra is a classic example of a meditative technique that combines the senses. Two senses are being used here: the sense of hearing as you listen to yourself repeating the mantra (either chanting it out loud or saying it in your mind) and the sense of touch as you pass the mala through your fingers to clock up the repetitions of the mantra.

Sit erect and relaxed in the safe environment of your meditation corner. Favourite mantras are "OM", "Peace and goodwill", "OM santi santi santi" (santi means "peace") or any short phrase that promotes healing and joy. Really feel the presence of the beads as you finger them gently but decisively.

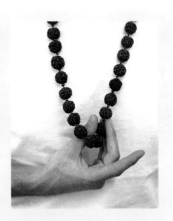

△ The mala is held in the right hand, and the positions of the fingers used to count the repetitions are symbolic: the thumb (cosmic consciousness) and the middle finger (sattva guna) move the beads, while the first finger (ego/personality consciousness) is kept well away from the action.

The Art of Visualization

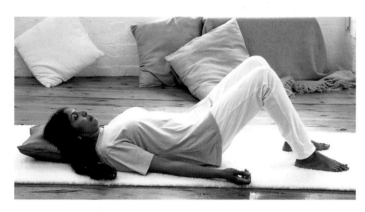

Visualization is a technique that brings the senses into full play, and enables us to build up a happy inner world. Relaxed visualization is a tool used in many different types of therapies. Its aim is to help us change our perception of the world by changing the way we feel inside ourselves. It can be done lying down or reclining just as well as sitting in an upright meditation pose. This means that we can help ourselves to feel better when we are tired and depleted, or ill in bed, or needing to create a calm and relaxed state to prepare for a peaceful night's sleep.

choosing an affirmation

You can use your relaxation time for your own greatest long-term benefit by using affirmations to create lasting change. The first step is to decide on an affirmation or resolve, known as a *sankalpa*, to repeat when you are in a state of deep relaxation.

You need to ask yourself what positive changes in your behaviour (life), perception (light) or attitude (love) would make you more like the person you would wish to be. The answer requires reflection and an honest appraisal of your personal qualities. Having decided on your sankalpa, you can set about creating a suitable visualization by using your imagination and all five senses to become fully present in a place of your choice where you feel naturally safe and relaxed. Once this scene is set you can go

△ For relaxation adopt a comfortable position lying on your back with your knees raised and feet flat on the floor. A cushion under your head keeps your neck from contracting at the back.

▽ Once you are deeply relaxed, focus your imagination and all your senses on being present in the place you want to be.

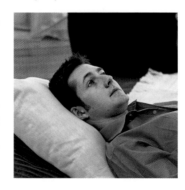

deeper and reinforce the changes in attitude, outlook and purpose that you have already decided to adopt. The unconscious mind is happy to respond to the suggestions put to it by the conscious mind, provided your nervous system is in a thoroughly relaxed and trusting state and that you express your intention in the following ways:
- Phrase your affirmation as clearly and as briefly as possible, with no "ifs" and "buts", descriptions or qualifiers.

CREATIVE IMAGINING

It has been said that nothing can be imagined that we have not already experienced – either at first or second hand. We have an almost infinite variety of memories to choose from. Our life happens in our heads, so we should create as harmonious an inner world as we possibly can. There is no need to put up with a haphazard and chaotic inner world once you know how to change it. The choice is yours and meditation techniques are the tools.

- Mention just one change. When that has occurred you can replace your sankalpa because it will have become redundant.
- Describe the change you wish for in the present tense, such as "I am ... [happy, healthy, confident, successful at .., or forgiving of ...]" or, "I am becoming more and more ... day by day." The unconscious mind lives only in the present and ignores the past or future. Tomorrow never comes and is of no interest to it.
- Express your sankalpa in positive terms only, for the unconscious mind becomes confused by negative words such as "not" and "never".
- Avoid any words like "try" or "work at" or "difficult" because they immediately put the nervous system on guard and undo all the good relaxation you have achieved up to now.
- Repeat your sankalpa three times slowly and decisively, so that your unconscious mind knows you mean business. In this way you are programming it to carry out your intentions all the time – even when the conscious mind is busy with other things. This is why the sankalpa has such a powerful effect.

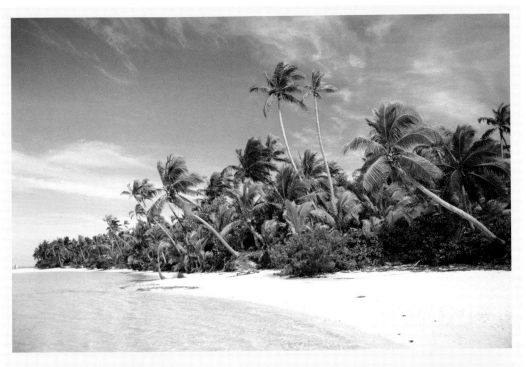

VISUALIZING A BEACH SCENE

You have become deeply relaxed, perhaps after some stretching and deep breathing exercises. Sit or lie down in a comfortable position and start to imagine yourself reclining on a beautiful beach. You are lying on soft sand near the water's edge on a pleasant sunny day. Use all your senses to appreciate all the details of the scene, so that you experience it fully.

You can feel the texture and dampness of the sand beneath you, dig your toes into it and let it run through your fingers. Look at the scenery around you, the deep blue of the sea and sky, the pale sand, the distant horizon, a few fluffy white clouds, seagulls flying overhead. You can hear the seagulls calling, the wavelets lapping across the sand and the sound of a gentle breeze moving the leaves of the trees behind you. You can smell the salt air and taste it on your

△ The beauty, warmth and peace of a tropical beach make it pleasing to all the senses, so it is an ideal subject for a visualization to help you create your happy inner world.

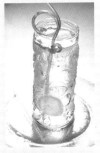

▷ The more detailed your visualization the more completely you will be able to experience the scene. Taste and feel the coolness of an iced drink on a hot day.

lips. What else can you feel, see and hear? Perhaps the air caressing your body, the intricate patterns of individual grains of sand and tiny shells, the sound of children laughing in the distance. Can you smell the sea, taste a half-eaten peach, feel the welcome coolness of the wind lifting your hair?

When you have built up all the details of this lovely scene, stay in it for a while feeling peaceful and contented, grateful and relaxed. The whole purpose of this visualization is to bring you to this inner place where you know that "all is well", now and always. Before you decide to leave the beach repeat your sankalpa (the affirmation or resolve you have already decided upon) slowly and clearly three times. Then gradually let the whole scene dissolve, knowing that it is always there for you to return to, no matter what is going on in the external world.

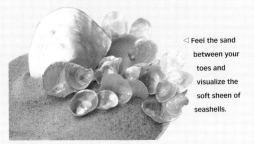

◁ Feel the sand between your toes and visualize the soft sheen of seashells.

Taking Imaginary Journeys

Visualizations while in deep relaxation are enjoyable and can reveal unexpected insights. They prepare for more structured traditional meditations.

The visualization described opposite takes you on a journey that starts with your everyday awareness and leads to a higher level of consciousness, as you walk slowly through the countryside and up a hill to your goal before returning more quickly by the same route. The Buddhist walking meditation, a practice in which the action of walking is itself the focus of awareness, can be a helpful preparation for your imaginary walk through the chakra fields. Remember to perform a grounding ritual at the end of your visualization to avoid feeling "spaced out" afterwards.

TELLING THE STORY
You may wish to make a tape of the visualization described opposite so that your voice guides you gently through it, with frequent pauses to build up the scene in your mind. Or get a friend to read it aloud to you. It should take about 20 minutes.

walking meditation

This popular Buddhist meditation combines the senses of touch, sound and sight. Walking in slow motion requires focus and concentration. Synchronize your breathing and mantra repetitions with your steps.

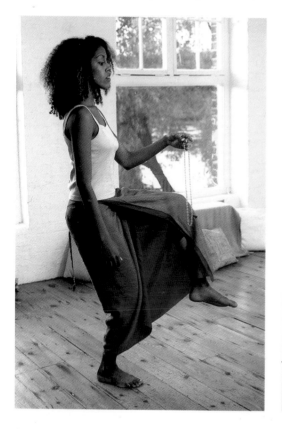

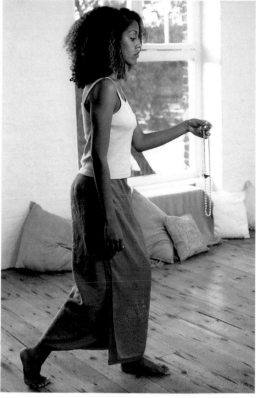

△ **1** Stand tall with your mala held in front of you at heart level. Very slowly raise one foot and step forward on to it, bending your back knee. As you step forward, keep your weight distributed evenly between both feet.

△ **2** Take your whole weight on to your front foot, lifting your back foot and standing as tall as you can. Gaze straight ahead all the time. Repeat the movements, saying your mantra with each step.

A WALK THROUGH THE CHAKRA FIELDS

Relax deeply, feeling your senses becoming very alert so that you notice every detail of your imaginary surroundings.

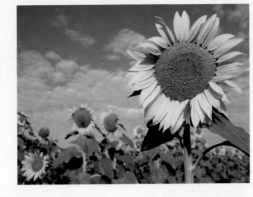

 Start by walking along a short lane that takes you to a stile giving access to a meadow. A sea of red flowers – perhaps poppies – grow in this field. They represent the vitality and growth of the base chakra. A footpath leads you gently uphill across this field to another stile. Follow this path, absorbing the vibrant redness, feeling the solid ground beneath you and the movement of your legs and feet as you walk. Inhale the natural earthy smell of living, growing plants.

The next stile takes you into a grove of orange trees laden with ripe fruit, representing the sensuality of the sacral chakra. Enjoy the abundance of nature and its glorious power to reproduce and sustain life. Eat some of the fruit, letting the delicious juices flow in your mouth. Dance your way along the path to the next stile.

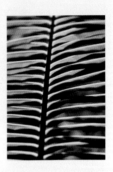

△ The sunflower's seeds store up the sun's energy, as the navel chakra stores our life force.

This leads you into a field of golden sunflowers, representing the light and heat of the navel chakra, which is often called the solar centre. Here we store our reserves of energy, or prana – just as the seeds of the sunflowers store the energy of life. Feast your eyes on the gold around you and let your skin soak up the warmth from the sun. Feel confident that your reserves of energy will always support whatever you set out to accomplish. At the end of the field is a gate in a wall.

This gate opens into a formal walled garden with a path that takes you under a long archway festooned with climbing roses in every shade of pink, luminous against their glossy green leaves and exuding heavenly scents. This beautiful garden represents your heart chakra, with its atmosphere of peace and joy. You touch the velvety petals and the roses lean down to share their beauty with you, inviting you to pick them. You take just one to keep as your constant companion, before passing through the gate at the end of the garden.

△ Notice every detail of the lush growth that fringes your path on your walk.

You find yourself on high ground under a wide blue sky across which birds are flying and calling to each other. The sky is reflected in pools of blue water from melting snows, and vivid blue gentians open their faces to the warm sun. This scene represents the throat chakra and the energies of pure space and sound. You hear your name being called and walk trustingly toward a high pass ahead of you.

Someone comes to meet you, offering to guide you onward and representing your own higher wisdom, found in your brow chakra. This chakra is often called the third eye: the "all-seeing eye" of the higher mind that unites the two hemispheres of the brain – logical intellect and creative imagination – to create insight. Your guide may tell you something or give you something to ponder upon later, before leading you over the pass.

Beyond is a grassy glade surrounded by trees. In the centre is a small white building – clearly a very special and spiritual place – that represents your crown chakra. Your guide gestures to you to enter alone, which you do very respectfully. There you sit and repeat your sankalpa, slowly and clearly, three times. You remain in this place, absorbing its spiritual energies, until you feel it is time to return to everyday awareness. You say "thank you" before rising and leaving to walk slowly back the way you have come, knowing that you can return here whenever you wish.

Back in the lane where you started your journey you become aware once more of your physical body. Take a few deep breaths, move your fingers and toes, yawn and stretch. Perform your grounding ritual to end your session, then get up slowly.

△ The endless blue sky represents the throat chakra, whose element is ether, or space.

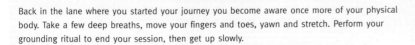

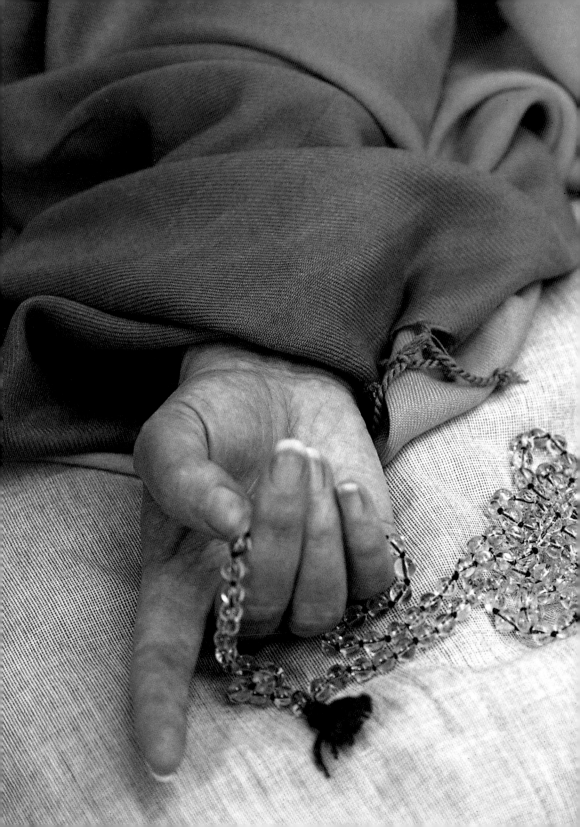

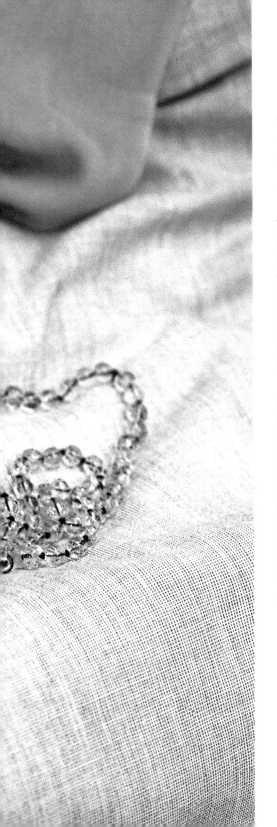

Everyday
Meditation

The ancient wisdom of both West and East offers tools to help us live in joy and peace, and can provide simple reasons to explain why and how people behave in the ways they do – so that we can better understand, accept and forgive ourselves and other people. When meditation becomes part of daily life, it can help us to improve the quality of all our interactions with the world around us.

For meditation practice we may set aside a time when we can focus our thoughts, free of the stresses and intrusions of the outside world, but meditation is not an escape from the world. Rather it is a way of expanding our consciousness to include the world, to become one with the infinite universe. Having established the habit of meditation, we can bring its mindful approach to bear on everything we do in our day-to-day existence, living our whole lives in a state of relaxed self-awareness.

Meditation in Daily Life

Many people think of the meditative state as being rather "otherworldly", something that they can only achieve if they divorce themselves from daily life. Although regular meditation practice requires that we set time aside to turn the attention inward, it can also be woven into daily life. We can turn mundane chores into a form of meditation by practising "mindfulness" – focusing all our thoughts on them; we can experience a sense of spiritual enlightenment from appreciating the beauty of everything around us; we can use meditative practices when trying to engage with and understand our emotions; and we can introduce meditative elements into the ways in which we relate to others.

▷ By focusing all your awareness on everyday activities such as eating, you can turn them into a form of meditation.

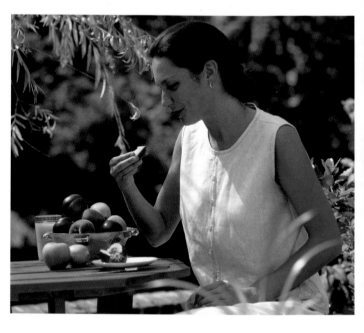

key elements

There are many ways in which you can bring meditation into every aspect of your day-to-day life:

• Focus your mind and body entirely on what you are doing at this moment, letting distractions wash around you.

• Live in the present moment as much as you can.

• Try to perceive the beauty and worth in everything (and everyone) around you, and in everything you do, no matter how mundane the task.

• Learn to use your senses to the full.

• Develop self-awareness, and work with the interplay between your emotional and physical self – noticing how certain breathing practices and positions affect your mental state, for example.

WORKING WITH YOUR FEELINGS

The following traditional technique, based on experiencing "opposites", allows you to become impartially aware of your feelings (many of which are usually below consciousness):

• Relax deeply – sitting, reclining or lying on your back.

• Imagine various "pairs of opposites" and notice the physical sensations that arise.

• Start with pairs that have little or no positive/negative emotional associations – such as hot/cold, hard/soft, light/dark – and observe

how you feel in your body while remaining deeply relaxed.

• Move on to a more emotionally challenging pair, starting with the positive side, and observe what feelings are evoked: birth/death, spacious/confined, happy/sad, delighted/angry and welcome/excluded are some examples.

• Still deeply relaxed, observe what feelings arise in your body as you contemplate the negative half of the pair – so that you can recognize and identify them from

now on and understand what "pushes your buttons" and how you feel out of sorts when your emotions are negative. You can then take appropriate action to make you feel better and defuse tension in and around you.

• Repeat the positive half of the pair before moving on to the next pair of opposites.

• End with your sankalpa and some gentle deep breathing before coming out of relaxation with a grounding ritual.

RELATING TO OTHERS

This Buddhist "loving kindness" meditation helps you to relate better to those around you. Breathe in universal love and kindness to help and support yourself, then breathe it out, directing it to a specific person or group. Repeat this meditation often, until it becomes second nature both to receive and to give loving kindness. Make it part of your daily life: any part of it can be used in any situation to promote peace and harmony.

- Relax deeply in a seated position with your spine erect.
- Breathe in, drawing "loving kindness" from the universe into yourself.
- Breathe out, directing that loving kindness with gratitude toward a particular person, or to all those who have taught you (given you light in many ways). Breathe more loving kindness into yourself.
- Breathe out, directing loving kindness with gratitude toward a particular person or to all those who have nurtured and nourished you (given you life in many forms). Breathe in...
- Breathe out, directing loving kindness with blessings toward a person or people you love dearly. Breathe in...
- Breathe out, directing loving kindness with blessings toward acquaintances, neighbours, people you work with. Breathe in...
- Breathe out, directing loving kindness with forgiveness to people who annoy or obstruct you, who are unkind or dismissive. Breathe in...
- Breathe out, directing loving kindness with forgiveness to anyone who has ever hurt or injured you in any way. Breathe in...
- Breathe out, radiating the prayer, "May all people everywhere be happy." Breathe in and give thanks for all the loving kindness you receive. Pause before coming out of your meditation and grounding yourself with a ritual.

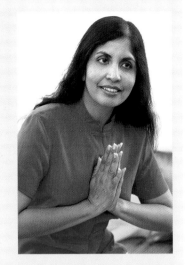

△ The traditional Indian greeting "Namaste", spoken with a bow while bringing the hands together at the heart chakra, acknowledges the presence of the divine in the heart of each person, conveying the sense that everyone is part of the unity of creation.

how are you feeling?

As a way of linking the physical and non-physical, it is important to get into the habit of noticing consciously what your senses are telling your mind. This makes it much easier to monitor your emotions as they arise, because you can feel them through your senses. In fact, there is no other way to feel how you are "feeling". For every emotion there is a corresponding physical sensation: we "see red" when angry, our legs "turn to jelly" when we are frightened, sadness makes the heart "ache" or we are "in the dark" when confused.

Once you learn to recognize how you are actually feeling you can avoid reacting negatively to everyday situations. Whenever you notice a negative feeling arising, pause for an instant (the proverbial "counting to ten"), relax and visualize the positive, opposite feeling. You can then respond in a positive manner instead, bringing what you have learned through the regular practice of meditation into your daily life.

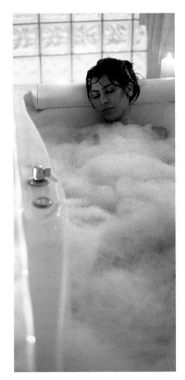

▷ Use the time you spend in the bath or shower each day to relax and enjoy the present moment.

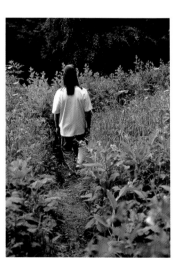

◁ When you take a walk among plants and trees, focus your whole mind and all your senses on the experience, noticing the beauty of everything you pass along your path. Plants teach us how to "just be".

Getting to Know Yourself

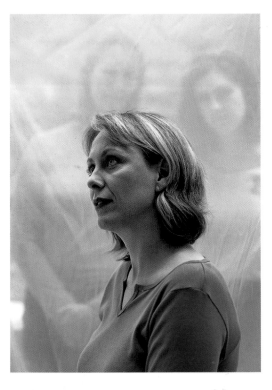

AVOIDING OVER-ATTACHMENT

It is a mistake to become too attached to any one of the three gunas – even the bright and beautiful sattva guna. The gunas are strands of nature, which is described as energy in flux, ever-changing and therefore never real. Traditional prayers are often chanted for dissolving our attachment to nature and the gunas, in order to focus on the eternal reality of consciousness (or spirit). The following mantras (translated from the Sanskrit) are frequently used for group and private meditation:

Lead us from the unreal to
the real,
From darkness to light
And from death to immortality.

▽ **We seek freedom from attachment rather like a ripe cucumber falling from the vine.**

... May Siva [supreme consciousness] liberate all beings. May he liberate us from death [the impermanence of nature and the gunas] for the sake of immortality [living in the eternal now] even as the ripe cucumber drops naturally from the vine [of attachments].

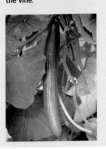

Everyone can benefit from getting into the habit of recognizing the various forces that make us think, feel and behave as we do in our daily lives. It is helpful to consider these forces working within us in terms of the chakras, koshas and gunas. Even when we are alone, our behaviour, thoughts and attitudes reflect the interactions between the koshas that are constantly taking place within the chakras.

correcting imbalances

Describing these inner processes in terms of the three gunas can help us to become aware of any imbalances. The three strands of the gunas are interwoven at every level: at the physical (anna maya kosha) levels, at energetic (prana maya kosha) levels, the instinctive mental (mano maya kosha) and intellectual (vijnana maya kosha) levels,

△ **Meditation allows you to quieten the constant background chatter of your thoughts to contemplate things clearly and impartially, fostering greater self-knowledge.**

and also at the level of feeling and purpose (ananda maya kosha).

We cannot escape the qualities of tamas, rajas and sattva, but through meditation we can learn to influence which one is dominant. In tamas we are stuck fast, going nowhere and achieving nothing. We need the desire and energy of rajas to get things moving, but too much makes us the slaves of passion. A balance of tamas and rajas – of rest and exertion – brings sattva, in which peace and balance can predominate. This is the state required for meditation: the preliminary practices such as stretching and breathing are designed to achieve and maintain sattva, in which a

balanced nervous system can respond appropriately to each moment as it arises.

Meditation allows us to stand back and observe ourselves impartially, as witnesses who are prepared to accept what we find, reflect on it and then create change. We can restore inner harmony whenever we feel it slipping from us, and live in the harmonious state of being that Patanjali described:

... the qualities of the heart are cultivated:
friendliness towards the joyful,
compassion towards the suffering,
happiness towards the pure
and impartiality towards the impure.
Yoga Sutras, Ch 1,
translated by Alistair Shearer

This is what is known to Buddhists as the "practice of the four virtues".

Lord Krisna's dance – developing harmony and balance

Krisna is the Hindu lord of love and the embodiment of divine beauty and joy. He expresses love's eternal flow through movement. The air moves through his reed flute to create enchanting music, and his body moves in joyful dance. This is an active balancing meditation that helps to bring about physical and mental harmony.

"Energy and consciousness reflect each other."

Traditional yogic wisdom

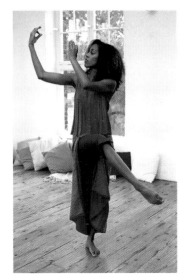

△ **1** Stand tall on your left leg, and slowly raise your right leg up and across to the left. Then turn your trunk to the right, raising both your arms to the right as if you are holding and playing a flute. "Hear" the music you are playing while "feeling" Krisna's lightness and joy.

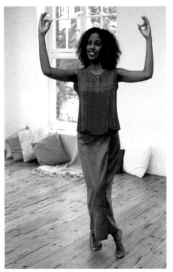

△ **2** Lower your right foot gracefully to the floor, stepping across the left, and turn to face straight ahead, keeping your arms raised. Transfer your weight to your right foot and raise your left leg to repeat the dancing step, turning your body to the left.

CHART YOUR STATE OF BEING

Remember that a degree of tamas and rajas is necessary in life – it is only unhealthy if one of these states dominates. We progress from tamas through rajas to the balanced state of sattva.

TAMAS

The quality of inertia in nature, tamas is a form of poverty and stagnation that can make us feel trapped and deprived. It constricts the flow of life-light-love, preventing us from experiencing and sharing natural spontaneity, inspiration and joy. It saps our energy, making us build emotional walls around ourselves.

Stuck in timetables and routine
Ignorance and prejudice
Timidity, fear, victim mentality
Dependency on other people
Low energy, self-neglect, poor diet
Illness, helplessness, pain
Grief, regrets, sadness
Hopelessness
Poverty

RAJAS

Here there is too much of everything – especially passion, spreading out of control like a forest fire. Rajas makes us restless and full of unsatisfied desire; we become aggressive and insensitive to the needs and feelings of others. When rajas is dominant we see other people only as objects that are there to be exploited and manipulated.

Self-centred impatience and disregard
Contempt for tradition, risk-taking
Self-confidence, arrogance, aggression
Ambition, wilfulness, domination
Greed, drive, eventual burnout
Determination to survive, lust for life
Concentration on the future
Feverish desire
Determination to succeed no matter what

SATTVA

The quality of balance or harmony in nature, sattva makes tamas and rajas become complementary and positive rather than destructive, creating light to dissolve both darkness and passion. The sattva guna is calm, pure and kind, but it is still part of the changing pattern of nature rather than unchanging consciousness or spirit.

Spontaneity and co-operation
Understanding and respect
Trust and willingness to share
Self-reliance and inner guidance
Healthy balanced lifestyle
Acceptance and living life fully
Living joyfully in the now
Faith in the process and divine plan
Content with "enough" and inner joy

Energetic Exercise as Meditation

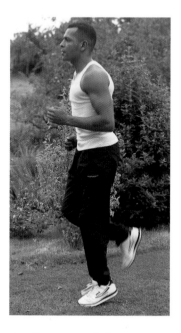

If you are bound up in a demanding working life it is easy to feel that you have no time to spare for relaxation or physical exercise. But trying to maintain a high level of mental activity throughout your waking hours soon becomes counter-productive, leading to stress, exhaustion and illness.

A regular exercise routine not only helps to keep the physical body fit and healthy, but also contributes to a balanced lifestyle, helping you to live a busy life with the minimum of stress. Vigorous exercise produces a natural feeling of wellbeing, even euphoria, because it stimulates the release of endorphins, the body's own painkillers, in the brain, making you feel good and releasing mental tension. When you are feeling tamasic – tired and

◁ Building exercise into your daily routine helps you to achieve a healthy balance between work, rest and exertion, raising your energy levels.

sluggish – vigorous exercise may seem a daunting prospect, but its rajasic nature can promote the balanced state of sattva if it becomes a regular part of your daily life.

This feeling of inner balance leads to meditation in action – while travelling, at work, at home, at play and in all relationships. Affection, openness, focus and witnessing become your predominant attitudes and frustration, irritability and mood swings are far less frequent.

exercise for relaxation

Energetic exercises, such as the examples shown on these pages, loosen contracted muscles, unwinding stress and unblocking the flow of energy in the body. Whether you choose yoga, dancing, swimming, jogging, go to the gym or play a team sport, the release of tension brought about by exercise allows you to relax fully afterwards, in preparation for the meditative state.

developing spatial awareness

If you practise yoga, a real understanding of the subtleties of the classical poses will help to develop your spiritual and physical awareness, which are vital for successful meditation. Insight can be gained by trying them out in different ways, as with Adho Mukha Svanasana (downward facing dog pose), a vigorous posture that gets the energy flowing.

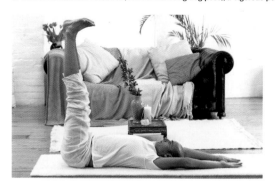

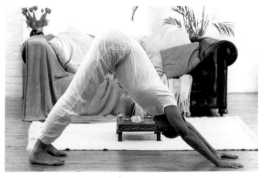

△ 1 The pose lying down: in this position, gravity presses your spine flat against the floor so that it is elongated and the chest is opened as you stretch your arms over your head, maintaining contact with the floor from shoulders to fingertips. Your legs are straight and exactly vertical, at right angles to the spine and with heels pushed to the ceiling. Notice where you are stretching and opening the body, and feel which muscles are working.

△ 2 The pose from standing: the classical pose is more vigorous, as you are pushing upward against gravity with your arms and legs. Make exactly the same right-angled shape with your body and maintain the feeling of the flat elongated spine and open chest that you experienced when lying down. Experimenting by inverting the pose will have made you far more aware of what it involves.

cross-crawl exercise

This is a series of vigorous dancelike movements that "wakes up" the brain as well as the body by requiring you to move in an unaccustomed way that requires conscious thought. When you always make certain movements in the same way, you develop neural "habit pathways". This kind of exercise is designed to challenge you to adapt to doing things differently. Similar well-known exercises include the tricks of patting your head with one hand while rubbing your abdomen in circles with the other, or making circles with one arm to a count of three and simultaneously circling the other arm to a count of four.

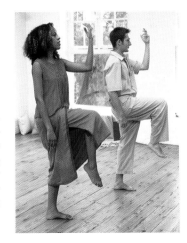

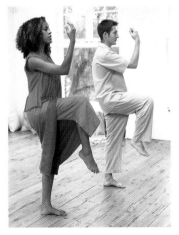

△ **1** Marching vigorously on the spot, raise your right thigh and left upper arm parallel to the floor for several beats.

△ **2** Without missing a beat, change to raising your right thigh and right upper arm together, followed by your left thigh and left upper arm. Continue marching on the spot for the same number of beats, then change smoothly back to step 1 and repeat.

ball of energy

This is a moving visualization that increases spontaneity and flexibility, and makes a good warm-up before vigorous exercise. It engages all the chakras, building firm yet springy strength in the life chakras (abdomen, legs and feet), openness and expansiveness and free expression in the love chakras (chest and neck) and focus and imagination in the light chakras (skull).

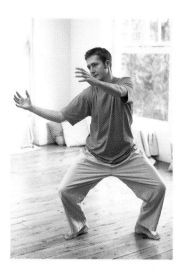

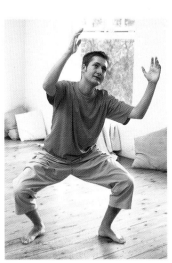

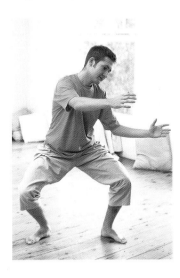

△ **1** Stand with the knees loose and springy, the spine stretched up out of the pelvis and the chest open. Start creating an imaginary "ball of energy" between your palms by pushing them lightly against resistance in a kneading motion. They will naturally find the right distance apart after a few moments as you begin to feel the energy passing between them.

△ **2** Toss the ball of energy up in the air and catch it again, stretching loosely and keeping your knees springy. Stay grounded by keeping your feet firmly in contact with the floor. Do not move them.

△ **3** Take the ball of energy to the side in a sweeping circle, then down, to the front and up the other side in a series of sweeping stretches of the upper body. Keep focused on it and enjoy playing with it. Feel the groundedness of your lower body contrasting with the freedom of your upper body and the spontaneity of your movements.

Repetitive Tasks as Meditation

Performing simple repetitive tasks can become an excellent form of meditation. Such tasks can be very soothing – it all depends upon your attitude. If you are feeling relaxed and in a sattvic frame of mind you can enjoy focusing upon the gentle rhythms of going for a walk, chopping vegetables, filing at the office, knitting, sewing, weeding the garden – even vacuuming the house or doing the washing up. If, on the other hand, you are feeling tamasic – tired and bored – such tasks seem like drudgery and make you feel trapped. In a rajasic mood you may feel impatient and frustrated and your mind will wander as you daydream about doing something or being somewhere more exciting.

mindfulness

By giving all your attention to a simple repetitive task you become aware of every detail of what you are doing, living fully in the present and bringing all your senses to bear on the experience. In this relaxed state of awareness, the mind simply witnesses all that you are doing and thinking, without judging or reacting to it. It stays clear, attentive and receptive.

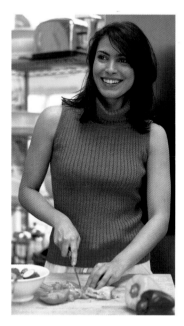

△ The caring act of preparing food can be an ideal focus for meditation if, unlike this woman, you do not let distractions intrude. As you peel and slice, use all your senses to become fully aware of the food's texture, colour, scent and form.

"Wherever we go we have to take ourselves with us."
Traditional wisdom

written mantras

Likhit japa is the traditional practice of writing or drawing a mantra over and over again rather than chanting it aloud. The mantra that is most often used in this form of meditation is the symbol OM, which is carefully drawn repeatedly on a page while repeating the sound silently in your mind with each repetition of the symbol.

Like other repetitive tasks, likhit japa is a way to keep the mind focused and still. It is considered a powerful form of mantra use because it reinforces the habit of silent repetition of the mantra. It is a very pleasant and creative task to do in a meditation group – perhaps after lunch when everyone

The Story of the Sweeping Monk

There was once a Zen Buddhist monk who was given the task of maintaining the monastery garden. It was typical of such gardens – a simple courtyard spread with raked gravel, with a few large stones and potted plants arranged to create an atmosphere of peace and harmony. There was also a stately tree in the garden.

The monk swept up all the leaves that had fallen from the tree, deadheaded and tidied the plants, then raked the gravel in smooth sweeping strokes as he backed out toward the entrance. Just as he closed the gate a single leaf fell from the tree right into the middle of the courtyard. His fellow monks commiserated with him: "What a shame! Just when it was so perfect."

"Not at all," replied the gardener with a radiant smile, "I am simply being given another opportunity to serve." He opened the gate and walked across the gravel, disturbing its smoothness with his footprints. He picked up the leaf and calmly proceeded to back his way out again, raking the gravel as he went – still smiling, still focused, still enjoying his own company, still enveloped in deep peace and joy.

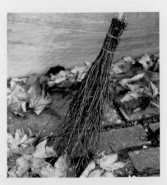

△ The story of the sweeping monk is an example of the spiritual enlightenment that can come from performing everyday tasks.

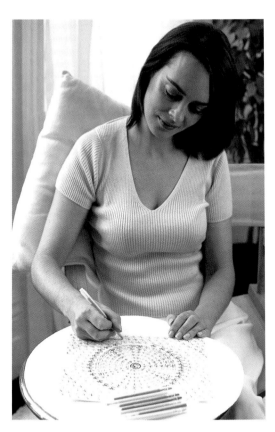

◁ When doing likhit japa, repeat the mantra silently in your head each time you draw the symbol, focusing your attention on its meaning. The aim is to preserve the rhythm of the repetitions, as if you were chanting the mantra.

▽ A written mantra such as the OM symbol can be used creatively, drawing with different coloured pencils to make a pattern or an original picture. Hindus sometimes write the symbols on birch bark or leaves, or use them to build up a picture of a deity.

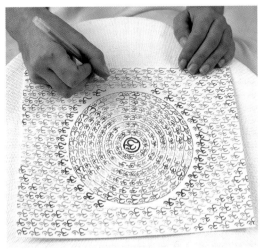

wants to relax – or at home alone as a way of unwinding.

The ways in which likhit japa can be performed seem infinite. Some Hindu monks keep a notebook and a pencil in their pocket and simply draw neat rows of OMs across the page whenever they have a spare moment. The aim is to fulfil a self-appointed task – such as drawing 100,000 OMs, perhaps aiming for a definite number on each page.

Other mantras can be copied out in a similar way, or you can use a phrase that is meaningful to you, such as "world peace", repeating it with intent that the world will become ever more peaceful as a result of your thought vibrations: every action starts with a thought, and if enough people think the same thought they can change the world. You can draw a symbol, such as a dove, to represent your repeated phrase, covering your page with a flock of birds that will continue to remind you of the thought that you sent out to bring

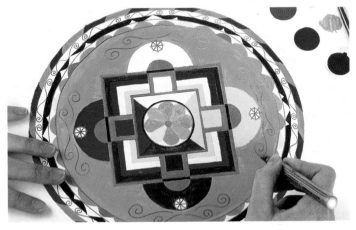

healing to the world while you were doing likhit japa meditation. There are many other familiar symbols that represent spiritual inspiration and which you could draw repeatedly in lines or patterns to reinforce the appropriate feelings in yourself – you might choose a rose to represent

△ Creating and contemplating a mandala, a symbolic representation of the universe, is another valuable form of meditation.

"unconditional love", a flame for "the divine presence within", or joined palms in prayer or greeting for "we are all one".

Hobbies and Skills as Meditation

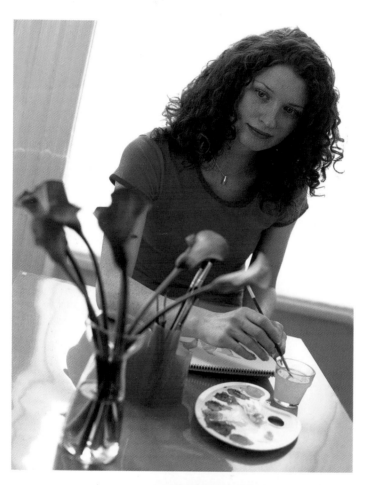

Like exercise and rest, spending time on skills and crafts we love is an important element of a balanced, harmonious life that can lead us away from the negativity of tamas and the self-obsession of rajas. Learning new skills simply for the pleasure of doing so, and spending time on hobbies we enjoy, are ways in which we can relax and develop a sattvic attitude to life, which is the way to higher consciousness and the state of meditation.

a state of self-forgetfulness

Once you experience the fact that it is not so much what you do as how you do it that leads to a state of meditation in daily life, endless possibilities become available. This is the essence of *karma* yoga – actions performed in a state of self-forgetfulness. The sattvic state induces relaxed concentration on the task in hand simply because it is there to be done and enjoyed for its own sake.

Both tamas and rajas increase self-centredness, whereas sattva is an open state of unconditional welcome to each moment as it arises and to all the relationships contained therein. It is a state in which you can lose yourself in what you are doing – and find that you enjoy your own company as a result. This is why hobbies are so satisfying and an excellent way to develop sattvic qualities.

Creative writing, for example, can be a very meditative experience. You are alone with your thoughts and really have to get to know yourself. An excellent way to start is by writing a spiritual diary, containing your feelings, dreams and insights, which helps to develop self-awareness. If you enjoy painting, you can spend many happy hours observing and recording the beauties of nature. Or you can let your imagination run riot, as children do, and see what appears on the paper – this can also be very psychologically revealing and further develop your self-awareness.

△ **Creative hobbies such as painting foster self-surrender: it is not how well you perform or the end result that matters, but your enjoyment of relating to your subject and materials.**

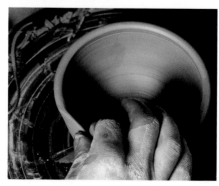

▷ **There is something intensely satisfying and releasing about the skill of making pots, where all your attention is concentrated on the symmetry of the shape you are creating and the feel of the clay.**

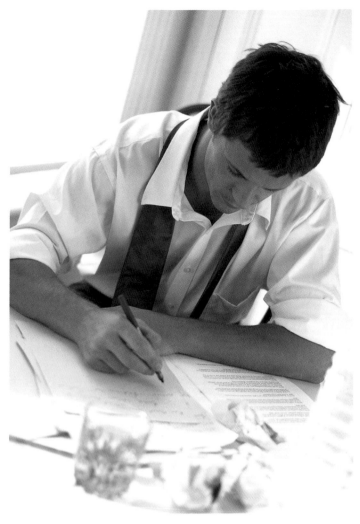

◁ Focus on the creative and enjoyable aspects of your job – making work into a form of stimulating play – and you will increase its rewards. Approach mundane or difficult tasks with an attitude of self-discipline, to help you achieve what you set out to do to your own satisfaction.

▽ Supporting each other in interesting and rewarding pastimes brings a great deal of mutual pleasure, raises energy levels, and helps to create a harmonious, sattvic home.

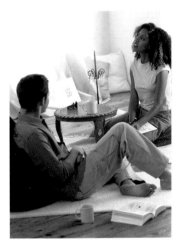

making work into play

With practice, you can even turn the work you are paid to do into your favourite "hobby" if you approach it with the right attitude, so that you can honestly say: "I am so lucky to be paid to do what I enjoy." Meditation practice can help you look for ways to get greater enjoyment from what you do for a living.

The reverse can also occur – an enjoyable hobby can become a tiresome burden if you feel under an obligation to deliver. The

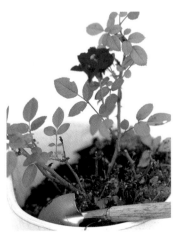

▷ Gardening brings the pleasure of watching plants grow and the feeling that you are working in harmony with nature.

most interesting job or the most skilful pastime may become a chore if it is approached with a negative attitude. Patanjali's three "preliminary practices" – self-discipline, self-awareness and self-surrender – can help you restore your interest and pleasure.

Self-discipline is a contract you make with yourself to complete what you set out to do, regardless of whether any demands are being made on you by others. Self-awareness is the art of recognizing unwillingness and procrastination as an aspect of tamas and taking steps to renew your enthusiasm for the project (balancing with rajas) so that you can start again with an attitude of self-surrender and self-forgetfulness (sattva). Like the gunas, Patanjali's three qualities resemble the interwoven strands of a single rope and without all three of them, little of real worth or enjoyment can be accomplished.

Focusing the Mind

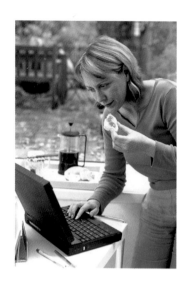

◁ Modern life is made even more complex by technology that allows us to do several tasks at once. Concentrate on one thing at a time.

▷ When the phone rings, focus on it briefly rather than grabbing it immediately, giving yourself time to settle and prepare your mind.

Centripetal force is energy that flows from the edges to the middle, as when you pick up sensations from the surface of the body and register them consciously in the brain. All the practices that prepare for meditation have the quality of drawing energies back into your central self, into a deep pool or store. Using this energy, you can respond richly to life in a sattvic, conscious, focused and loving manner, directing your full attention to each task.

directed attention

"Alternating current" flowing between a subject (me) and an object (you) is a simple way to describe all relationships. This current needs to be focused rather than dissipated

if relationships are to be nourishing and creative. The Sanskrit word for this is *ekagrata*. It means "one-pointedness" and refers to the process of gathering attention in from the periphery and then directing it on to a specific object. Ekagrata is a

The demands of modern life can tempt you to attend to several things at once – with the result that nothing is done with full awareness, your attention is fragmented and you lose your sattvic outlook on life. Regular meditation practice helps you to recover a focused approach, dealing with each moment as it arises calmly and giving it your full attention.

pulling in opposite directions

According to the teachings of yoga the mind tends to function in two opposing ways: centrifugally and centripetally.

Centrifugal force is when energy is drawn away from the centre to the periphery, where it is dissipated and loses its force. This is what happens when you allow worldly attachments to grab and hold your attention, hang on to negative emotions and prejudices, or try to do everything at once. Spreading yourself too thinly without refocusing squanders your energies, letting them drain away like water being scattered across sand, so that you end up feeling depleted and unfulfilled. Wasting your vital forces in this way leads to stress, exhaustion and eventually to illness.

▽ As you water a plant, focus on its beauty and the care you are giving it. Bringing the whole of your attention to each action is a form of meditation in itself, and makes any routine daily task more rewarding.

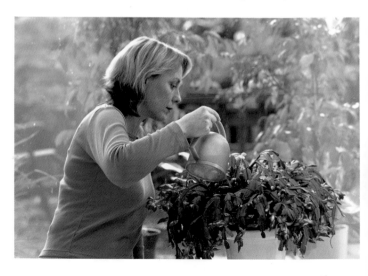

"TIME OUT" PREVENTS "BURNOUT"

Most of us need more time for ourselves and this can usually be achieved by following Patanjali's advice. Self-discipline enables you to say "no" and keep certain periods of the day sacrosanct for your own recharging and deep healing. With self-awareness, when you feel you are losing your focus you can stop to stretch, breathe, or repeat a mantra to bring you back into sattvic balance before proceeding. Self-surrender enables you to let go of all unnecessary or negative concerns, feelings or thoughts and to simplify your lifestyle, trusting in the divine guidance and support within yourself that is just waiting for you to draw upon it. Your "higher self" will never force its attentions upon you – it is up to you to seek within, to ask for help and to make time to be receptive to your inner voice through meditation.

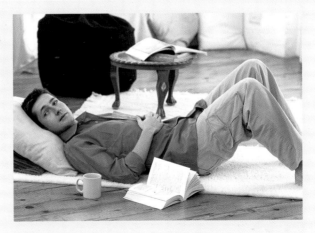

△ When taking time out, find a private space and don't let yourself be distracted by other people, near and distant noises or worrying about other demands on your time. Cultivating self-awareness will give you the confidence to take a break when you need one.

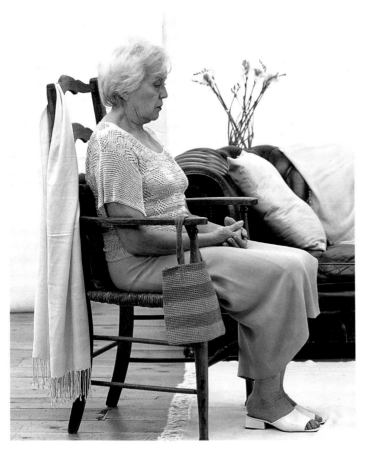

rhythmical two-way mental process similar to the physical process of breathing in and out, and the emotional process of receiving sensations and responding appropriately. We are seldom fully aware of how much energy is tied up in long-term attachments, hopes, fears, plans and resentments that bind us to the past or future and prevent us from living fully in the present.

coping with life's demands

Modern technology often makes it possible to do several tasks at once. In the office you may be listening to instructions, designing a spreadsheet on a computer and taking a telephone call, but it is all too easy to forget part of the instructions, mess up the spreadsheet and be unhelpful to the caller. Domestic situations can dissipate energy in the same way – absentmindedly answering a child's questions while driving a car in heavy traffic having left late for an appointment, then forgetting to pick up the cleaning. The more you can release energy tied up in supporting negative emotions and thought patterns, the more will be available to support your busy life instead.

◁ Before going out to keep an appointment, a short meditation will help you to centre your energy and clear your mind.

Using the Language of Mudras

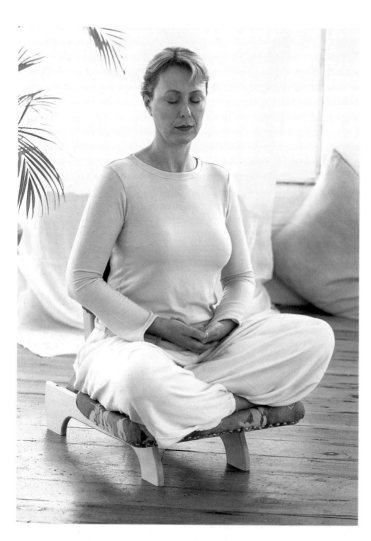

◁ The traditional postures for meditation are designed to promote the flow of energy through the koshas, but with regular practice the position you adopt becomes a trigger that helps you gain the meditative state. As you settle yourself into your customary position (or mudra) your breathing slows and deepens, mental chatter is stilled and you can begin your journey inward.

also create a different mood within. When you are feeling dull or irritable, pause to breathe deeply and relax and see how your mood improves.

the purpose of mudras

If you are in a sattvic mood you will radiate relaxation and peacefulness simply by the way you stand, move and sit. When you hold your body in a sattvic pose, breathing peacefully, alert yet relaxed, you actually become sattvic – and this is the general purpose of mudras. They alter the flow of prana through the koshas and balance the nervous systems. They use body language to achieve specific results.

hand mudras

Hand positions (*hasta mudras*) reveal a great deal. Many everyday positions demonstrate a sattvic attitude: for example, a handshake signifies trust and friendship (by offering the hand in which you would traditionally have held a weapon) and joining your palms at your heart with a bow to accompany the Indian greeting "Namaste" signifies respect and love for another person.

Many energy circuits terminate at the fingertips, as is well known in therapeutic disciplines that "move" or "rebalance" energies, such as acupuncture, shiatsu and reflexology. By positioning the hands in certain ways we can, therefore, reduce negative feelings and enhance positive ones by creating a positive flow of energy.

To begin with you may need to hold a hand mudra for half an hour or so to feel its subtle effects, but once you have practised

---

The Sanskrit word *mudra* means "attitude" or "gesture". It refers to a physical position that reflects our mood, changes our breathing pattern or alters our state of consciousness. The attitudes we strike, often unconsciously, constitute our "body language", which other people recognize and respond to. They reveal how body and mind are a unity: thought (mood) affects energy and energy (movement) affects thought.

body language and the gunas

Someone in a tamasic mood will slouch and droop, looking tired or bored or unco-operative. A person in a rajasic mood will show anger or excitement by thrusting the chin forward aggressively, waving arms about, or clenching fists. In each case a change of posture can help to change the mood. A different stance not only conveys a different message to other people, but can

There are a great many hand mudras that can help you to remain in a peaceful sattvic state in any situation.

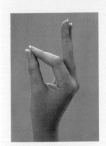

◁ *Gyana mudra*: This mudra is used for practising meditation. The tip of the thumb (cosmic consciousness) is joined to the tip of the index finger (individual or personality consciousness), so that the energies are harmonized. Often the fingernail of the index finger is pressed into the cleft between the root of the thumb and the rest of the hand to represent letting go of the ego in surrender to the greater good. This mudra can help you to restrain your self-centred impulses whenever you feel threatened.

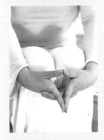

◁ *Yoni mudra*: Join your palms, then clasp the middle (sattva), ring (rajas) and little (tamas) fingers together, so that the energies mingle. Open the palms, keeping the index finger and thumb tips joined, with the index fingers (ego) pointing down and thumbs (cosmic consciousness) pointing up. This mudra protects you by taking your energies inward and back to the source (*yoni* means "womb"). Use it in crowded places, when you are travelling or wherever there are angry or disturbed energies.

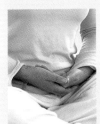

◁ *Bhairava mudra* (for men), *bhairavi mudra* (for women): The Buddha is often portrayed using this mudra. Men place the right palm over the left, and women the left over the right, both palms facing up with fingers relaxed. The thumb tips may touch to close the energy circuits. This mudra focuses your energy for meditation or to maintain inner peace when relating to others. The *anjali mudra* is similar, but with the hands more open in a gesture of prayerful pleading.

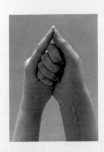

◁ *Sankha mudra* (the conch shell): Fold the fingers of your right hand around your left thumb, covering the back of the right hand with your left fingers. Touch your right thumb tip to your left index fingertip and place your hands in your lap. A conch shell, when placed to your ear, makes a sound like the sea – it is one of the sounds of nada, the inner vibration. When you blow into a conch shell it sounds like OM, the primordial vibration, recalling the vibrational basis of all phenomena.

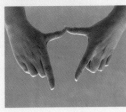

◁ *Sakat mudra*: This mudra is used to control anger. Spread the palms and point the index (ego) finger of each hand downwards to release pent-up tension that might otherwise escape in angry words. Press the thumb tips (cosmic consciousness) together to unblock the preoccupation with what is unimportant in the greater scheme of things.

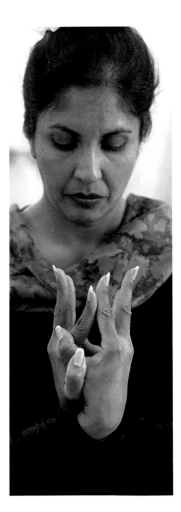

△ Once you are practised in using hand mudras, try creating meditative sequences from a range of different positions, or invent mudras of your own. You could devise a graceful "hand dance" that promotes a serene, contemplative state.

and become thoroughly familiar with it, adopting it will immediately produce the desired sattvic effect.

You can use a hand mudra unobtrusively, as an instant trigger that changes your energies. An example is the use of a mala (or Christian rosary or Muslim worry beads). If you practise regularly it is enough, in difficult situations, to simply visualize yourself passing your mala beads through your hand (using your inner senses of sight and touch) to evoke a sattvic mood and feel centred and at peace.

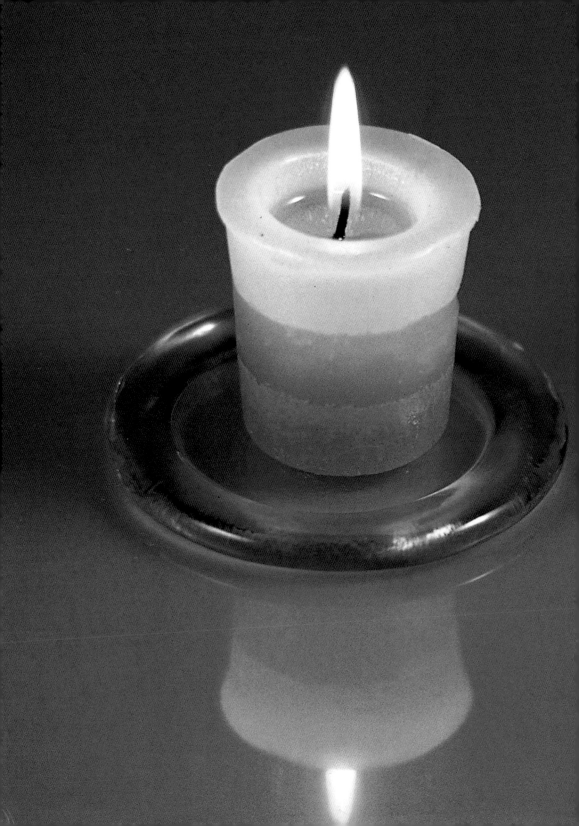

Sample Meditations

The meditations in this chapter are designed to help you to a deeper understanding of your own evolutionary path into the wisdom and love of your soul nature. The previous chapters have shown why it is so important to become balanced at all levels, and how the traditional "good" qualities are the natural expression of our higher selves.

Practising the meditations described on the following pages can help to bring healing to your relationships and even to the planet. The subjects suggested for contemplation include some of the precepts on which the sage Patanjali based his system of yoga – such as *ahimsa*, the principle of non-violence that is at the core of "right living" – and an exploration of the chakra system that governs the body, mind and emotions.

Meditation may be silent or accompanied by sounds such as the chanting of a mantra. It may be practised alone or in a group: the loving co-operation of the members generates a powerful energy that we can tap into to find healing and wholeness.

Meditating on: the Five Yamas

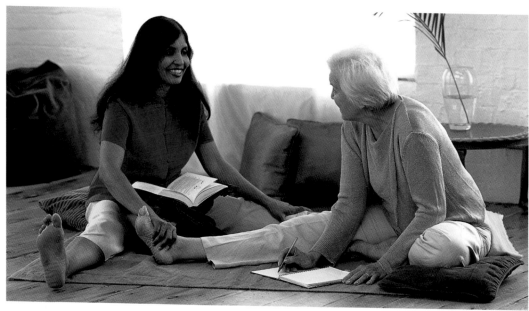

Patanjali, the great master of classical yoga, based his system of eight limbs on the ethical foundation of the yamas. These five precepts deal with personal integrity, self-restraint and respect for other people and all forms of life, and Patanjali presents them as "abstentions" to be practised in thought, word and deed. If we could return instantly to a state of sattva every time rajas or tamas became inappropriate we would automatically be practising Patanjali's yamas, known collectively as "the great vow" or "rules for living".

By making one of the yamas the focus of a contemplative meditation, we can explore the ideas it presents and gain insights that we can continue to reflect and act on after the meditation, thus improving our interactions with the wider world and with other people.

ahimsa

Together we form "society", yet exploitation of the weak and vulnerable, causing infinite pain and distress, underlies the competitive structure of our modern materialist society and is responsible for much of the misery in the world. *Ahimsa* is abstention from violence, aggression, domination and harm to any living thing, including human beings, and this first precept, which is central to the concept of "right living", is common to all the world's great religions and underpins the other four yamas.

△ The essence of the five yamas is that they promote an attitude of acceptance, respect and love for people around you as they are, rather than as commodities for exploitation.

satya

The principle of *satya* is abstention from falsehood, deceit, concealment and economy with the truth. Global advertising, big

DISCURSIVE OR CONTEMPLATIVE MEDITATION

The meditation on the yamas featured on these pages is a contemplative, or discursive, kind of meditation. With this type of meditation awareness is focused upon a concept – rather than a sensation or a physical object – to bring new understanding. The thoughts that arise concerning the chosen idea are observed without judgment and can be written down as they occur to you without disturbing either the focus or the train of thought. Have paper and pen beside you before you start the meditation so that you can record your insights immediately or soon after meditating, before they have faded from your mind. You will be surprised at the depth and clarity of your new ideas: they may change your whole attitude to concepts or feelings that you were previously unaware of, or took for granted.

contemplative meditation

Allow at least half an hour of uninterrupted time for contemplative meditation on one of Patanjali's yamas. Later you may wish to spend longer. A timer can be useful, so that you know when to start coming out of your meditation, leaving enough time to ground yourself and write down the insights you have gained in order to reflect upon them later.

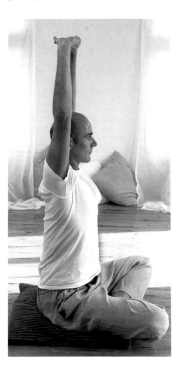

△ **1** Sit with your spine erect and stretch and settle your body into a relaxed, alert position by stretching the arms overhead, with the fingers intertwined.

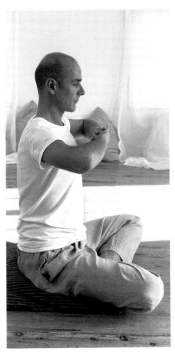

△ **2** Lowering your elbows to shoulder level, concentrate your attention on your breathing, lifting and opening the chest.

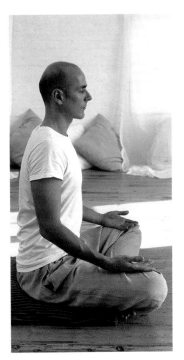

△ **3** Open your hands and let them rest, palms up, on your knees. You may like to repeat a mantra for a few moments, or the name of the yama you plan to explore, to settle yourself into a sattvic state.

business, politicians and the media break this abstention at every turn. The desire to hoodwink others – purposely eroding the boundaries between truth and falsehood – arises from a lack of respect for them. Patanjali's practice of self-awareness, which helps us to see and accept ourselves as we are, allows us to see more clearly through self-deception and intentional distortion wherever they occur, to be less seduced by glamour and hype and more focused on values that are genuine.

asteya

Self-interest and the profit motive stem from the belief that "what is yours is mine and what is mine is also mine". *Asteya* is abstention from theft, taking advantage,

giving less than is due, getting something for nothing and all other forms of exploitation. Patanjali's practice of self-surrender loosens the grip of "me and mine" until we realize that we own nothing: we enter the world at birth without possessions and leave them behind when we die. Everything that we use and enjoy in life is only on loan.

brahmacharya

This is abstention from lust and greed, which are disrespectful and rajasic and cause us to dissipate our life energies. Modern society is increasingly obsessed with sexual gratification, and we are encouraged by liberalism and advertising to feel entitled to take whatever we desire. *Brahmacharya* is

associated with sexual abstinence, but actually concerns lust and greed of all kinds. It is about respecting the life force within ourselves and directing it toward personal evolution rather than personal gratification. Loving partnership supports life and evolution, whereas lust does not.

aparigraha

The fifth yama is abstention from acquiring and hoarding possessions for their own sake, seeing ourselves in terms of what we have rather than who we are. Keeping life simple prevents us from tying up time, money and energy worrying about mere things. It frees us to focus on more rewarding pursuits and relationships and upon living fully rather than on the pursuit of lifeless things.

Meditating on: Opposing Qualities

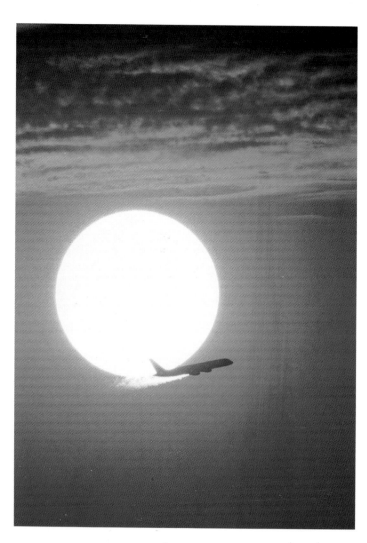

◁ The ultimate aim of meditation is the transcendent state of samadhi, in which the truth is clearly seen. It has been likened by the scholar I.K. Taimni to the experience of a pilot flying out of a cloud bank into bright sunlight.

through sharing. Bad feelings in the light chakras result from confusion and a sense of disconnectedness, whereas good feelings come with understanding and access to higher wisdom.

Transcendence depends upon cultivating and maintaining good feelings and a positive outlook on life. Gratitude, acceptance, respect and personal responsibility are just some of the positive qualities of the yamas. Positive qualities make us feel good – even to reflect on them brings peace and joy, helping to lead us inward toward a state of deep meditation, which we can experience in the balanced, contented sattvic state. Having entered the meditation in a sattvic state the chosen object of meditation can further deepen our good feelings.

meditating on opposites

Taking one obstacle that is currently hindering you as the focus of a contemplative meditation can be very helpful, provided you can accept that it is just "one face of the coin" – the negative face – and aim to bring it into balance so that it no longer disturbs you. Ask yourself what is its opposite face – the positive and sattvic aspect? Having established that, and having truly felt the positive as keenly as you previously felt the negative, you are ready for the most important question: what is the "substance" of the coin that is now showing you its two complementary faces?

Opposites are always complementary parts of a greater whole, the poles that connect the energy of a continuum – nothing either good or bad exists in isolation. This type of meditation brings a much wider perspective on life and frees you from the "slavery of the opposites".

Meditation increases self-awareness, but this alone is not enough to achieve lasting change and spiritual evolution. If we are to transcend the programming created and reinforced by our genes and conditioning, we also need to engage self-discipline and self-surrender. All the different kinds of energy in the chakras need to be balanced and working together.

good and bad feelings

We feel bad in the life chakras if we are hungry (feeling lack), embarrassed (feeling fear of criticism) or angry (feeling thwarted) and we experience good feelings when eating a delicious meal, socializing happily or moving toward a goal. Bad feelings in the love chakras arise from self-centredness and blocked self-expression, and good feelings

PAIRS OF OPPOSITES

Patanjali describes the yamas in terms of abstention from certain forms of behaviour that are all at the negative end of a spectrum. In order to follow his precepts, we need to understand the positive forms of behaviour that are their opposites, at the other end of the spectrum:

- **Ahimsa** is abstention from **violence** – harming or hurting any living being.

  The opposite of violence is gratitude, acceptance, respect and personal responsibility for looking after all forms of life.

- **Satya** is abstention from **falsehood** – distortion of the truth as we understand it.

  The opposite of falsehood is gratitude, acceptance, respect and personal responsibility for expressing the truth as clearly as we can.

- **Asteya** is abstention from **theft** – taking what we are not entitled to.

  The opposite of theft is gratitude, acceptance, respect and personal responsibility for managing with the resources allocated to us.

- **Brahmacharya** is abstention from **incontinence** – squandering life energies through lust.

  The opposite of incontinence is gratitude, acceptance, respect and personal responsibility for the forces of life within us and the enjoyment of our senses.

- **Aparigraha** is abstention from **acquisitiveness** – coveting and hoarding material things.

  The opposite of acquisitiveness is gratitude, acceptance, respect and personal responsibility for the processes of life-light-love.

coin meditation

This meditation starts with experiencing opposites and then discovering the quality that encompasses them both – the substance of the coin itself. Simple examples include hot/cold, the two faces of temperature; rough/smooth, the two faces of texture; love/hate, the two faces of a relationship. The deeper the qualities of the opposites the more likely it is that their substance proves to be love.

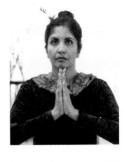

▷ **1** Prepare yourself for meditation so that you are in a sattvic state.

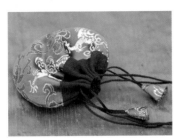

△ **2** Imagine that you have a bag containing coins. Each unknown coin has two faces, one representing a negative quality and the other its positive opposite.

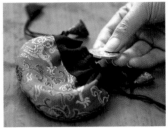

△ **3** Take out a coin and stroke one side of it, allowing any feeling – one of a pair of opposites – to develop. Whatever arises, stay with it. Then experience its opposite quality equally intensely, before discovering the quality that encompasses both "faces" of the coin. Come out of meditation slowly. After the meditation make sure that you stretch and ground yourself thoroughly.

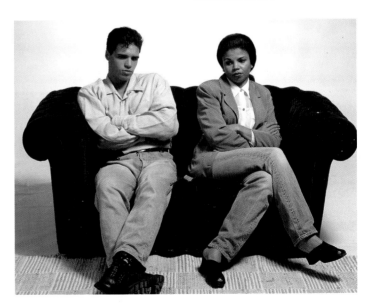

△ Negative feelings stand in the way of self-awareness and self-expression, and can isolate us from one another. A meditation on opposites can help to remove emotional obstacles by helping us to understand how all such feelings are only a part of a larger whole.

Meditating on: the Path to Freedom

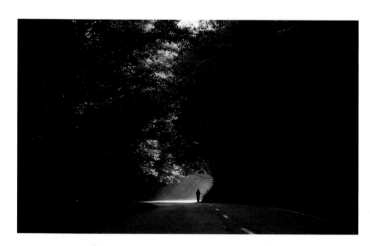

◁ The meditative journey of spiritual evolution leads us away from the darkness of fear toward the light of unclouded truth.

The transcendent state of total liberation of mind and body is known by different names in different religious traditions – samadhi, the state of unclouded truth, union with the divine, and so on – but the meaning is always the same. It is a serene state in which the ultimate truth of existence is revealed and the soul becomes one with universal, unchanging consciousness. We can step on to the path that leads to this spiritual freedom when we decide to change ourselves, whatever our circumstances – rather than blaming the rest of the world for our problems.

overcoming obstacles and distractions

Patanjali teaches that the practice of meditation is the "royal path" to samadhi because it weakens the obstacles that lie in the way of change and spiritual growth: illness, fatigue, doubt, carelessness, laziness, attachment, delusion, failure to achieve and failure to maintain progress.

All these familiar obstacles are manifestations of tamas and rajas. We know from our own experience that they can all agitate the mind, weaken the body and obstruct the spirit, distracting us from following the true path.

focusing on uplifting states

Once we have erased our negative states through meditation, we need to move on to contemplation of those uplifting states that Patanjali assures us precede the ultimate state of samadhi:

• **Trust** (an aspect of self-surrender). Spiritual masters tell us that only two emotions – fear and love – really exist, and that of these two fear is an illusion that we can simply drop when we are ready to do so. Letting go of fear is the great surrender, and enables us to surrender all the other needs that hold us back, such as:
  – **staying in control**, together with all the rajasic effort this involves
  – **protecting ourselves**, instead of co-operating cheerfully with life's natural processes
  – **promoting ourselves** – and attaching too much importance to success in the eyes of the world
  – **needing to justify our existence**, when our existence is really justification in itself
  – **holding on to limiting perceptions of who we are**, instead of revelling in being essential to the glory and wholeness of life, light and love.

• **Perseverance** (an aspect of self-discipline), with regular practice and a daily routine, enables us to maintain our enthusiasm and determination.
• **Recollection** (an aspect of self-awareness) reinforces what we have learned, as we test our new skills and insights at every opportunity in daily life. Driving instructors often tell their pupils that they only really start learning to drive after passing their test and the same is true for meditators. Every "test" becomes an opportunity.
• **Tranquillity** (the state of sattva) becomes second nature once we can combine self-discipline with self-awareness and self-surrender.
• **Wisdom** (through meditation) brings us to the end of our spiritual path – for in the state of boundless freedom there are no paths at all.

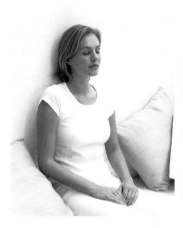

△ Others can tell us how they have discovered their own truth through meditation, but we have to realize for ourselves that we can choose to let go of fear and embrace freedom.

"Do not believe anything because you have heard it – even from the wise – or read it in any book. Believe it only if it accords with your own experience."

Buddha

the seagull: soaring toward freedom

These movements will help you to free yourself from distractions and focus upon the heart chakra, where you embrace uplifting states, accept and balance emotions, heal past traumas, forgive others and yourself and let go of all hurt, anger and resentment. The seagull lives totally in the present moment, as it soars through the skies. Visualize yourself flying high in the blue sky and let all negativity go, releasing it as you breathe out and filling the space in your heart with fresh glory on each breath in.

▷ **1** Sit between your heels in Virasana (hero posture) and bring your palms together at the heart chakra in Namaste mudra.

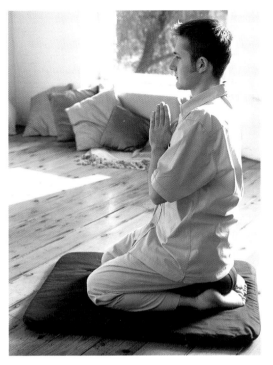

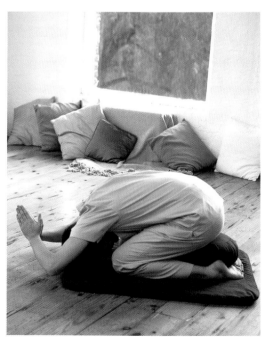

△ **2** As you breathe out, bend forward and place your forehead on the floor, keeping your hands and elbows as high as possible and stretching your chest. Surrender and empty your lungs.

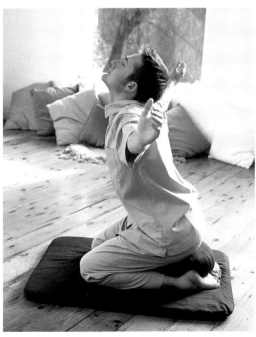

△ **3** As you breathe in, sit up, lift your sternum and stretch your arms like wings wide to the sides. Look up and joyfully surrender to the air, the moment and the movement. Surrender and fill your lungs. Repeat for several minutes.

Meditating on: the OM Mantra

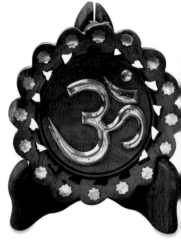

Patanjali begins his list of meditations with: "Complete surrender to the almighty Lord … who is expressed through the sound of the sacred syllable OM. It should be repeated and its essence realized." (From Alistair Shearer's translation of the Yoga Sutras.) OM, or Aum, is recognized in many cultures as the primordial sound, whose vibration brought the universe into being. Daily repetition of the OM mantra, chanted aloud, whispered or repeated silently, has a cumulative and profoundly beneficial effect.

When chanted aloud (intoned rather than sung), the OM sound – pronounced as in "home" – should be deep and full, with the vibrations resonating in the life chakras, then moving up into the chest and the love chakras, and finally closing with a long,

humming "mmm" in the head and the light chakras – all on one deep steady note. Overtones may sometimes be heard. These are the faint sounds of the same note at higher octaves, as when groups of Buddhist monks chant in a deep resonant rumble, with the overtones wafting above like celestial choirs.

a–u–m

The syllable can also be divided into three sounds – A (the created beginning), U (the sustained now) and M (the dissolution of creation). This trinity corresponds to sat-chit-ananda. A is the beginning of life, time and forms; U is maintained through the relationships of cosmic love; M comes when we experience personally that all is spirit – and the rest is mental illusion.

△ The Sanskrit symbol of the sacred syllable OM is often used as an object on which to focus. Place it on a low table so that you can concentrate your gaze on it during your meditation practice.

chanting with a mala

The mala has 108 beads. It should always be held in the right hand and passed between thumb (representing universal consciousness) and middle finger (representing sattva guna). One bead is passed with each repetition of the mantra. Start from the larger bead (*sumeru*) and, when you come round to it again, do not cross it but turn the mala and go back for another round.

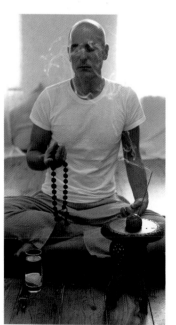

1 Sit in a meditation pose and settle your body and breathing.

◁ 2 Hold the mala in a comfortable position (traditional positions are near your heart or on your right knee).

3 As you breathe in chant OM silently. As you breathe out chant OM aloud (or silently), then move to the next bead on the mala and repeat 107 times. If your mind wanders bring it back gently to the mantra.

4 Sit for a few moments and feel the vibrations of the sound within you, before grounding yourself. The sensation of these vibrations creates a trigger for you – recalling them at other times will take you back instantly to the sattvic state you were in while chanting.

"This Self, beyond all words, is the syllable OM.
This syllable, though indivisible, consists of three letters – A–U–M
[representing three states of being] …The fourth [state], the Self,
is OM … the supreme good, the One without a second.
Whosoever knows OM, the self, becomes the Self."

Mandukya Upanisad

chanting the mantra in a group meditation

This meditation is particularly effective when done in a group. Each person sounds his or her own note, all taking a breath in together (as indicated by the leader) and then chanting A, U, or M on the slow breath out. The meditation ends with everyone chanting OM on their own note and in their own rhythm, so that the sounds mingle together until a natural pause occurs. Silence follows until the meditation ends with a grounding ritual. The more people who join in the OM chanting the more powerful the effects become and the longer the subsequent silence is likely to continue.

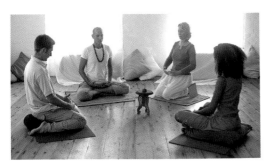

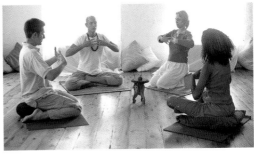

△ **1** Sit in a circle in a comfortable meditation pose with spine erect and sternum lifted. Place the hands in front of the body with palms facing the lower abdomen and fingertips just touching. Breathe in together and chant A (aah ...) on a deep note on the breath out, to resonate in the life chakras in the abdomen. Repeat this sound at least twice more, to energize and remove blockages.

△ **2** Move the hands up, with palms in front of the heart and fingertips just touching. Breathe in together and chant U (oooh ...) on the breath out to resonate in the love chakras. Notice the different quality of the sound and the vibrations. Repeat twice more, feeling your own sound resonating within you.

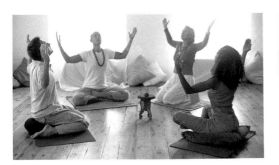

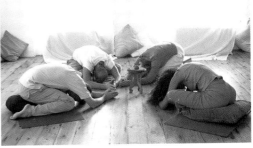

△ **3** Move the hands overhead, stretching up and out in a joyful expression of complete freedom, palms facing forward. Look up (without compressing the neck) and breathe in together. Breathe out to chant M (mmm ...) into the skull cavity and the light chakras, experiencing the sound within. Repeat twice more, then bring your hands down and remain silent. Finally chant OM, each in your own rhythm and pitch, until the group naturally falls silent. Sit in this silence for a while.

△ **4** Finish by bringing hands and forehead to the floor in a gesture of grounding and complete surrender.

DHARMA AND KARMA

OM is said to be the sound of creation, harmony and order. The eternal being expressed through the sound of OM is not the personal deity of any religion but the super-conscious organizing principle that sustains *dharma* (the divine order) by means of *karma* (cause and effect), and whose wisdom is available to all human beings as "the teacher of even the most ancient tradition of teachers".

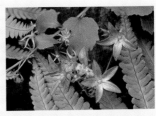

▷ **OM is the sound vibration that underlies every part of the universe, down to the smallest detail.**

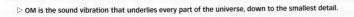

Meditating on: the Chakras

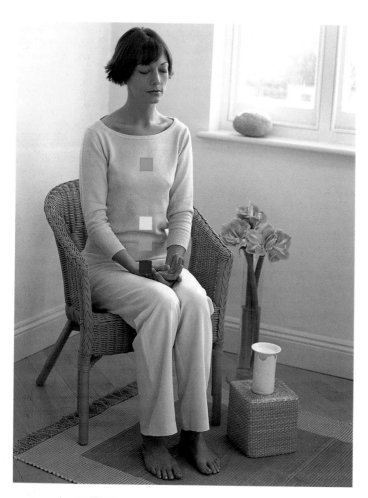

◁ Most of us have a dominant type of chakra energy, and traditional correspondences can help to define the basic character of the chakras. Each of the four lower chakras corresponds to one of the four elements.

The chakras, which exist at the energy level, can be thought of as transformers that process the energy from all the koshas through our bodyminds into the physical world. The body, mind and emotions are all extensions of chakra function. Changes at one level will bring automatic changes at every other level.

The chakras are vortices of energy within our own being that we can become aware of for ourselves and then work with to balance and activate all levels of our being. We can gain a wealth of psychological insight by using meditation to explore the qualities traditionally attributed to each of the major chakras.

awareness of the chakras

To gain true insight into yourself, you need to understand the current state of your own chakra system – and this means becoming aware of it. To help you do this, work through the series of three meditative breathing routines that follows. You should bring focused awareness and discrimination to your exploration, so that, whatever your meditation may reveal, you can remain an impartial observer and learn from the experience, rather than getting carried away by it – especially if emotional responses catch you unawares.

As you explore your chakras during the meditation, try to feel each one's individual brightness or dullness. All the chakras spin, giving off light, colour, sensation and sound, and it is by picking up these subjective phenomena that you can assess if or when a particular chakra is under- or overactive within the system as a whole.

"Balance comes when we can accept and get along with everyone without compromising what we believe in. The balancing of the chakras and the flowering of each one brings us to Patanjali's 'state of unclouded truth' and heaven on earth."

Author

CHAKRA CORRESPONDENCES

Each of us has a mix of influences, but one particular influence is usually dominant. Like each sign of the astrological zodiac, each chakra is associated with an element, which can help us to recognize its basic character. The four lower chakras display the following characters:

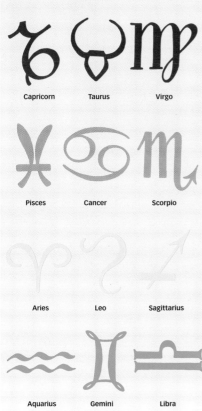

Capricorn   Taurus   Virgo

Pisces   Cancer   Scorpio

Aries   Leo   Sagittarius

Aquarius   Gemini   Libra

1 The base chakra (muladhara) corresponds with the element of earth – as do the star signs of Capricorn, Taurus and Virgo. Their characteristics ensure survival, and among them are practicality, reliability, tenacity, logic, and a generally materialistic and no-nonsense approach to life. An earth weakness can be a rigid and unimaginative outlook, unless it is tempered by other influences. If earth is blocked we fail to ensure that we have the wherewithal to survive and if it is overactive we are obsessed with protecting ourselves by acquiring possessions.

2 The sacral chakra (svadisthana) corresponds to the element of water – as do the signs of Pisces, Cancer, and Scorpio, whose characteristics ensure social bonding. Among them are empathy, enjoyment, sensuality, homemaking and caring for others. A water weakness can be a tendency to tearfulness, emotional sensitivity and slipping into overindulgence to avoid facing facts. If water is blocked we may become outcasts from society, upon whose acceptance our lives depend, and if it is overactive we may become addicted to substances, pleasures or people.

3 The navel chakra (manipura) corresponds to the element of fire – as do the signs of Aries, Leo and Sagittarius, whose characteristics enable us to achieve personal success. They include warmth and friendliness, enthusiasm and zeal to inspire others to believe in themselves and their opinions. A fire weakness is the tendency to burn out through overconfidence and ignoring obstacles. If fire is blocked we lack the energy to plan or achieve anything and drift helplessly through life, and if it is overactive we develop inflated egos.

4 The heart chakra (anahata) corresponds to the element of air – as do the signs of Aquarius, Gemini and Libra. Their main characteristic is to reach beyond the ego to other people, beauty and harmony, ideas and ideals. Air is a property shared by all, and air signs understand that we are all interactive parts of a greater whole. An air weakness is a tendency to be disorganized and unrealistic, though well-meaning. If air is blocked we are imprisoned by our ego and if it is overactive we do not recognize boundaries.

Chakras 1–3 are the life chakras that combine to maintain physical life for the individual. Chakras 1–4 can be perceived as forming the base that supports the three "higher" elements: ether (or communication), mind (the organ of consciousness) and spirit (the link with the whole).

1 chakra awareness: "switching on the light"

First, settle yourself into a suitable position for meditation practice to promote a sattvic state. Awareness is a function of ajna, the brow chakra, so this meditation begins by "switching on the light".

▷ A good "switching on" practice is tratak – focused gazing for a few moments upon an object such as a candle flame, flower or crystal. This balances the nervous system and focuses energy in the centre of the head to light up the mind. Alternatively, you could perform a short breathing practice, such as alternate nostril breathing.

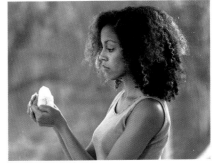

2 chakra awareness: breathing up and down the spine

This sequence will make you sensitive to the energy pathway upon which the chakras are located, like roundabouts or junctions on the busy highway that lies within the spinal cord.

1 First breathe in and "drive" up the motorway from the tailbone to the top of the head.

▷ **2** Breathe out and drive back down again. Alternatively, you can imagine drawing light up on the breath in and letting it release back down on the breath out – like mercury rising and falling in a thermometer. You may like to feel the flow of breath with your hands as you practise this exercise.

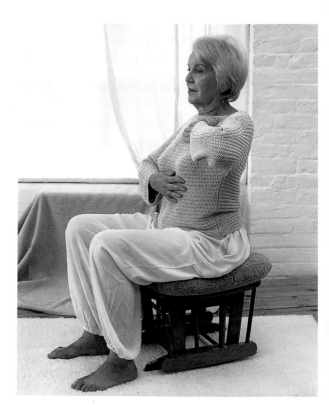

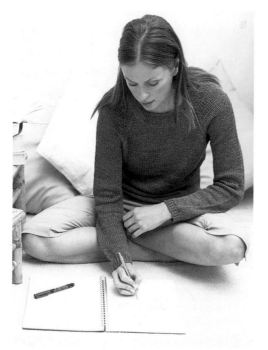

3 chakra awareness: stopping at each chakra

You should really feel the quality of each major chakra as you practise the following meditation.

1 At the base of the spine breathe in and out of the base chakra. Energy is concentrated at this point on the breath in and radiates outward as it is released on the breath out. Repeat twice more before moving up to the next chakra point, the sacral. Again, breathe in to focus energy in the chakra and breathe out to allow it to radiate outward.

2 Continue up the spine with three breaths to activate each chakra point. After breathing into the crown chakra three times, pause and rest, letting its energies inspire and heal you, then start the downward journey, beginning with the crown chakra. After reaching and breathing in and out of the base chakra three times, pause and rest again – feeling the nurturing support and safe solidity of the physical plane upon which you live. The aim is to restore balance between the chakras by understanding and putting right what is causing imbalances.

3 Repeat the whole process once or twice more in a slow, relaxed and observant manner. Then come out of your meditation gently and ground yourself throroughly.

◁ **4** Once out of the meditation, you may like to record your experience to help you reinforce your increasing sensitivity to the different "feel" of each chakra.

chanting the chakra bija mantras

Once you have located your chakras and can breathe in and out of them easily, you may like to explore chanting to brighten them up or nourish them. Each chakra has its own sound (see box below). These are *bija*, or "seed" mantras, which have no literal meaning but are designed to plant the seed of a concept in the mind. They should each be chanted three times on a low, slow note that vibrates in tune with the chakra's own vibratory rate. The Sanskrit sound *am* is soft – somewhere between "ham", "hum" and "harm".

▷ **1** Start at the base chakra and chant in each chakra all the way up. Pause after chanting in the crown chakra, then start again at the crown chakra and move down, pausing again after chanting into the base chakra.

2 Repeat the whole cycle twice more before coming out of the meditation. The bija mantras are represented by Sanskrit letters placed within a symbol that you may also like to visualize.

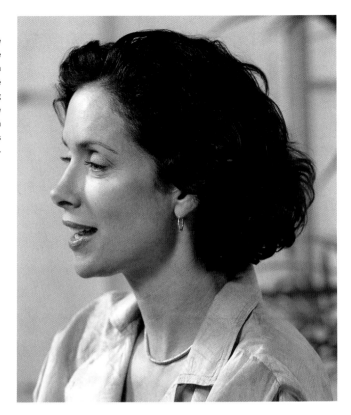

THE SOUNDS OF THE CHAKRAS

As you chant these sounds, think of the qualities of each chakra, expressed perfectly by their particular symbol.

- **LAM** for the **base chakra (muladhara)**, placed within a **yellow square** (the compact quality of earth).

- **VAM** for the **sacral chakra (svadisthana)**, placed within a **blue-white crescent moon** (the moon governs the waters).

- **RAM** for the **navel chakra (manipura)**, placed within a **red triangle pointing downwards** (fire spreads upwards and outwards from a single point).

- **YAM** for the **heart chakra (anahata)**, placed at the centre of **two interlaced triangles** (the colour varies, as does the colour of air, which joins heaven and earth together).

- **HAM** for the **throat chakra (visuddhi)**, placed within a **white circle** (ether or space pervades the entire universe).

- **OM** for the **brow chakra (ajna)**, placed within a **grey or mauve circle between two petals**. This is the "command centre" where all opposites (the two petals) merge and are transcended through awareness and understanding.

- **OM** (or the entire Sanskrit alphabet) for the **crown chakra (sahasrara)**, at the **centre of a sphere of light** radiating in all directions – spirit pervades all creation.

Meditating on: Hearts and Minds

"Placing the mind in the heart" is a famous Buddhist concept, shared by every spiritual tradition. The mind is a marvellous tool – processing sensual information and directing the body to act accordingly, observing, reflecting, learning from our past experiences, judging and making decisions, planning for the future. It is the activities of the heart, however, that make the world go round, as love is expressed as relating, interacting, sharing, giving and receiving.

the divine spark

The energy of the heart lies at the core of our existence, and our heartfelt attitudes drive our lives. In modern society the mind, with its ability to create technical marvels, is afforded our ultimate respect and the qualities of the heart are downgraded – yet the mind is always subservient to the heart and we "follow our heart" even when it leads us in a direction contrary to our better judgment. The teachings of every spiritual tradition insist that our minds (light) and our ego personalities (life) exist to serve the divine spark in us all that resides within our hearts (love).

▷ The eternal flame – the divine spark within the heart of every being – is the subject of the meditation on the cave of the heart.

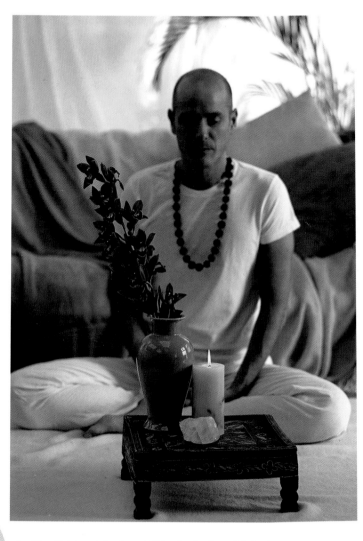

"The ancient effulgent being, the indwelling Spirit, subtle, deep-hidden in the lotus [chakra] of the heart, is hard to know ... Smaller than the smallest, greater than the greatest, this Self forever dwells within the hearts of all. One who is free from desire, with mind and senses purified, beholds the glory of the Self and is without sorrow."

Katha Upanisad

meditation on the "cave of the heart"

Our "heart home" is a sacred haven, untouched by any negativity, where we can feel safe, supported and healed. This meditation will help you to find this home.

1 Get settled into a still and peaceful state and prepare to visualize.

2 Imagine seeing yourself from a distance, sitting in your meditation pose within a luminous bubble that is suspended in space between heaven and earth. The sphere is your aura. A silvery cord attaches it firmly to heaven, then passes through your body seated in the centre of your aura and attaches it firmly to the earth.

3 Now look within your aura. The silver cord that passes through your body has your chakras strung along it like beads on a necklace.

4 Imagine yourself breathing deeply, seated inside your aura. As you breathe in you are, at the same time, drawing light down from the heavenly end of the cord and life up from the earthly end of the cord. As you breathe out, you puff this mixture into your aura, as though into a balloon, so that it gets brighter and bigger. Continue pumping both light (consciousness) and life (vitality) into your aura until it feels radiant and healthy.

5 See yourself sitting in your "mind space" in your skull, which is like a room with a front wall of mirrored glass. You can look through it to see the external world, but it also reflects back to you your own thoughts and mental pictures.

6 Imagine yourself standing up to leave your "mind space" and going down, either by a lift or a staircase, to the level of your "heart space".

7 On this level is a door. Open it reverently and walk into the "cave of your heart", where you see a low table, upon which a small lamp is burning – the eternal divine flame, the symbol of who you really are. This is who we all are, at heart.

8 Around the table are low benches. Sit down and gaze into the flame, letting its warmth and joy permeate and heal you at every level. Feel connected to your divine self.

9 When you are ready, let the scene dissolve and give it to the earth by breathing out deeply. Let it all go – a gift of peace and joy from you to our beleaguered planet.

10 Come out of meditation slowly, grounding yourself and perhaps writing down your experience. Repeat this meditation until it becomes so familiar that you can "take your mind into your heart" whenever you wish, and rest in the healing presence that abides there.

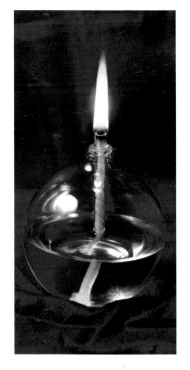

△ **Visualize your essential, eternal self as a lamp burning steadily in the cave of your heart.**

UNCONDITIONAL LOVE

Ananda maya kosha – the soul body – is the kosha of our highest wisdom. It contains our past experience and knows our future purpose. Unlike the mind, it experiences only unconditional love, however negative we may be feeling at our mental and emotional levels. It can be very helpful to invite into your heart the soul of a person who is causing you difficulties at the personality level. Since all souls love each other, deep healing can occur when two souls meet in the divine presence of the eternal flame, even though the other person is unaware of this meeting at a conscious level.

▷ **The practice of meditation allows us to gain access to our highest levels of consciousness, where our souls meet in loving kindness.**

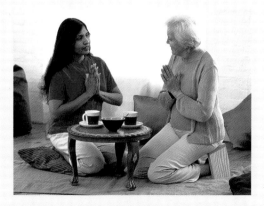

Meditating on: Living Life at Soul Level

It is through meditation that we truly experience our "soul level". We learn to listen to our own souls, and to reach out to other souls and the world around us – as in the group meditation on these pages.

the inner teacher

When we feel in need of help or guidance in our journey to the soul, we can call upon a source of higher wisdom. This can be our higher self, or a great master such as the Buddha, or any appropriate figure from our belief system. Whoever we invite may enter the privacy of our heart and answer our questions. By learning to ask, listen to this guidance and trust our innermost promptings, we can channel this higher wisdom into our lives.

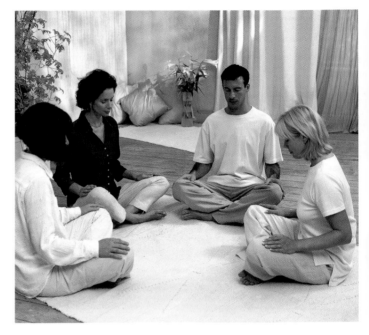

▷ A group meditation is a powerful expression of universal oneness, uniting all the members in loving co-operation. It is usually directed at a specific goal, such as healing.

healing group meditation

This meditation directs group energy to heal a specific person, the whole group or the whole planet. It can last 10–20 minutes and be led silently by one person sitting in the group, who rings a small bell to start each section, so that everyone proceeds as one.

1 Sit in a circle facing a candle in the centre – this represents the person or group in need of healing, or the whole planet and all living beings. Allow the group time to get settled.

2 Light the candle to begin the meditation.

3 Section 1: Each person connects with above (light) and below (life) and, on each breath in, draws light down and life up simultaneously into the group aura, like a huge balloon that encompasses the whole group and the flame at its centre.

4 On each breath out this group aura becomes filled with love energy, and grows ever brighter. Continue this section of the meditation for a few minutes, strengthening the group aura.

5 Section 2: Breathe light and life in as before and breathe love out, directing it specifically into the flame at the centre of the group, while visualizing total healing. Continue to direct healing energy for a few minutes.

▷ **6** Section 3: Give thanks for the healing received and channelled by each member of the group. Let the images slowly dissolve, breathe deeply and take your energy down into your feet to ground yourself, before opening your eyes and extinguishing the candle flame to end the meditation.

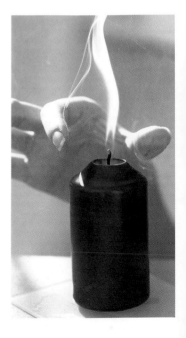

meeting your own soul

In this meditation, visualize yourself wearing soul robes of shimmering energies that both symbolize and veil the brightness of the spirit.

▷ **1** Get settled into a still and peaceful state, ready to visualize.

2 See yourself wrapped in your protective aura, which is firmly attached by a silver cord to the heaven (light) and earth (life) poles and suspended between them. This cord passes through your chakras within your aura.

3 Breathe in both light (from above) and life (from below) at the same time, so that they mingle as love. Breathe this out into your aura.

4 See yourself leaving your "mind space" and walking down into the area of your "heart space".

5 Settle reverently in front of the eternal flame that burns in a tiny lamp on a low table at the centre of your heart home. Gaze into this flame of love and enter a state of peace.

6 After a while look around your heart home and notice how it contains objects or images that remind you of those, alive or dead, with whom you share a bond. Love's bonds are eternal. Take comfort and support from this understanding.

7 Look down at yourself – you are wearing your soul robes of swirling energy. What colours do you see? They are your personal "energy signature".

8 You may finish your meditation at this point. Remember to give thanks for the healing of attitudes and relationships, and for any other help and guidance you have received. Look around you – your heart home will become adorned, as your loving relationships leave their impressions behind in the form of beautiful images. Let the images dissolve before grounding yourself thoroughly and possibly writing down your experiences. Alternatively, before finishing, you may wish to invite another soul (such as a beloved relative) to share your space before the eternal flame. They will appear quietly on a seat beside you and wait for you to become

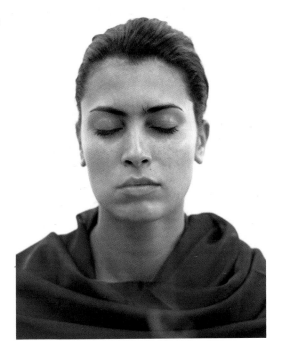

aware of their presence. Enjoy this meeting, thank them for responding and let their images dissolve before coming out of the meditation.

9 Once you have gained confidence you may wish to invoke a soul whose personality in this lifetime has been in conflict with your own, knowing that at soul level you share only love without any attempt to justify yourself or criticize another. It can be very helpful to "talk" about the attitudes and perceptions of your respective personalities. True souls are always in a state of peace. The ongoing healing effects upon both personalities can be truly amazing.

KARMA

The Eastern spiritual traditions assume that we all live a series of lives, gradually balancing out our negative and positive karma (the effect of our actions). The seeds of all past experiences lie buried deep in our souls. People we have interacted with before may be with us again now, as we evolve together through love and forgiveness, aided by meditation. Our actions in this life create the circumstances for our next incarnation, as we either take or ignore opportunities to release others from their negative karma through our unconditional forgiveness. By learning – often despite ourselves – to make choices dictated by love we spiral together toward the perfect freedom of existence (sat), consciousness (chit) and bliss (ananda) where life and light become one in love. It has been said that this freedom depends upon all of us for, since we are all one, there is ultimately only one of us to be liberated. This truth is becoming painfully obvious as regards the survival of our species and possibly even our planet.

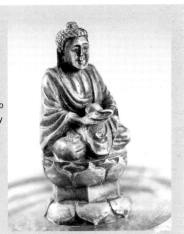

▷ **Buddhist meditation follows the Buddha's own precept: "Look within, you are the Buddha."**

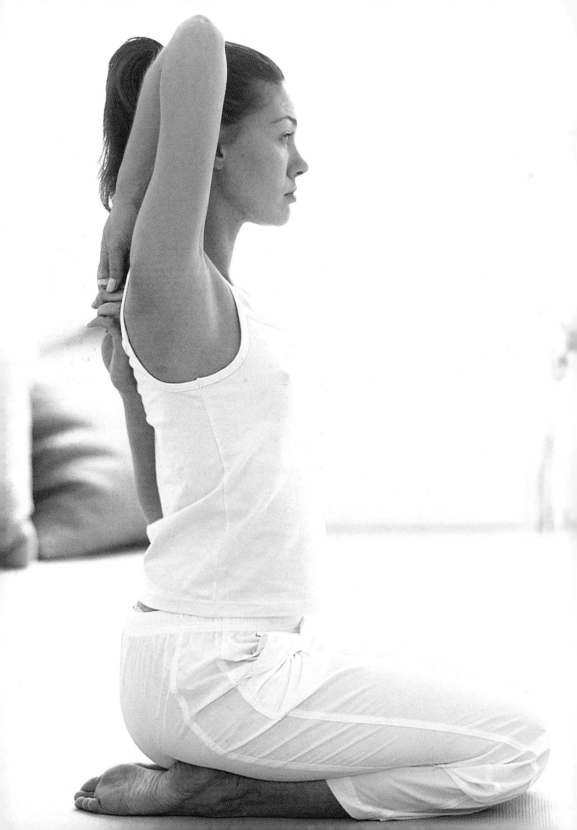

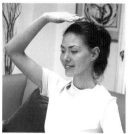
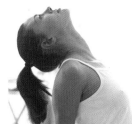
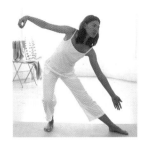
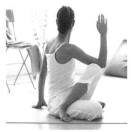

Working with the Chakras

Sages of the ancient East identified certain vortices of energy in the human body and named them "chakras", and the chakra system now features in many contemporary healing techniques. The seven major chakras resemble gateways that allow us to access different states of consciousness, and the subtle equilibrium of the chakras governs our health and well-being.

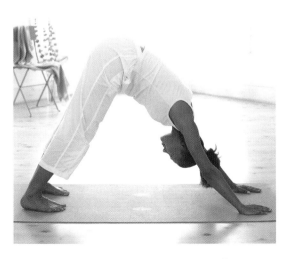

Balancing the Chakra System

The chakra system is complex and interrelated – each chakra, both major and minor, can be thought of as a cog in a machine. A change in the movement of one will create changes throughout the whole structure. There will be an efficient flow of energy when all parts are locked together in their activity, working harmoniously together. If one chakra becomes damaged or has its normal range of activity restricted this inevitably puts strain on its closest neighbours, which will also begin to suffer.

A chakra that becomes unbalanced in the system has become stuck at an inappropriate level of activity. It is either working with insufficient energy for its task, or it is working too hard. In either circumstance the other chakras will have to compensate by changing their levels of energy. This means that the system as a whole will be working at one level when it may be more appropriate for it to function at another.

overall balance

The chakra system, like the rest of the body, responds to the circumstances of its environment. In some circumstances a particular chakra will tend to take a larger role, but it should still operate in a balanced way within the normal working parameters of the system.

Different jobs and lifestyles need special areas of expertise, and the dynamics of the chakras need to adjust accordingly. For example, a singer will naturally need to have an especially active throat chakra to keep the voice healthy. The heart chakra, too, will need to have plenty of energy to foster a depth of feeling,

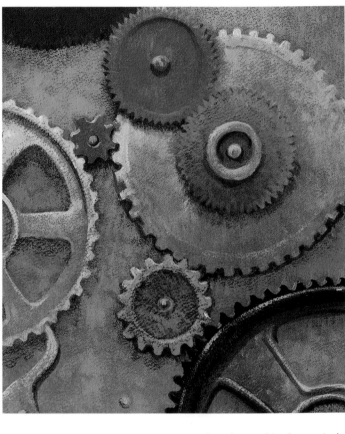

△ All parts of the chakra system respond to changes in every other part. Releasing stress from one area will help to relax the whole system, making everything run better.

empathy and personal involvement in the work. In such a person, an observer who was sensitive to energy fields would see a lot of activity at those two centres. Only if too much energy is focused in one area will problems start to show, beginning in

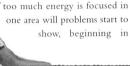

▷ False equilibrium is where a temporary stability has been achieved. However, even a slight change will bring about a breakdown in order. When this occurs in the chakra system, illness may develop.

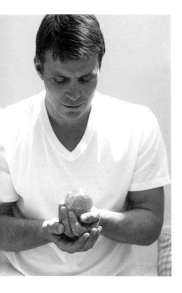

◁ Crystals, with their brilliant colour and unique structures are very effective ways to bring balance to the chakra system.

considerations

In learning about the symptoms of chakra imbalance presented here and in other books, it is important not to become disheartened about your own state of energetic health. At one time or another most of us will experience extremes of under- and overactivity in all our chakras. It is more important to recognize the common tendencies that are repeated through our lives. Once the most prevalent states are known they can be worked on and necessary alterations can begin to be made.

A physical balancing technique can have a beneficial effect on an emotional chakra stress, and a mental visualization exercise can allow positive change to happen at a physical, everyday level. So use those techniques and exercises that you find most helpful and that fit most comfortably into your everyday life.

Many traditional systems of spiritual development take into account the differences between individuals and their lifestyles, providing different sorts of practices to suit their needs. Today we are lucky in having a wide range of chakra balancing techniques from all around the world. Even the most hectic lifestyle can accommodate sufficient practices to help to reduce the burden of stress that overloads the chakra system and will eventually lead to health problems. The only thing that is needed is for us to set aside a little time dedicated to our own repair. This is largely a process of developing a habit. At first, all sorts of

distractions may arise until the routine becomes a natural part of our day. Most balancing practices need a little effort and dedication in the beginning – not only to bring in a new routine, but also because we are beginning to make changes in our energy systems.

Correcting a false equilibrium requires skill and patience. Like a tightrope walker who has been working for years with a pole that has a large weight at one end and nothing on the other end, we adjust to the weight of stress we have accumulated in our lives in order to continue as best we can. Removing all the stress in one go may seem to be the best solution but, like the tightrope walker, we need to familiarize ourselves gradually with the new state of balance at each step. If not, the risk increases that we will feel less secure than we did when we had all the stress.

Like kicking an addictive habit, the biggest problem most of us face is that habitual patterns of behaviour feel comfortable and part of our true personality. Working with a balancing system that focuses on the different levels of body, mind and emotion can be helpful in maintaining an even development of chakra healing. Traditional methods like yoga, Tai Chi and Chi Kung all have outer, physical activities that release stress from the body. They also have mental techniques that involve meditative states, or visualizations that help to clarify the subtle energies of the mind and emotions. It is important to pay attention to all these different levels of practice. For example, it will be of limited value to have a body that is supple and toned if you are still emotionally insecure or stuck in some past trauma.

Contemporary techniques, such as crystal therapy, colour therapy and flower essences, can help to remove specific stresses in chakra centres as well as bringing the whole body into a better state of balance.

those places where there are natural weaknesses as a result of past stresses or current overuse.

The chakra system will change gear with a change of activity. Meditation requires a different sort of energy from cooking the dinner; playing a musical instrument requires different skills from listening to an orchestra; escaping from a stressful situation uses different resources from gazing at a serene sunset. Problems arise when, through stress of one sort or another, the chakra system fails to change gear and becomes stuck in a single mode of functioning.

Throughout our lives, stresses of many sorts accumulate in all our systems, from physical to spiritual. These stresses can be like grains of sand or grit that create a little roughness in the workings of our chakra cogs, or they can be like a spanner that seriously throws the whole mechanism out of alignment.

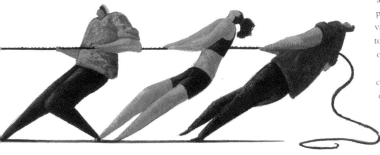

Cycles of Nature

In the classical Indian texts the chakras are related to a series of milestones in life. Each chakra and its function represent a stage of development and growth. Each stage can be seen as a time in which certain skills are developed. The precise shift from one stage of development to another will vary from individual to individual. The stages may overlap, but in some cases, where stress or trauma disrupts the chakra energy, this may create an underlying problem for subsequent growth. If one function remains underdeveloped, all the others dependent on it will have a built-in dysfunction.

conception and birth

The base chakra relates to the creation of the physical body, so it represents a stage of growth that begins at conception and continues until around the age of one year. The immediate, powerful energy of the base chakra is evident in the speed of growth and the primary need to survive. An infant during this time is dependent on others for its food, warmth and shelter. This period helps to anchor the individual into the physical world.

the developing baby

The sacral chakra begins to activate consciously at about six months and its effects last to around the age of two years. The feedback in this time comes from pleasure and gratification. The distinction between the child and the mother begins to become more apparent. Being given space to explore existence without negative reinforcement or verbal reprimand helps to build confidence in being a separate individual.

▽ All chakras are present in the growing child but during natural development energy focuses at certain centres.

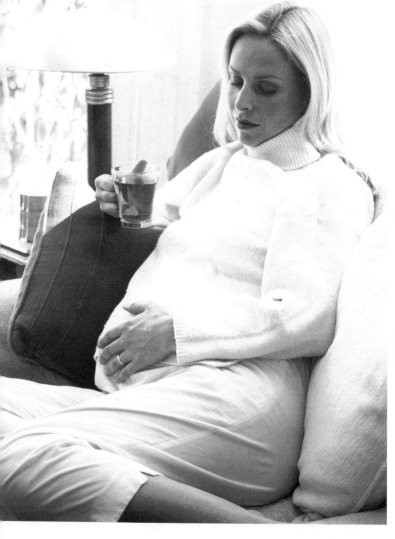

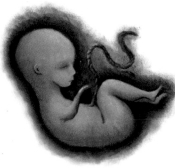

◁ From the moment of conception, consciousness coalesces around the energy of the chakras. The primary needs of survival and nutrition are the first focuses of each new life.

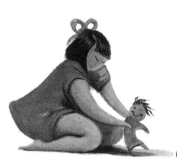

◁ Play exercises all the chakras, no matter what the age: it fosters a sense of security, energy, a desire to explore, confidence, ability to relate to the world, self-expression and imagination.

the small child

The onset of the activity of the navel chakra is commonly referred to as the "terrible twos". It starts at around 18 months and lasts until the child is about four years old. This is when language develops, together with an understanding of the passing of time. Maintaining the balance between freedom and discipline is crucial at this age. Lack of restraining discipline creates an overpowering, egotistic child, whereas too much control will stop any sense of autonomy developing.

the child

The heart chakra covers the period from four to seven years and is characterized by relationships outside the immediate family. Relating helps to build self-esteem and self-acceptance. If love and relationships are always seen as being conditional – that is,

▽ Shared, co-operative creativity flourishes when the sacral and throat chakras have developed in a balanced way. Problems can arise if other chakras do not work in harmony.

having an emotional price-tag attached – the underlying feelings of guilt and grief caused by not receiving enough love can create great difficulties through life.

the pre-pubescent

The development of the throat chakra between the ages of seven and 12 marks the beginning of the stage of self-expression. If the lower chakra energies have been integrated to a reasonable extent, confidence can be gained from a firm emotional base. Through the throat chakra, this is given back to the community and family, sometimes in plays and performances.

the adolescent

The brow chakra covers the adolescent years, when the young person should be encouraged to reflect on the patterns in their own and others' lives. This is the first of several key stages when it is possible to re-invent and readjust the role that an individual sees themselves playing in the world.

the adult

The crown chakra becomes active between 20 and 27 years, as the individual fully reacts and interacts with the world. Sometimes this stage stays dormant, because it relates to questions like "Why am I here?" and statements like "There must be more to life than this." These issues may never be looked at. On the other hand, the action of exploring them may be the beginning of a radical change of life and work. Having gone through a whole cycle, the

process begins again with the base chakra. Just as, in musical scales, each octave returns to the start note, the chakra cycle can repeat many times in a single life. The fact that this cycle renews itself periodically gives us opportunities to heal and repair ourselves. This enables us gradually to strengthen the energy within our chakra system and express more of our potential.

▷ As adults, we pass through successive cycles of the chakra system, continuing our own spiritual growth while also perhaps fostering the development of children.

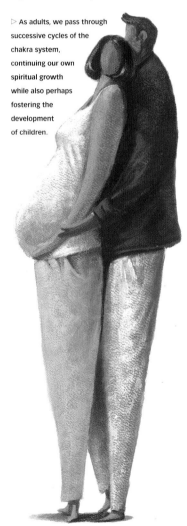

Discover Your Own Chakra Energy

Chakra energies are forever changing, interacting, balancing and rebalancing. From hour to hour and minute to minute as our activities alter, we move from concentration, to remembering, to physical coordination skills, to relaxing. As we do so, different chakras become more or less dominant. As individuals we each have a predisposition to certain chakras being more dominant than others. If we enjoy physical activity and have a practical, hands-on job, this will focus our energies at the first and second chakras. On the other hand, with an occupation that focuses on organizational skills and ideas, the solar plexus and brow chakras will inevitably become more significant.

Our life circumstances also alter the flow and interactions the chakras have with each other and with the environment. For example, if we are naturally comfortable working in socially complex interpersonal relationships – a heart chakra state – and then have to spend time where there is little chance to interact with others, or where our relationship skills are not valued, then this inevitably requires us to "change gear" and focus our chakra energies in different ways. If we can identify the chakras that need

▽ **Give yourself time to think about the questions before you choose your answer.**

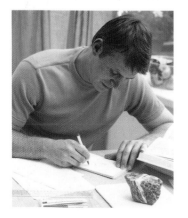

balancing, we can help ourselves a great deal in our journey towards our full potential and well-being.

Chakra dominance is not in itself a problem. However, where a major imbalance occurs, one or more chakras begin to take over the roles more properly belonging to others. This overburdens the dominant chakras and atrophies the others. We can survive for a long time in this false equilibrium, but it is like having a toolkit where only the hammer is used whatever the job. Often it is an accumulation of stresses and trauma in a chakra that reduces its effectiveness. If this is not remedied the system will naturally compensate by diverting energy to areas that are still working. This is the state of false equilibrium that most people cope with in their lives.

the questionnaire

In the following questionnaire there are seven options open to you for each question posed. Jot down the number of each reply on a sheet of paper. Pick more than one choice if it seems appropriate.

Now see how many times you recorded each number. Each refers to a chakra: 1 the base chakra, 2 the sacral chakra, 3 the solar plexus chakra, 4 the heart chakra, 5 the throat chakra, 6 the brow chakra and 7 the crown chakra. If you look at your score, you will be able to see which chakras are dominant for you.

For example, if you have two answers of number 1, two of 2, six of 3, two of 4, three of 5, one of 6 and three of 7, you will see that the third chakra, the solar plexus, is dominant. This is where most of your energy is focused. Although dominant, the solar plexus chakra needs the most attention and healing. Chakras 1, 2 and 6 (base, sacral and brow) have little focus of attention, so they too, may need healing and energizing.

▷ **If some of your chakras are overburdened your system will not be functioning properly.**

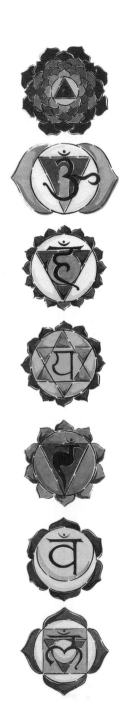

THE QUESTIONNAIRE

1 Which area(s) of your body concern you the most?
❶ feet and legs
❷ between waist and hips
❸ waist
❹ chest
❺ neck and shoulders
❻ face
❼ head

2 Which area(s) of your body do you dislike?
❶ feet and legs
❷ between waist and hips
❸ waist
❹ chest
❺ neck and shoulders
❻ face
❼ head

3 Which area(s) of your body are you proud of?
❶ feet and legs
❷ between waist and hips
❸ waist
❹ chest
❺ neck and shoulders
❻ face
❼ head

4 Which area(s) of your body are affected by major health issues?
❶ feet and legs
❷ between waist and hips
❸ waist
❹ chest
❺ neck and shoulders
❻ face
❼ head

5 Which area(s) of the body are affected most by minor health issues?
❶ feet and legs
❷ between waist and hips
❸ waist
❹ chest
❺ neck and shoulders
❻ face
❼ head

6 Which colour(s) do you like the most?
❶ red
❷ orange
❸ yellow
❹ green
❺ blue
❻ dark blue
❼ violet

7 Which colour(s) do you like the least?
❶ red
❷ orange
❸ yellow
❹ green
❺ blue
❻ dark blue
❼ violet

8 Which are your favourite foods?
❶ meat/fish/pulses
❷ rice/orange fruits
❸ wheat/yellow fruits
❹ green fruit and
   vegetables

9 Which sort of exercises or interests attract you?
❶ fast action
❷ dancing/painting
❸ crosswords/puzzles
❹ anything outside
❺ drama/singing
❻ mystery/crime novels
❼ doing nothing

10 What sort of people do you look up to or admire?
❶ sportspeople
❷ artists/musicians
❸ intellectuals
❹ conservationists
❺ speakers/politicians
❻ inventors
❼ mystics/religious figures

11 What sort of person do you think of yourself as?
❶ get on with things
❷ creative

❸ thinker/worrier
❹ emotional
❺ chatterbox
❻ quiet
❼ daydreamer

12 What emotions do you consider are uppermost in your life?
❶ passionate
❷ easy-going
❸ contented
❹ caring, sharing
❺ loyal
❻ helpfully distant
❼ sympathetic

13 What emotions do you have that you would like to change?
❶ temper
❷ possessiveness
❸ confusion
❹ insecurity
❺ needing things to be
   "black or white"
❻ feeling separate from
   others
❼ not saying "no"

14 If you get angry, what is your most common reaction?
❶ rage/tantrums
❷ sullen resentment
❸ get frightened
❹ blame yourself
❺ keep quiet
❻ withdraw
❼ imagine nothing happened

15 What are you most afraid of?
❶ dying
❷ lack of sensation
❸ things you don't
   understand
❹ being alone
❺ having no-one to talk to
❻ losing your way
❼ difficult situations

16 Which of these describes the way you prefer to learn?
❶ fast
❷ slowly
❸ quickly but forget
❹ through feelings
❺ by rote
❻ instinctively
❼ can't be bothered

17 What best describes your reaction to situations?
❶ enthusiastic
❷ go with the flow
❸ think things through
❹ see how things feel
❺ ask a lot of questions
❻ see the patterns then act
❼ drift along

18 If you are criticized or reprimanded, what is your usual response?
❶ anger
❷ resentment
❸ fear
❹ self-blame
❺ verbal riposte
❻ think about it
❼ denial

19 How would you describe your favourite books, films, video games?
❶ combat action
❷ art
❸ skill, intellectual
❹ romances
❺ courtroom dramas
❻ detective stories
❼ spiritual or self
   development

20 Which category best describes your friends?
❶ competitive
❷ creative
❸ intellectual
❹ loving
❺ idealistic
❻ rebellious
❼ spiritual

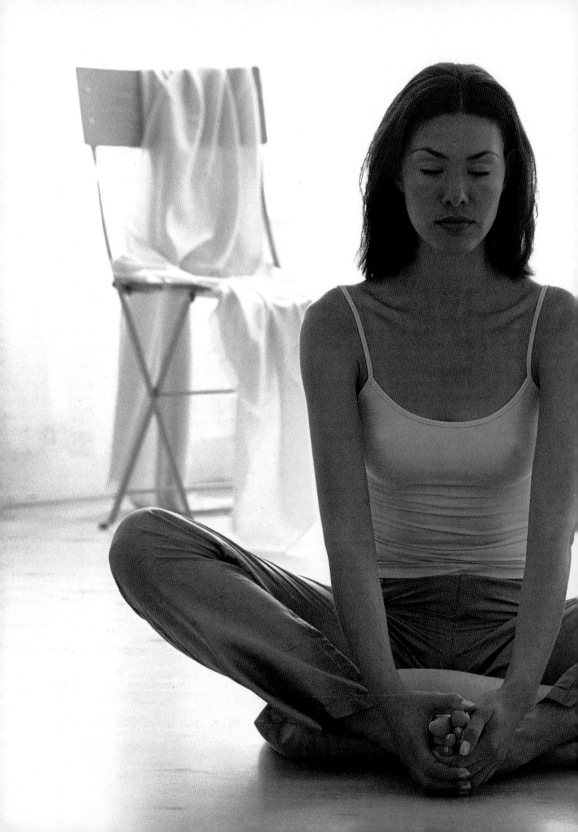

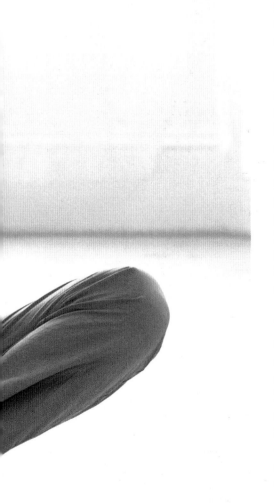

The Chakras and Well-being

Whatever their correlation to physical structures in the body, chakras are entirely non-physical. The mind, rather than the sense organs, is the traditional tool for accessing and balancing the energy of the chakras.

Once you have completed the questionnaire on the previous page you can use the following pages to find appropriate ways to heal and balance parts of the chakra system that you feel need attention. Each of the seven main chakras is characterized in relation to our physical and spiritual well-being. To energize the chakras and heal imbalances, appropriate therapies are drawn not only from yoga but from many other traditions, reflecting the importance of the chakra system in the spiritual practices of many cultures around the world.

The life chakras – the base, sacral and navel chakras – ensure the stability of the individual at the physical level and in society. The heart and throat chakras are the love chakras, integrating our energy with others around us and governing communication. The last two are the light chakras: the brow chakra brings clarity of perception and intuitive insight, and the crown chakra unites the individual with the whole of creation.

Base Chakra – Foundation of Energy

Matter requires stability and structure in order to exist. Energy must be organized and maintained in the face of all sorts of opposing forces in the universe. The force of gravity is the energy of compression and its focus is the basis of the first chakra, located at the bottom of the spine. This is the rock upon which the whole of the chakra system, the subtle energies and the physical body rely, and without which disorder would soon arise.

The Sanskrit name for the base chakra, muladhara, means "root", and the foundation of our life is the physical body

▽ The muladhara chakra ensures our physical existence, nourishing and energizing the whole chakra system.

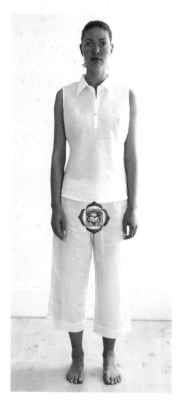

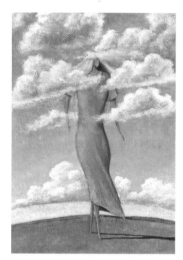

△ Placing too much value on thought processes, of knowing rather than feeling, can create an imbalance that isolates us from the planet.

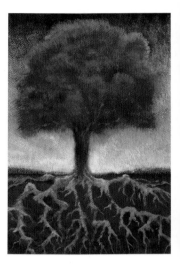

△ Our sense of self, and desire to live, are the hidden roots of our existence; this is the ground of our being that sustains us constantly.

and its ability to use energy to sustain itself. Survival is the key activity of the base chakra, which deals with life at the level of practicality. The base chakra is the closest energy centre to the earth and it links us to the planet itself.

head in the clouds

The base chakra is what links 'us' – the consciousness sitting up there in the head commenting on everything that's going on – with our bodies. Many ancient cultures saw the mind or soul as located in the heart. The West puts emphasis on the head, the seat of the rational thinking mind, and often views the body as an awkward nuisance. With such a dissociation, the natural connections with physical reality and the sense of being a part of creation can be lacking. This induces a false sense of detachment, disinterest or even disdain, where nothing is truly valued and nothing is appreciated. Life can quickly become dull and meaningless.

reactions

The base chakra relates to physical solidity and support, especially to the skeletal structure of the body and its flexibility. It is no use having a strong physical base if there is no flexibility. In order to survive any sort of stress, body and mind must be responsive. In an emergency, we must react quickly in an appropriate way, resisting or giving way as necessary. This instinctive feel for survival is the "fight or flight" response of the adrenal glands just above the kidneys, which are responsible for preparing us for rapid action when faced with the threat of danger.

Like the adrenal glands, the base chakra has a relationship with the circulatory system and the blood supply. It also influences the skeletal muscles of the arms, legs and torso that allow us to move through the world. The base chakra is linked to the colour red and is responsible for maintaining the body's heat – the core temperature that allows chemical reactions to take place in the cells at the correct rate.

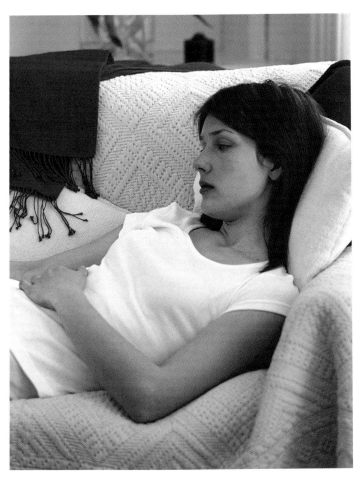

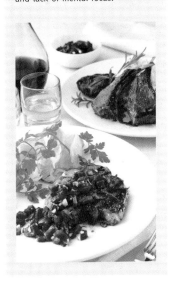

⊲ Both the inability to sustain energy levels and the need for continual excitement or stimulation can indicate imbalance in the base chakra.

TO ENERGIZE THE BASE CHAKRA

Exercising the sense of touch, attending to practical matters, gentle movement and exercise can help to energize and re-connect us to the base chakra. Any of the following will help:
• A warm bath.
• Massage, aromatherapy or reflexology.
• Walking, running, jumping or stamping the feet improves the circulation, co-ordination and our link to the planet.
• Eating, especially high protein foods. Taking a good mineral supplement may also help. A shortage of zinc is one of the commonest causes of "spaciness" and lack of mental focus.

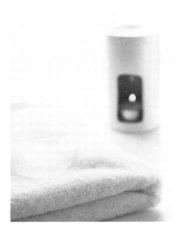

▽ Any activity, such as bathing, that emphasizes physicality and stimulates the senses – especially smell – helps to balance the base chakra.

Imbalances in the base chakra can show up in many ways. Characteristic symptoms include a chronic lack of energy, with exhaustion following even slight exercise, problems with stiffness and painful movement, particularly in the hips, legs and feet. When poor physical co-ordination or poor circulation (a tendency to have cold hands and feet) is present, the base chakra is worth looking at.

The base chakra may also need healing and energizing when someone is uncomfortable with their body. This can lead to a sense of confusion or unreality and may show in a lack of drive or motivation and an aversion to getting involved in practicalities or physical exercise. Conversely, an imbalance in the base chakra can also cause excessive tension or excitability, with a continual need for stimulation.

Sacral Chakra – the Pleasure Principle

The sacral chakra is the second energy centre. It is located in the area below the navel and above the pubic bone, at the front of the pelvis. Physically this chakra is involved with the organs of the lower abdomen – the large intestine, the bladder and the reproductive organs.

Detoxification is one of the key functions of the sacral chakra, at every level, from the physical through to the spiritual.

▷ The sacral chakra is the reservoir of our life energy, from which energy, or chi, is channelled or directed through the rest of the body.

▽ The sacral chakra, located in the area below the navel and above the pubic bone, is the second energy centre.

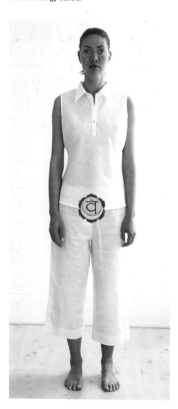

Traditionally this chakra is connected with the element of water and has its characteristics of flow, cleansing and movement. The symbol of the chakra is a white, blue or silver crescent, which is also a reminder of the moon's influence on all things watery, including the ebb and flow of the emotions.

So while the defining characteristic of the base chakra is the element of earth, representing solidity, focus and the structure of the skeletal system, the sacral chakra represents the polar opposites of these: flow, flexibility and the emptiness or hollowness of the body's organs – bladder, intestine, womb and so on.

The whole pelvic region is shaped like a bowl, in which the energy focus of the sacral chakra lies. The pelvis is shaped to support the legs and the many different muscles that control their movement. Any strain or tension here can create a whole range of symptoms, from lower back pain, irregular or painful menstruation, constipation and sciatica to problems with fertility, impotence and fluid balance in the body.

Any disease state that features poor balance of fluids or flexibility will correspond to an imbalance within the second chakra. Water

▷ Belly-dancing is an ideal activity to balance the sacral energies. It strengthens the pelvic and abdominal muscles and it encourages flexibility.

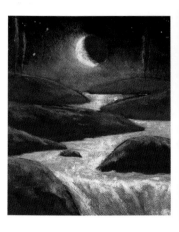

△ The sacral chakra is associated with the energy of the moon and with the emotions and fluids of the body.

absorption is an important function of the large intestine, while control of the mineral and water balance in the blood is regulated by the kidneys. If the functions of these areas are impaired, the balance of chemicals in the body is upset, and it becomes more difficult to eliminate toxins and waste products, which effectively poison the body.

It is the job of the sacral chakra to keep things moving. Any rigidity of the joints, such as in arthritis and other similar conditions, can also reflect unbalanced energy at this centre.

balance and flow

The area of the sacral chakra within the pelvis is also our centre of gravity. It rules our sense of movement and balance, and gives grace and flow to our activity. It is the reservoir of what the Indians call prana and the Chinese call chi – the life-energy that infuses every living system, the subtle substance within the breath that is so important in the spiritual disciplines of the

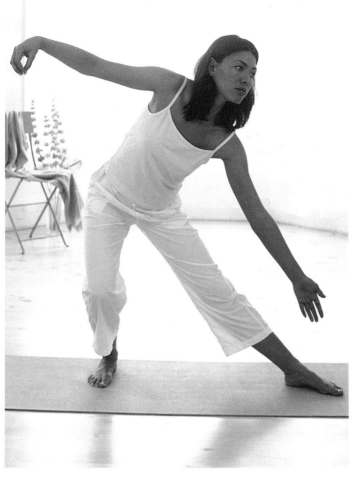

WU CHI

One way of energizing and balancing the sacral chakra is to take up belly dancing. Another is to perform this standing posture exercise, called *wu chi* in Chinese. Begin by holding the posture for 2–5 minutes, then increase the time gradually.

1 Stand with your feet apart, directly under your shoulders.

2 Let your hands hang loosely by your sides and allow your shoulders to drop.

3 Imagine your whole body is hanging by a thread attached to the top of your head, suspending you from the ceiling.

4 Allow yourself to relax, making sure your knees are not locked. Breathe normally.

Watch as you become aware of the tensions in your muscles and the internal chatter of your mind. Let them go.

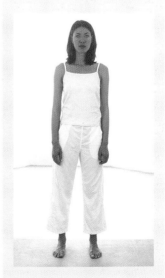

△ The slow, graceful movements of Tai Chi and Chi Kung stimulate the flow of *chi,* visualized as a subtle substance with a consistency and speed of flow similar to those of honey.

East and in the martial arts that developed among the elite monks of the Hindus, Buddhists and Taoists.

Today the West is familiar with the disciplined exercises of Tai Chi and Chi Kung. They have developed over thousands of years as an effective way to control and direct the flow of the subtle force of chi through the body and even beyond, into the environment. One of the main centres for gathering and distributing chi is known in Chinese as *tan tien.* It is equivalent, though not identical, to the sacral chakra. The same place is called the *hara* in Japanese, the centre of the life force. From this reservoir chi can be channelled and directed through the rest of the body to maintain health and give great amounts of strength and endurance, or to open up states of awareness.

It is only from a flow outwards from ourselves that we can begin to explore and experience the world that is not us. Remaining centred and solid within the security of the base chakra, our awareness can reach beyond the immediate, stretching out a curious hand to things just beyond our grasp. Movement and curiosity is required. The grace and balance of the sacral chakra's smooth flow of energy helps us succeed. Here we begin to experience the energy of the world around us.

Navel Chakra – the Organizer

The third chakra, situated behind the navel at the solar plexus, is a fusion of many different energies. It is the centre of inner power and drive, and is associated with the personality, defining the boundaries of the individual. The physical attributes of the navel or solar plexus chakra fall into three main areas: the digestion, the nervous system and the immune system.

digestion

The process of digestion and assimilation of nutrients is vital to sustain life. The organs linked to the solar plexus are the stomach,

▽ The navel chakra, below the ribcage, is the main organizing principle affecting all parts of the body and mind.

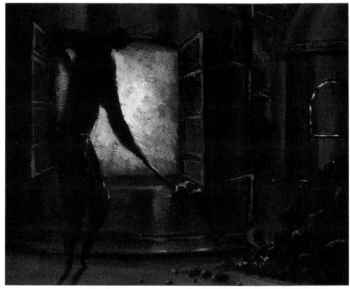

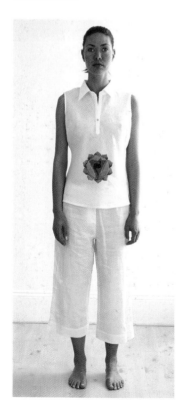

△ The navel chakra is associated with the element of fire, not only because it creates physical heat in the body, but also because it takes raw materials and transforms them.

▽ The navel chakra is often referred to as the fusebox of the body. In this area are large concentrations of nerve tissue that, if disrupted, can affect the whole nervous system.

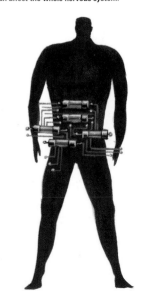

liver, gallbladder, pancreas, duodenum and small intestine. For digestion and the assimilation of nutrients to be successful, all these organs have to work in harmony. This involves a series of chemical reactions using a great many different catalysts. From the alkaline enzyme-rich saliva in the mouth, food moves to the acidity of the stomach. Here it is churned, thoroughly mixing the natural acids and enzymes. It then passes into the duodenum, where bile from the liver, via the gallbladder, begins to break down fats, and more enzymes from the pancreas begin to act on sugars and carbohydrates. As the mixture moves through the small intestine, the valuable nutrients from the food are absorbed through the wall of the intestine into the bloodstream. Failure to digest food efficiently means that nutrients are not absorbed.

▷ If the ability of the body to recognize nutrients is impaired, so that absorption does not take place, eating healthily will make little difference.

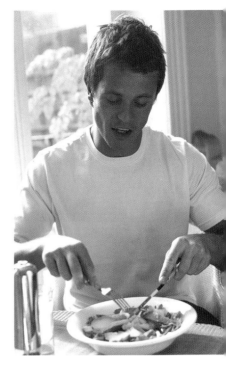

immune system

The immune system works like a library or a computer. It stores and categorizes information about everything the body encounters. For instance, on meeting a virus, the body recognizes it as an enemy and activates the defence mechanisms to fight and overcome the infection. If the body later encounters the same virus again it has the information to prevent a serious invasion.

Problems with this identification process often show up when the body reacts to harmless or even beneficial substances as if they are dangerous. This is experienced as allergy or intolerance. The opposite malfunction happens when the body harbours an infection for a long time because it fails to recognize its presence and so neglects to fight it at all. Difficulties also occur when the body fails to recognize its own enzymes, hormones or neuro-transmitters, and sometimes there is an inability to recognize minerals and vitamins that should be absorbed by the small intestine. These problems surface as deficiencies but do not respond to increased intake because the problem is not lack, but a failure to recognize the substance.

The navel chakra is put under great pressure by the way we live today. Its physical functions are strained by the types of food we eat, the pace of life and new toxins in our environment. It is not surprising that many of the diseases in our society today are a sign of some dysfunction in the navel chakra.

ARDHA MATSEYANDRASANA
This exercise, the spinal twist, tones the whole of the solar plexus. The more upright you keep your spine, the easier it is to twist.

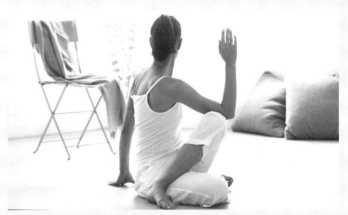

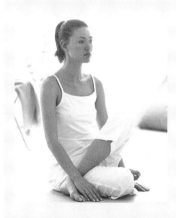

1 Kneel down on a blanket or thick mat, resting on your heels. Slide your buttocks to the right of your feet. Lift your left leg, so the left foot is across the right knee.

2 Shuffle your bottom around to get comfortable and to keep your spine straight. Bring your left arm round behind you, resting your fingers on the floor to steady yourself. Bring your right arm to rest on the outside of the left leg, the elbow bracing against the knee. Breathe in, then as you breathe out, lift your spine and twist round to look over your left shoulder. Breathe normally.

3 When you feel ready to release the pose, breathe in, then as you breathe out, unwind yourself. First bring your left arm back around to the front and follow its movement with the head, naturally straightening the spine. If you are unable to stretch into the full twist, simply hold the knee instead of bracing it with an elbow. Repeat on the other side, mirroring the steps.

Heart Chakra – Embracing the World

The heart chakra is located near the centre of the breastbone or sternum. The physical organs and parts of the body linked to this chakra are characterized by their actions of expansion and contraction, drawing in and pushing away.

physical attributes

The heart, with its rhythmic expansion and contraction, is the powerful muscular pump that sends oxygenated blood to all parts of the body. By its movement, the diaphragm, the powerful muscle below the lungs, creates changes in pressure, allowing us to breathe in fresh air. As the diaphragm contracts, the

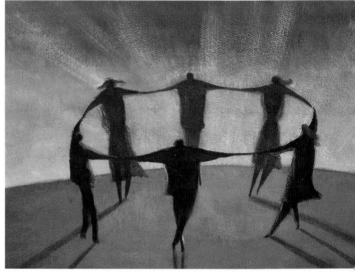

△ The heart chakra governs our interactions as we reach out to touch and embrace other people.

▽ The heart chakra is at the centre of the main chakras and is the balance point for the system.

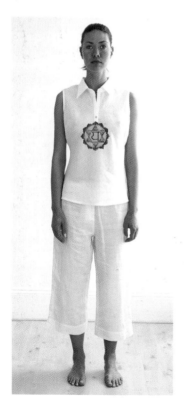

outbreath expels carbon dioxide from the body. The lungs are composed of tree-like air ducts that bring air into contact with the bloodstream. The blood picks up oxygen from the air, releasing back into it carbon dioxide and other waste products as it returns from its journey through the body.

These processes of expansion, interchange and contraction are reflected in our relationship with the world. The heart chakra regulates our interaction, making sure that we become neither too involved nor too remote from the world around us. The relationship is in constant motion: if it stays stationary all balance is lost. Reaching out and physically touching helps us to gather information. As we gather information we respond and begin to relate.

The action of the arms can be one of enfolding, enclosing, embracing and absorption. Equally, the arms can defend, push away and protect. The degree to which we keep the physical balance between what is outside us and our inner being is often reflected in the way we hold our upper torso and arms. Tension and rigidity suggest stasis and defensiveness. A relaxed stance and flowing movement not only shows ease with the world, it reduces the stress levels on the heart and lungs.

▽ Arms and hands are the executors of the heart chakra energy. They reach out to hold or ward off the world around us.

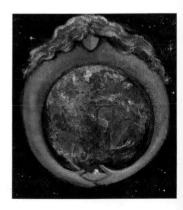

GOMUKHASANA

This posture extends the muscles and cavities of the chest and stretches and energizes the shoulders and arms. If your hands do not meet at first, ease into the pose by holding a 25–30cm/ 10–12in length of cane or wood.

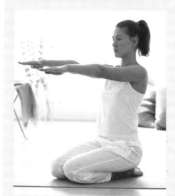

1 Kneel on the mat, sitting back on your heels. Stretch both arms out in front of you.

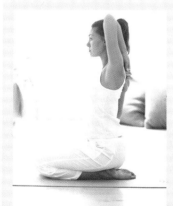

2 Raise your left arm over your head, bending it at the elbow so the left hand rests near the top of your back.
3 Sweep your right arm round to the right side, bending it at the elbow, sending the right hand up your back.
4 If your hands meet, lightly clasp your fingers, otherwise hold each end of the piece of wood.

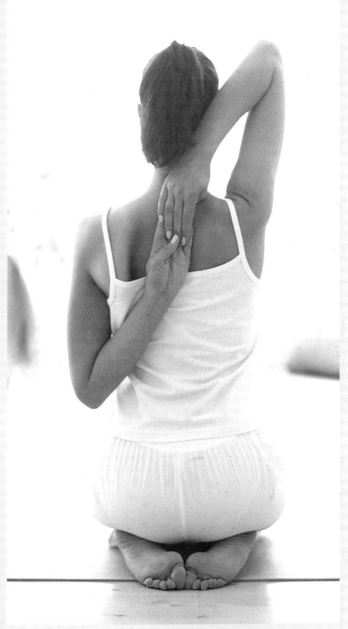

5 When you have a grip on your hands, or the wood, take a breath in and bring your hands closer together, expanding your chest. Breathe normally. On an outbreath, loosen your grip then repeat, starting by raising your right hand above your head and mirroring the above stages.

Brow Chakra – Seeing the Picture

The chakra located in the centre of the forehead is called ajna, meaning command. It is directly related to the senses of sight and hearing, although all three upper chakras – the throat, brow and crown – are physically close together and share many correspondences. Throat chakra influences extend to the mouth and jaw and up to the ears, while the brow has more links with the face, eyes, nose and forehead. The neck and base of the skull can be influenced by both brow and throat energies. Crown chakra energies relate to the cranium, the bones of the top of the head at and above the hairline.

▽ **The brow chakra is the seat of understanding, from where we picture how the world is.**

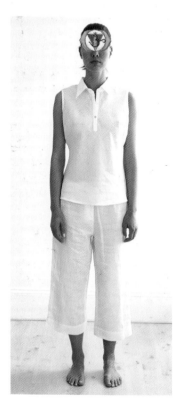

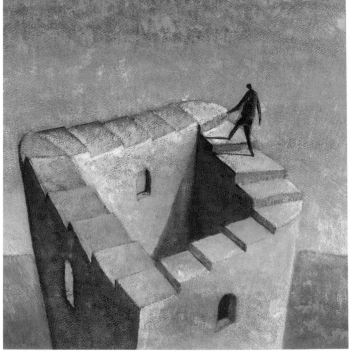

△ **Perception is understanding how different parts come together to make a whole. It is the job of the brow chakra to interpret clearly.**

thoughts

Our everyday awareness is located in the area of the brow chakra, from where our higher sense functions scan the world around us. The consciousness of self, of the unique personality of the mind, is felt to be seated here, like a commander at his control post. We are very much in our heads – more than, say, in our heart or our solar plexus. The physical body belongs to us but we do not think of it as being "us" in the same way.

We relate to our own thoughts, our interpretations and inner conversations, continually assessing the information that feeds in through the senses. We relate to others by focusing attention on the face – the eyes and the subtle changes of expression, feeling that the "real person" is somewhere in there. This arises from the awareness that here at the brow chakra we begin to make sense of and interpret the world. The brow chakra is all about seeing, not just seeing with the eyes, but seeing with the mind – making sense of and understanding what is being perceived.

eyesight

We do not see what the eyes see. The eye focuses light through the lens and an upside-down image is thrown on to the retina at the back of the eye. However, only one tiny spot, the fovea, has a concentration of light-sensitive cells great enough to produce a complete focused image; the rest of the eye receives a vaguer, more blurred picture. Rapid movement of the eyes adds more

CLEAR SEEING

Seeing clearly depends on the co-ordination between the mind and the eyes. Confusion in understanding (seeing) arises when blocks in the brow chakra disturb the complex relationship between eye movements and nerve impulses as they travel to the centres of visual comprehension in the brain. Getting confused shows that stress is affecting co-ordination. Practice will re-open these pathways, increasing your ability to focus and understand the world around you. This simple exercise helps both the muscles controlling eye movement and the balance between the left and right hemispheres of the brain.

▽ Seeing is not simply a sense of perception. We use "I see" to mean "I understand". Seeing relies on the flexibility of the mind as well as the sharpness of the eyes.

1 Sit in a relaxed position with an upright head. Gaze forwards with your eyes relaxed.
2 Turn your eyes upwards and as high as they will go, making sure your head does not move. Now slowly and attentively roll your eyes in a clockwise direction.
3 When you return to the top again, relax and gaze forward for a moment.
4 Now repeat the exercise, but this time move your eyes anticlockwise, in the opposite direction to before. Make sure your head remains still and that your eyes move as slowly and evenly as possible.
5 Repeat each cycle a couple of times unless you feel some strain. If you want to check your eye-brain co-ordination, do this exercise while you are saying a nursery rhyme or counting numbers.

of memories, the brain organizes the visual information so that we can understand and really "see". Perception is the art of creating order from potential chaos, from random impulses. Perception is the main function of the brow chakra.

Balancing this chakra can help physical problems with the eyes, but more than this, it will help remove confusion caused by an inability to distinguish important things from insignificant ones; in visual terms, the foreground from the background. Clear seeing, understanding and perspective are all mental skills that are needed to interpret visual data, as well as the mental pictures that are our thoughts, memories and ideas.

Seeing the picture allows us to move within the orderly, familiar patterns of life. Without the brow chakra making sense of information received by the brain, we would be paralysed by confusion and indecision.

▽ Pattern-making is essential for the mind to understand what it is being shown by the eyes. Whenever possible a pattern will be seen, even in a random display of colours.

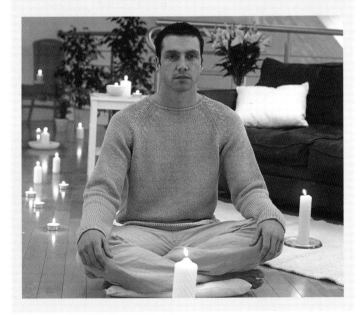

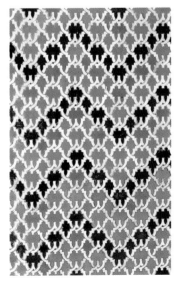

information, scanning the field of vision to allow us to get a clearer set of images. When these images travel to the brain they are switched, so that information from the left eye travels to the right hemisphere of the brain and vice versa.

breaking the code

The brain interprets the flurry of electrical nerve impulses and fills in all the gaps itself. Recognizing familiar shapes and relationships between things, creating patterns that mean something from its store

Crown Chakra – The Fountain Head

The Sanskrit name for the crown chakra is sahasrara, meaning "thousand-spoked". This description refers to the image of the thousand-petalled lotus which, in Hindu thought, represents cosmic consciousness. The chakra is described as being positioned just above the head.

the pituitary gland

The gland most often associated with the crown chakra is the pituitary, though some texts quote the relevant gland as being the

▽ The crown chakra is the main coordinating centre of the body and ensures that the individual is also connected to universal sources of energy.

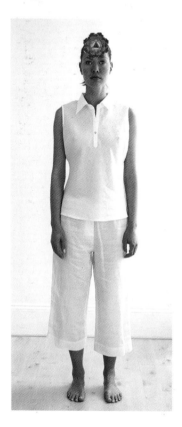

pineal. The pituitary gland is located at the base of the brain. It has two sections, the anterior and posterior, which are each responsible for releasing particular hormones. The pituitary is often referred to as the "master gland" because it affects so many other glands and body functions.

the brain

The brain is a most complex organ with four main sections and billions of nerves. One section of the brain, the cerebrum, is involved with sensation, reasoning, planning and problem solving. The diencephalon contains the pineal gland, the thalamus and the hypothalamus, which are referred to collectively as the limbic system. This controls body temperature, water balance, appetite, heart rate, sleep patterns and emotions. The brain stem, midbrain, pons and medulla oblongata control breathing, heart rate and blood pressure. The cerebellum controls posture, balance and the co-ordination of the muscles that are associated with movement.

co-ordination

From the viewpoint of physical health, the crown chakra is mostly concerned with co-ordination. Co-ordination is needed at all levels. Individual cells within the pituitary gland and the diencephalon have to co-ordinate to ensure the smooth running of the bodily functions. The cerebellum is responsible for helping us to co-ordinate our muscles to achieve balance, posture and movement.

Co-ordination skills are learned at an early age – and reinforced by crawling on all-fours. Research in the last 30 years has shown that children who do not crawl on all-fours in infancy often experience co-ordination difficulties as they grow up. It has been found that returning to this early form of locomotion, even as an adult, can assist the cerebellum in gaining full muscle control. It has also been discovered that

LITTLE YOGA NIDRA

This exercise, yoga sleep, combines visualization with the flow of energy through the body. Sit or lie in a comfortable position and allow your breathing to slow.

1 Bring your attention to your left big toe: don't move it, just be aware of it as a focus for the mind.
2 Shift the focus in turn to your second, third, fourth and fifth toes. Then to the ball of the foot, instep, top of the foot and left heel.
3 Carry on to the lower leg, back of the knee, top of the knee, top of the thigh, back of the thigh and left buttock.
4 Take your attention to your right big toe and work up the right leg as before.
5 Take your attention to the left side of your back, left side from hip to armpit and left side of the chest. Then to the right side of your back, right side from hip to armpit, right side of the chest.
6 Focus on your left thumb. Then first finger, second, third and fourth; your palm, back of the hand, wrist, inside elbow, outside elbow, upper arm, left shoulder.
7 Then to your right thumb; first, second, third and fourth finger; palm, back of hand, wrist, inside of the elbow, outside of the elbow, upper arm and right shoulder.
8 On to your head and neck; left side of your face, right side of your face; left ear, right ear; left eye, right eye; mouth, inside the mouth.
9 At the end you should be feeling totally relaxed. You can repeat it if you are particularly tense or find it hard to relax.

ADHO MUKHA SVANASANA

The downward facing dog posture helps to balance energy between the feet and the crown chakra.

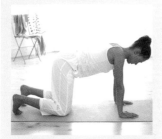

1 Kneel on a non-slip mat on all-fours, making sure your knees are in a straight line under your hips. Make sure your hands are in a straight line under your shoulders and spread your fingers. Tuck your toes under.

2 Breathe in, lifting your pelvis and straightening your legs, keeping your head low.

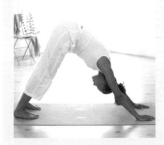

3 Breathe naturally. As you stay in the posture, imagine your bottom is lifting upwards, but your heels are lowering to the floor, stretching your back.

4 When you decide to release the posture, breathe in, then as you breathe out, lower yourself back on to all-fours.

5 Slide yourself back until you are sitting on your heels, rest your forehead on the floor and relax for a few moments.

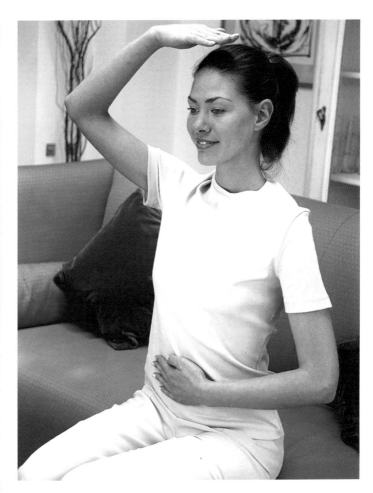

△ The well-known test of rubbing your stomach while tapping your head is a good example of body-mind co-ordination.

▽ Activities such as balancing and juggling require whole-brain co-ordination. Balance in life demands whole-chakra co-ordination.

many types of learning difficulties can be helped by exercises that utilize opposite parts of the body, confirming that brain co-ordination and function can be improved.

Co-ordination problems can occur on many levels throughout life. Physical difficulties like poor balance or clumsiness are quite obvious manifestations of the problem. Dyslexia often results from poor co-ordination between brain hemispheres, as the eyes move across a page of writing or scan down a text. On a less obvious level, co-ordination with the world as a whole is also a function of the crown chakra. Finding yourself at the right place at the right time, or just happening to meet the one person you were needing to speak to, having lucky coincidences and strange sequences of events that all work out very well, are signs that your crown chakra is feeding you good information.

Useful Addresses

RETREATS
Jean Hall
www.yogajeannie.com

Free Spirit Travel
www.freespirityoga.co.uk

Yoga Italy
www.italyyogaretreats.com

UNITED KINGDOM
Yogahome
Lightsite, 14 Allen Road,
London N16 8SD
Tel. 020 7249 2425
yogahome.com

Battersea Yoga
2 Kite Yard, Cambridge Rd,
London SW11 4TA
Tel. 020 7978 7995
www.batterseayoga.com

Triyoga
57 Jamestown Rd
Camden NW1 7DB
Tel. 020 7483 3344
www.triyoga.co.uk

Sivananda Yoga Vedanta Centre
51 Felsham Road
London SW15
Tel. 020 8780 0160
www.sivananda.org

**Satyananda Yoga
Centre**
70 Thurleigh Road
London SW12
Tel. 020 8673 4869
www.syclondon.com

Iyengar Yoga Institute
223A Randolph Avenue
London W9
Tel. 020 7624 3080
www.iyi.org.uk

The British Wheel of Yoga
25 Jermyn Street, Sleaford
Lincolnshire NG34 7RU
Tel. 01529 306 851
www.bwy.org.uk

The Life Centre
15 Edge Street
London W8 7PN
Tel. 020 7221 4602
Fax 020 7221 4603
nottinghill@thelifecentre.com
www.thelifecentre.com

USA
The Ashtanga Yoga Center
1905 Calle Barcelona
Carlsbad, CA 92009
Tel. (760) 632-7093
info@ashtangayogacenter.com
www.ashtangayogacenter.com

Manju Pattahbi Jois
(son of Sri K. Pattabhi Jois)
www.manjujois.com

Ashtanga Yoga Studio
5117 MacArthur Blvd N.W.
Washington, D.C. 20016
Tel. (202) 556-0371
info@aysdc.com
www.aysdc.com

Ashtanga Yoga Shala
295 E 8th Street
New York, NY 10009
Tel. (212) 614-9537
info@aysnyc.org
www.ashtangayogashala.net

Ashtanga Yoga Seattle
New Seattle Massage
4519 1/2 University Way
Northeast
Seattle WA 98105
ashtangayogaseattle@gmail.com
www.ashtangayogaseattle.com

Ashtanga Yoga Shala
1213 State Street
Santa Barbara, CA 93101
Tel. (805) 965-7175
yogashala324e@yahoo.com
www.ashtangasantabarbara.com

SF Ashtanga
701 Eleventh Avenue
San Francisco, CA 94118
Tel. (415) 221-9644
sfashtanga@gmail.com
www.sfayoga.com

Namaste Berkeley Studio
3229 Lakeshore Ave
Oakland, CA 94610
Tel. 510-832-9642
info@ilovenamaste.com
ilovenamaste.com

Yoga Source Santa Fe
901 W. San Mateo Road
Santa Fe, NM 87505
Tel. (505) 982-0990
Fax (505) 982-4072
staff@yogasource-
santafe.com
www.yogasource-santafe.com

Chicago Yoga Center
3047 N. Lincoln Avenue
Chicago
IL 60657
Tel. (773) 327-3650
info@yogamind.com
www.yogamind.com

AUSTRALIA
Ashtanga Yoga Moves
30 Alma Street
Paddington
2021 NSW
www.yogamoves.com.au

Ashtanga Yoga Byron Bay
P.O. Box 1443
Byron Bay
2481 NSW
Tel. 266 849299
centreofbalance@hotmail.com
www.dena.net.au

Absolute Astanga Yoga
P.O. Box 220
Cooroy
4563 Queensland
Tel. 07544 25060

Ashtanga Yoga Shala
10 Moreton Street
Paddington 4064
Queensland
Tel. 7342 01010
www.ashtangayogashala.com.au

Studio Cirq
19 Meyers Place
Melbourne 3000
Victoria
Tel. 9654 9994
www.studiocirq.com.au

NEW ZEALAND

Te Aro Astanga Yoga
110 Cuba Street
Wellington, 6011
Tel. 021 0272 2362
info@astanga.co.nz
www.astanga.co.nz

The Yoga Academy
190 Federal Street
Central City
Auckland
Tel. 9 357 0750
yoga@yoga.co.nz
www.yoga.co.nz

FURTHER READING

Light on Yoga, B.K.S. Iyengar
Yoga Mala, Sri K. Pattabhi Jois
Hatha Yoga: The Hidden Language, Swami Sivananda Radha
The Shambhala Encyclopedia of Yoga, Georg Feuerstein
Asana Pranayama Mudra Bandha, Swami Satyananda Saraswati
Ashtanga Yoga, Lino Miele
Heart of Yoga, Developing a Personal Practice, T.K.V. Desikachar
A Systematic Course in the Ancient Tantric Techniques of Yoga and Kriya, Swami Satyananda Saraswati
When Things Fall Apart: Heart Advice for Difficult Times, Pema Chödrön
Old Path, White Clouds: Walking in the Footsteps of the Buddha, Thich Nhat Hanh
Chakras: Energy Centres of Transformation, Harish Johari

ACKNOWLEDGEMENTS

With endless thanks to all those who have given me so much love and support: John, Val, Clare, Fran, Karen, Kay, Jack, Gill, Seamus, Kirsty, Jane, Beth, little Jack and Bee. My deepest respect and gratitude to the past and present teachers of the yoga tradition who share and pass on their wonderous insight, wisdom and knowledge, in particular Sri K. Pattabhi Jois, B.K.S. Iyengar, T.K.V. Desikachar and Swami Satyananda Saraswati. My teachers, in particular Gill Clarke who has been a continuous source of inspiration, Tessa Bilder for illuminating the inner journey, Anya Evans for giving me the value of discipline. *Jean Hall*

The authors and publishers would like to thank the models: Steve, Sandra and Grant for the Astanga yoga postures, and Neil Casselle, Anna Ford, Patricia McLoughlin, Antony Malvasi, Priya Rasanayagam and Nina Zambakides for modelling in the Meditation section of the book. Thanks for the loan of props to Paul Walker at Yoga Matters, suppliers of yoga mats, props and clothing. 32 Clarendon Road, London N8 ODJ, 020 8888 8588 fax 020 8888 0623 www.yogamatters.co.uk (www.yogapropshop.com). Thank you to Stuart Mackay at Beyond Hope for supplying the prAna clothing. Contact www.prana.com for stockists. Our thanks also go to Mariananda Azaz and colleagues at the Self-Realization Meditation Healing Centre, Yeovil, Somerset, UK, for the loan of their lovely portable meditation stool, and Meditation Designs, Totnes, Devon, UK, for supplying a marvellous selection of special meditation cushions and mats. Thanks to Penny Brown for the chakra symbol artworks that appear on page 25b, p27, p155b, p178bl, p189l, p219b and p232r.

Extracts from *The Yoga Sutras of Patanjali* by Alistair Shearer, published by Rider, are quoted by permission of the Random House Group Limited. For editions sold in the US and Canada: extracts appear from *The Yoga Sutras of Patanjali* by Patanjali, translated by Alistair Shearer. Used by permission of Bell Tower, a division of Random House, Inc. The extracts from T. S. Eliot's *Little Gidding* are quoted by permission of Faber and Faber Ltd.

PICTURE CREDITS

Thanks to the following agencies and individuals for permission to reproduce their images:

t=top, b=bottom, r=right, l=left
akg-images/British Library: p147r; Peter Anderson: p194r; The Art Archive/British Library: p13bl, p25tr; Bettmann/Corbis: p147tl; Stephen Brayne: p200b; Nicki Dowey: p16; Jean Hall: p13br; Alistair Hughes: p175br, p211b; National Museum of Karachi/Bridgeman Art Library: p150t; Craig Knowles: p149tr/br; Don Last: p147bl, p193bl, p199b; Araldo de Luca/Corbis: p146b; Kevin R. Morris/Corbis: p146t; Fiona Pragoff: p178t, p219t, p224t; The Purcell Team/Corbis: p156; Nathan Rabe: p10tr/bl; Gary Walton: p228–9b, p230br, p231, p236t, p238t/br, p240t/br, p242t/br, p244t/br, p246r, p249br. Werner Forman Archive: p247br.

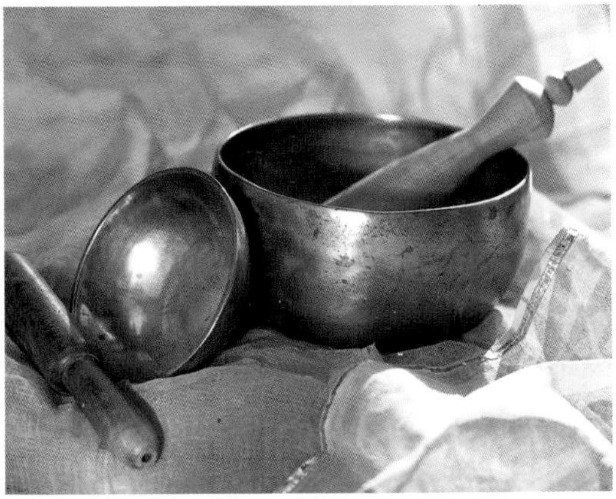

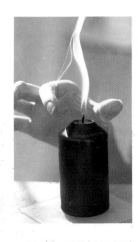